AF680241

Cystic Fibrosis: Diagnosis and Management

Cystic Fibrosis: Diagnosis and Management

Editor: Fredrick Robinson

MURPHY & MOORE
www.murphy-moorepublishing.com

www.murphy-moorepublishing.com

MURPHY & MOORE

Cataloging-in-Publication Data

Cystic fibrosis : diagnosis and management / edited by Fredrick Robinson.
p. cm.
Includes bibliographical references and index.
ISBN 978-1-63987-149-0
1. Cystic fibrosis. 2. Cystic fibrosis--Diagnosis. 3. Cystic fibrosis--Treatment.
4. Genetic disorders. I. Robinson, Fredrick.
RC858.C95 C97 2022
616.37--dc23

© Murphy & Moore Publishing, 2022

Murphy & Moore Publishing,
1 Rockefeller Plaza,
New York City, NY 10020, USA

ISBN 978-1-63987-149-0 (Hardback)

This book contains information obtained from authentic and highly regarded sources. Copyright for all individual chapters remain with the respective authors as indicated. All chapters are published with permission under the Creative Commons Attribution License or equivalent. A wide variety of references are listed. Permission and sources are indicated; for detailed attributions, please refer to the permissions page and list of contributors. Reasonable efforts have been made to publish reliable data and information, but the authors, editors and publisher cannot assume any responsibility for the validity of all materials or the consequences of their use.

Trademark Notice: Registered trademark of products or corporate names are used only for explanation and identification without intent to infringe.

Contents

Preface

This book was inspired by the evolution of our times; to answer the curiosity of inquisitive minds. Many developments have occurred across the globe in the recent past which has transformed the progress in the field.

Cystic fibrosis is a genetic disorder that is inherited in an autosomal recessive manner and characterized by coughing up mucus and difficulty in breathing as a result of frequent lung infections. It mostly affects the lungs but can also affect the liver, kidneys, pancreas and intestines. Other signs and symptoms of cystic fibrosis are poor growth, clubbing of fingers and toes, fatty stool, sinus infections and infertility in most males. Degrees of symptoms may vary from person to person. Cystic fibrosis can be diagnosed by genetic testing or sweat test. There is no permanent cure for this disease; however, lung infections can be treated with antibiotics. Most of the topics introduced in this book cover the advancements in the diagnosis and management of cystic fibrosis. It includes some of the vital pieces of work being conducted across the world, on various topics related to this disease. This book is meant for students who are looking for an elaborate reference text on cystic fibrosis.

This book was developed from a mere concept to drafts to chapters and finally compiled together as a complete text to benefit the readers across all nations. To ensure the quality of the content we instilled two significant steps in our procedure. The first was to appoint an editorial team that would verify the data and statistics provided in the book and also select the most appropriate and valuable contributions from the plentiful contributions we received from authors worldwide. The next step was to appoint an expert of the topic as the Editor-in-Chief, who would head the project and finally make the necessary amendments and modifications to make the text reader-friendly. I was then commissioned to examine all the material to present the topics in the most comprehensible and productive format.

I would like to take this opportunity to thank all the contributing authors who were supportive enough to contribute their time and knowledge to this project. I also wish to convey my regards to my family who have been extremely supportive during the entire project.

Editor

1

Respiratory Virus in Cystic Fibrosis

Dennis Wat

Abstract

Life expectancy in Cystic Fibrosis (CF) has improved dramatically in the last few decades; this is very much due to the emergence of disease-modifying treatments, optimisation of nutritional status and the inception of specialist CF units. However, progressive obstructive lung disease characterised by chronic inflammation, bacterial colonisation and recurrent infections of the lung, resulting in irreversible pulmonary damage, remains the major cause of mortality in individuals with CF. Historically, bacterial infections are the major pathogens accounting for clinical deterioration in CF. More recently, there has been emerging evidence to support respiratory viruses being accountable for the colonisation of bacteria and progression of lung disease in CF. This chapter sought to provide an overview on the impact of respiratory viruses in CF lung disease, the interaction between viruses and bacteria, the preventative and therapeutic measures that are currently available for the management of viral lung disease in CF.

Keywords: Cystic fibrosis, respiratory virus, bacteria, Pseudomonas aeruginosa

1. Introduction

Cystic Fibrosis (CF) is the most commonly inherited potentially lethal disease amongst the Caucasian ancestry. The prevalence of CF is reported as 0.737 per 10,000 in 27 European Union countries [1]. The United States (US) Cystic Fibrosis Patient Registry reports a similar prevalence of 0.797 CF patients per 10,000 people [2]. It is an autosomal recessive disease and is caused by mutations in the Cystic Fibrosis Transmembrane Conductance Regulator gene (CFTR) [3]. The most common mutation is caused by deletion of phenylalanine at position 508 (Delta F508) of the CFTR on chromosome 7, which accounts for approximately 70% of CF cases. The primary function of CFTR in many tissues is to regulate and participate in the transport of chloride ions across epithelial cell membranes. To date, more than 1,900 mutations have been described in this gene.

CF is a multisystem disease as CFTR is expressed in different organs [4]; however, the lungs are the predominant organs that bear the brunt of the disease [5]. Recurrent pulmonary infections may start at very early stages in the lives of patients with CF. It has been hypothesised that low airway surface liquid volume and impaired mucociliary clearance are responsible for the pathogenesis of lung infections. These in turn lead to impaired bacterial clearance from respiratory epithelial cells [6]. Pulmonary infections remain the greatest cause of poor life quality, morbidity and mortality in CF that eventually lead to premature death in this condition [7].

Apart from chronic lung disease with recurrent exacerbations, exocrine pancreatic insufficiency is also a feature that leads to malabsorption and subsequently growth retardation and maturation. Endocrine pancreatic insufficiency is another feature of CF with the manifestation of diabetes. Obstructive azoospermia in male CF patients leads to male infertility.

The median survival from CF has taken great strides over the past 40 years as a consequence of the introduction of specialist centre care, nutritional optimisation, prevention and aggressive management of pulmonary exacerbations [8]. In the United Kingdom (UK) CF population in 2012, the median survival was reported as 43.5 years, compared to 38.8 years for the population in 2008 as per the UK CF Registry [9]. It has been postulated that the continuing improvement in survival of CF patients in successive cohorts means that the previous prediction of patients with CF living beyond a median age of 50 years is not impossible. The recent introduction of Ivacaftor to the management of CF patients with G551D CFTR mutations may further enhance the overall survival [10].

Historically, bacteria have been the predominant cause for respiratory exacerbations. The presences of some organisms including *Staphylococcus aureus, Pseudomonas aeruginosa* and *Burkhoderia cepacia* in the airways have been shown to lead to clinical deterioration [11-13] and may subsequently lead to morbidity and mortality. Pulmonary exacerbations are associated with acquisition of new organisms and increased concentration of airway flora [14]. The new acquisitions of *P. aeruginosa* in CF have been demonstrated to occur in the winter months coinciding with the peak of respiratory viral infections [15, 16]. In the event of a pulmonary exacerbation the absence of pyrexia, raised inflammatory markers and systemic response, pathogens other than bacteria can be the potential cause. Respiratory viruses have been implicated by a number of studies in the last 30 years as potentiators for CF exacerbations [17-29]. *Influenza* is a substantial health threat; it is associated with approximately 36,000 deaths and 220,000 hospitalisations in the USA on an annual basis [30]. The recent emergence of novel *influenza virus (H1N1)* further heightened the awareness of influenza-like illness. CF Pulmonary exacerbation rates have also been shown to be significantly increased during the winter months and are highly associated with the influenza season [31]. Respiratory viruses that are associated with the exacerbations of CF include *influenza A and B, respiratory syncytial virus (RSV), parainfluenza virus (PIV) types 1 to 4, rhinovirus, metapneumovirus, coronavirus* and *adenovirus*.

In the last 30 years, there have been a number of published studies depicting the impact of respiratory viruses in CF. A number of studies have also demonstrated the relationship between respiratory viruses and bacteria in the pathogenesis of CF exacerbations [15, 32]. The introduction of molecular diagnostic technologies has further enhanced the awareness of respiratory viral aetiology in CF exacerbations as they have much higher detection rates than traditional methods. However, further understanding is required to appreciate their relationship in order to allow the development of potential novel treatment. If indeed respiratory virus does lead to secondary bacterial infection in CF, viral vaccinations and anti-viral therapies would be important therapeutic options for CF. On the other hand, the currently commercially available vaccines and anti-virals for the prevention and treatment of respiratory viral infections are limited; they are primarily for influenza infection. The potential development of new vaccines and anti-virals is an exciting field which may offer alternate therapeutic opportunities for CF exacerbations.

This chapter will focus on the literature regarding respiratory viruses in CF and their clinical implications, the detection techniques for viruses and their differences in sensitivities, the interaction between viruses and bacteria, and the management of viral infections.

2. Viral respiratory infections in CF

Early studies looking at respiratory viruses in CF relied on repeated serological testing, either alone [20] or in combination with viral cultures for viral detection [21-25]. These methods are relatively insensitive and more recent studies have utilised molecular-based methodologies [18, 26-28, 33-36]. All these studies produced different results in terms of prevalence of respiratory viruses in CF. The differences can be due to different methodologies, different sampling methods; the differences can also be accountable by different populations studied as the prognosis for CF has improved with each successive birth cohort.

Wang et al. [25] described the relationship between respiratory viral infections and deterioration in clinical status in CF almost 30 years ago. In this 2- year prospective study [25], viruses were identified through serology and nasal lavage in 49 patients with CF (mean age 13.7 years) on a quarterly basis and at the onset of exacerbations. Although the CF patients had more respiratory illnesses than sibling controls (3.7 versus 1.7/year), there were no differences in virus identification rates (1.7/year). The rate of proven virus infection was significantly correlated with the decline in lung functions, nutritional status, radiology score, and frequency and duration of hospitalisation.

More recent studies suggest no difference in the frequency of either upper respiratory tract illness (URTI) episodes [22] or proven respiratory viral infections [24] between children with CF and healthy controls, but children with CF have significantly more episodes of lower airway symptoms than controls [22, 24]. Ramsey et al. [24] prospectively compared the incidence and effect of viral infections on pulmonary function and clinical scores in 15 school-age patients with CF aged between 5 and 21 years and their healthy siblings. Over a 2-year period, samples were taken at regular two monthly intervals and during acute respiratory illnesses (ARI) for pharyngeal culture and serology for respiratory viruses. There was a total of 68 ARI episodes that occurred in the patients with CF and in 19 episodes there was an associated virus identified. A total of 49 infective agents were identified either during ARIs or at routine testing in the patients with CF; 14 were identified on viral isolation (*rhinovirus* on 11 occasions), whilst 35 were isolated on seroconversion (*PIV* on 12, *RSV* on 9 and *M. pneumoniae* on 6 occasions). At the time of an ARI, the virus isolation and seroconversion rates were 8.8% and 19.1%, respectively, in children with CF compared to 15.0% and 15.0%, respectively, for the healthy siblings. In contrast, the rates of virus isolation and seroconversion at routine 2 monthly visits were 5.6% and 16.2%, respectively, for children with CF and 7.7% and 20.2%, respectively, for the healthy siblings. There was no significant difference in the rate of viral infections between the patients with CF and their sibling controls, as measured either by culture or serology. The rate of viral infections was higher in younger children (both CF and controls); however, the rate of decline in pulmonary function and severity score was both lower in the younger children with CF and the ones with more viral infections. The authors concluded that there were no significant adverse effects with viral infections in CF.

Likewise, Hiatt [22] assessed respiratory viral infections over three winters in 22 infants less than 2 years of age with CF (30 patient seasons), and 27 age-matched controls (28 patient seasons). The average number of acute respiratory illness per winter was the same in the control and CF groups (5.0 vs. 5.0). However, only 4 of the 28 control infants had lower respiratory tract symptoms in association with the respiratory tract illness, compared with 13 out of the 30 infants with CF (Odd ratio – 4.6; 95% confidence interval 1.3 and 16.5; p-value <0.05); 7 of the infants with CF cultured *RSV*, of whom 3 required hospitalisation. In contrast, none of the controls required hospitalisation. Pulmonary function measured by rapid chest compression technique was significantly reduced in the infants with CF after the winter months and was associated with two interactions; *RSV* infection with lower respiratory tract infection and male sex with lower respiratory tract infection.

From previous reports, two viral agents appear to have the greatest effect on respiratory status in CF, namely *RSV and influenza*, possibly because the uses of viral culture and serology have underestimated the effects of rhinovirus. In younger children, *RSV* is a major pathogen resulting in an increased rate of hospitalisation. Abman et al. [37] prospectively followed up 48 children with CF diagnosed through newborn screening and documented the effect of *RSV* infection. Eighteen of the infants were admitted into hospital a total of 30 times over a mean follow-up of 28 months (range 5-59]. In 7 of these infants *RSV* was isolated, and their clinical course was severe with 3 requiring mechanical ventilation and 5 necessitating chronic oxygen therapy. Over the next 2 years, these infants had significantly more frequent respiratory symptoms and lower Brasfield chest radiograph [38] scores than *non-RSV*-infected counterparts.

In older children and adults with CF, *influenza* seems to have the greatest effect. Pribble et al. [23] assessed acute pulmonary exacerbation isolates from 54 patients with CF. Over the year of the study, 80 exacerbations were identified, of which 21 episodes were associated with an identified viral agent (*influenza A* – 5 episodes; *influenza B* – 4 episodes; *RSV* – 3 episodes) with most agents identified on serology. Compared to other respiratory viruses, infection with *influenza* was associated with a more significant drop in pulmonary function (FEV_1 declined by 26% compared with 6%). There were also a higher proportion of patients with a greater than 20% drop in FEV_1 within the *influenza* infected cohort. A retrospective study in older patients with chronic *P. aeruginosa* infection reported an acute deterioration in clinical status in association with *influenza A* virus infection, which was confirmed by serology [39].

Over a 1-year period, Smyth et al. [27] prospectively investigated 108 patients with CF (mean age of 7.9 years) using a combination of viral immunofluorescence, culture and seroconversion to identify respiratory viruses. With the exception of *rhinovirus*, a semi-nested reverse transcriptase PCR technique was used. During the study, 76 subjects had 157 respiratory exacerbations (1.5 episodes/patient/year) and a viral agent was identified in 44 episodes, 25 of which were *rhinovirus* and an equal distribution of other viruses was identified almost always on seroconversion. Rhinovirus identification was associated with significantly more days of intravenous antibiotics, whereas, those children in whom a non-rhinovirus was identified had a significantly greater decrease in FEV_1 over the year of the study. When all viruses were considered as a whole, patients had significantly greater decline in Shwachman score [40] and days of intravenous antibiotics use.

Collinson et al. [26] followed 48 children with CF over a 15-month period using viral cultures for viral detection, with the exception of *picornaviruses* where polymerase chain reaction (PCR) was used; 38 children completed the study and there were 147 symptomatic upper respiratory tract infections (URTIs), 2.7 episodes/child/year, with samples available for 119 episodes. *Picornaviruses* were identified in 51 (43%) of these episodes, of which 21 (18%) were *rhinoviruses*. In those children old enough to perform spirometry, there was significant reduction in both FVC and FEV_1 in association with URTIs, with little difference in severity of reduction whether a picornavirus was identified or not. Maximal mean drop in FEV_1 was 16.5%, at 1-4 days after onset of symptoms, but a deficit of 10.3% persisted at 21-24 days. Those with more URTIs appeared to have greater change in total Shwachman score [40] and Chrispin-Norman score [41] over the study. Six children isolated a *P.aeruginosa* for the first time during the study, 5 at the time of a URTI and only 1 was asymptomatic at the time of first isolation. However, the data from this study have to be handled with care as the term 'URTI' does not necessarily imply a positive viral isolation.

Punch et al. [42] used a multiplex reverse transcriptase PCR (RT-PCR) assay combined with an enzyme-linked amplicon hybridization assay (ELAHA) for the identification of seven common respiratory viruses in the sputum of 38 CF patients; 53 sputum samples were collected over 2 seasons and 12 (23%) samples from 12 patients were positive for a respiratory virus (4 for *influenza B*, 3 for *parainfluenza type 1*, 3 for *influenza A* and 2 for *RSV*). There were no statistical associations between virus status and demographics, clinical variables or isolation rates for *P. aeruginosa, S. aureus or A. fumigatus.*

Olesen and colleagues [28] obtained sputum and laryngeal aspirates from children with CF over a 12-month period in outpatient clinics. They achieved a viral detection rate of 16%, with *rhinovirus* being the most prevalent virus. FEV_1 was significantly reduced during viral infection (-12.5%, p=0.048), with the exception of *rhinovirus* infection. The authors were not able to demonstrate a positive correlation between respiratory viruses and bacterial infections in their studied population as the type or frequency of bacterial infection during or after viral infections were not altered. They also concluded that clinical viral symptoms had a very poor predictive value (0.39) for a positive viral test.

Our group in 2004 [36] utilised 'real-time' multiplex Nucleic Acid Sequenced Based Amplification to examine the role of respiratory viruses in CF children. Over an 18-month period, a viral detection rate of 46% was achieved during reported episodes of respiratory illness. The results compared favourably with previous studies and it may be that earlier studies relied heavily on repeated serological testing, either alone [20] or in combination with viral isolation [21-25]. The viral detection rate was 18.3% from routine nasal samples. However, this was comparable to the seroconversion rate of 12.3% as reported by Wang et al. [25]. Ramsey and colleagues [24] also achieved a similar seroconversion rate of 16.2% from asymptomatic samples. These results suggest that a laboratory method with a higher sensitivity for viral detection does not increase the detection rate in asymptomatic samples, implying that false positives are not necessarily more common than less sensitive diagnostic methods. *Influenza A and B* viruses were the major viruses in causing respiratory exacerbations in CF and both viruses are more commonly detected during pulmonary exacerbations; 22 of 88 [23%) viruses found in this study were *influenza viruses (A & B)*. The result is consistent with majority of the previous studies which showed that *influenza* virus represented between 12% and 27% of all viruses detected. However, the findings are in contrast with other studies where rhinovirus is the major virus in CF exacerbations [26, 28, 43]. The *influenza* vaccine uptake rate during the study period was up to 70% [36]. It is possible that the detection rate for *influenza* virus could have been higher had the vaccine coverage not been this high.

Asner et al. [44] performed an observational cross-sectional study of CF children from a large paediatric referral centre investigating the association between respiratory viruses and pulmonary exacerbations by taking mid-turbinate swabs, sputum and throat swab samples that were tested by a direct immunofluorescent antibody assay and a multiplex PCR panel. Forty-three patients were recruited into the study. Pulmonary function tests, quality of life and severity scores were recorded. Sputum cell counts, bacterial density and cytokines were measured. Twenty-six (60.5%) subjects were tested positive for at least one respiratory virus by any diagnostic method applied to any sample type. Of the 26 virus positive subjects, 17 (65.4%) were positive for one virus and the remaining 9 (34.6%) were positive for two or more viruses. *Coxsackie/echovirus* was the most commonly identified pathogen (29.4%) amongst the 17 subjects that were positive for one virus. Virus-positive patients were younger (p=0.047) and more likely to be male (p=0.029). They were also more likely to present with fever (p=0.019), have higher CF clinical severity (p=0.041) and lower quality of life scores (p=0.022). However, virus-positive and negative patients had similar IL-8, neutrophil percentage, elastase levels and 26 additional cytokines levels between both groups. The authors reported a higher rate of viral detection with mid-turbinate swabs than with sputum samples. The study was primarily conducted in the outpatient setting and subjects may have milder form of exacerbations which may in turn explain the lack of inflammatory response in virus-positive subjects. There was also a significant median age difference between the virus-positive and negative groups (6.9 vs. 13 years, $p=0.047$), with respiratory viral infection being more common in younger children presumably related to the delay maturation of the immune system.

A CF centre in Milan (Italy) led by Esposito and colleagues [43] showed that human *rhinovirus* was the most frequently isolated virus from CF patients <25 years of age during respiratory exacerbations and when subjects were clinically stable over a 1-year period. Molecular techniques were utilised to isolate viruses from nasopharyngeal samples. The authors demonstrated that human *rhinovirus* was more common among patients with pulmonary exacerbations than among clinically stable patients. The human *rhinovirus* viral load was however similar in subjects with or without acute respiratory exacerbations ($p=0.46$). There were no correlations between the associated clinical condition and viral load as well as between bacterial colonisation, colonising bacterial, and viral infections between the 2 groups. This finding is similar to de Almeida et al. [17] who did not show a difference in viral infection between the exacerbation and clinically stable groups. Therefore, this raises a possibility that isolation of *rhinovirus* from nasopharyngeal swabs does not always indicate that it is a cause of exacerbation as it may be explained by a coincidental upper airways infection, a carrier state, or prolonged shedding of a pathogen that caused a previous infection [45].

In 2009, a novel swine pandemic *influenza A virus (H1N1)* was identified. Nash et al. [46] showed that the symptoms of CF patients infected with H1N1 tend to be mild. There was no significant reduction in FEV_1 % predicted, FVC % predicted and body mass index regardless of whether the patients were positive or negative for *H1N1*. Colombo et al. [47] performed a multi-centre survey showing that diagnostic testing did not identify clinical characteristics specifically associated with *H1N1* infections. Similarly, they did not show a significant decline in lung function associated with this infection. To date, the significance of *H1N1* infection in CF remains undefined.

In contrast, the data regarding respiratory viral infection in adults is sparse. An observational study conducted by Hoek et al. [48] over a 1-year period amongst adult CF patients yielded a viral isolation rate of 33% [8/24] utilising molecular techniques and conventional methods. Etherington and colleagues [18] from an adult CF centre published a retrospective case control study looking at the prevalence of respiratory viruses during exacerbations. Viral throat swabs were taken from all patients presenting with an acute pulmonary exacerbation requiring intravenous antibiotic treatment over a 12-month period. Viral isolation was performed by PCR. There were 432 pulmonary exacerbations in 180 adults. In total, there was a total positive viral isolation in 42 exacerbations indicating a prevalence of 9.7%. *Rhinovirus* was the commonest isolated virus and was found on 29 occasions (69%). *Influenza A/H1N1* was isolated in seven patients (16.7%). They demonstrated a measurable impact of viral infections in CF as exacerbations associated with a positive viral PCR had a greater fall in lung function at presentation with higher levels of inflammatory markers. These patients also received more days of intravenous antibiotics, showed less response to treatment and had a shorter time to next pulmonary exacerbation compared to matched controls.

Flight et al. [35] followed up 100 adult CF patients prospectively for 12 months. Sputum, nose swabs and throat swabs were collected every 2 months and at the onset of pulmonary exacerbation for virus detection. PCR assays for *adenovirus, influenza A&B, human metapneumovirus, parainfluenza 1-3, respiratory syncytial virus* and *human rhinovirus* were performed on each sample. Symptom scores, spirometry and inflammatory markers were measured at each visit. Overall, virology results were available for 626 of 649 completed study visits. Of these, 191 (30.5%) were positive for a respiratory virus including 9 episodes of dual viral infection. Human *rhinovirus* accounted for 72.5% of viruses. Overall incidence of viral respiratory infection (VRI) was 1.66 (95% CI 1.39 to 1.92) cases/patient-year. VRI was associated with increased risk of pulmonary exacerbation (OR=2.19; 95% CI 1.56 to 3.08; $p<0.001$) and prescription of antibiotics (OR=2.26; 95% CI 1.63 to 3.13; $p<0.001$). Virus-positive visits were associated with higher respiratory symptom scores and greater C-reactive protein levels. Virus-positive exacerbations had a lower acute fall in FEV_1 than virus-negative exacerbations (12.7% vs. 15.6%; $p=0.040$). The incidence of exacerbations, but not VRI, was associated with greater lung function decline over 12 months (-1.79% per pulmonary exacerbation/year; 95% CI -3.4 to -0.23; $p=0.025$).

Experimental data on the effects of viral infections in CF are limited. Toll-like receptors (TLRs) have recently been identified as key mediators of the innate response and they recognise pathogens through detection of conserved microbial structures that are absent from the host. Kurt-Jones et al. [49] found that *RSV* persisted longer in the lungs of infected TLR4-deficient mice compared to normal mice. Haynes et al. [50] also demonstrated that TLR4-deficient mice when challenged with *RSV* exhibited impaired natural killer cell trafficking and impaired virus clearance compared to normal ones. Limited human studies have demonstrated the important role of TLRs in host response against many major groups of mammalian pathogens [51]. The relationship between TLR and respiratory virus including *RSV* in humans will require further studies before it can be established.

Some studies have suggested a higher viral replication when there is an impairment of the innate host defence in CF. *Influenza* titres were significantly increased in a mouse model which were chronically infected with *P. aeruginosa* compared to control model [52]. This in turn led to an increase in susceptibility to fatal streptococcus pneumonia infection. Increased virus replication was also found after *PIV* infection of CF human airway epithelial cells, compared to controls [53]. One of the possible causes of increased virus replication and of virus persistence might be a reduced production of respiratory nitric oxide (NO), which is a vital part of innate antiviral defence mechanism [54]. Increased production of NO protects against viral infections. In CF patients, expression of the NO producing enzyme NO synthase type 2 (NOS2) is considerably reduced.

Xu et al. [55] showed that CF cells that were infected with influenza A had less IFN-related antiviral gene induction at 24 h but more significant inflammatory cytokine gene induction at 1 h after infection. Therefore, the lesser antiviral and greater early inflammatory response may explain the severe respiratory illness of CF patients with viral infections. Sutanto and coworkers [56] showed that CF airway epithelial cells had a marked increase in IL-8 production, a reduction in apoptosis and an increased viral replication compared with airway epithelial cells from healthy children following exposure to human rhinovirus. This is despite the fact that CF and healthy airway epithelial cells have similar basal and stimulated expression of IL-8 in response to pro-inflammatory stimuli. The increment of IL-8, together with a reduction of apoptotic responses by CF cells to human rhinovirus, could contribute to augmented airway inflammation in the setting of recurrent viral infections early in life.

Azithromycin has previously been shown to offer anti-rhinoviral activity in bronchial epithelial cells and, during rhinovirus infection by increasing the production of interferon-stimulated genes [57]. However, the role of anti-viral properties of Azithromycin in CF is not clearly defined. Schögler et al. [58] showed that primary bronchial epithelial cells from CF children that were pre-treated with Azithromycin had a seven-fold reduction in rhinovirus replication without inducing cell death. Azithromycin also increased RV-induced pattern recognition receptor, IFN and IFN-stimulated gene mRNA levels when measured by real-time quantitative PCR. Therefore, it is likely that Azithromycin pre-treatment reduces RV replication in CF bronchial epithelial cells, possibly through the amplification of the antiviral response mediated by the IFN pathway.

3. Detection of respiratory viruses

The diagnostic accuracy and sensitivity of respiratory viral detection is determined by several factors:

1. Appropriate respiratory specimen for testing – Nasal swabs, nasopharyngeal aspirates, nasal swabs and mid-turbinate sampling are reasonable sampling methods in young children who may not be able to expectorate. However, in older patients, sputum is easy to obtain, painless and quick. Bronchoalveolar lavage (BAL) is a useful intervention to obtain specimen in the distal airways but it is more invasive. However, it can provide useful information regarding the activities of respiratory viruses and bacteria in the distal airways.

2. Appropriate specimen transport method – There are recognised procedures for transporting clinical specimens for diagnostic virology testing. These procedures should be adhered to closely to enhance the chances of isolating the viral organism. For instance, nasal swabs should be transported in viral transport medium and all specimens should be refrigerated if there is a delay of more than 2 hours in reaching the laboratory.

3. Detection methods – Molecular techniques have superseded many conventional methods such as viral culture and serology as they are far more sensitive and specific; in addition, they have a more rapid turn-around, allowing diagnostic technology to have an immediate impact on clinical management. The advantages of such technology will allow the appropriate utilisation of anti-virals, many of which are virus-specific; it may play a role in complying with hospital infection control policy; finally, it can provide useful infor-

mation to public health authorities such that public health policies can be adjusted accordingly, e.g. the outbreak of SARS and influenza H5N1 virus.

4. Utilisation of real-time multiplex amplification technique allows multiple viruses being quantified even if the copy number of the viral target is low.

More recently, Virochip has been shown to be a pan-virus microarray platform that is capable of detection of known as well as novel viruses in a single assay simultaneously [59]. Probes chosen for Virochip can identify nodes in the viral taxonomy at the family, genus and species levels. As the Virochip probes are updated regularly, the extent of probes that can be covered are ever increasing, up to 36,000. It has a diagnostic sensitivity comparable to PCR for detecting respiratory genomes at levels as low as 100 genome copies. At the present time, Virochip is very much a research tool, and several issues must be addressed before it can be used as a routine test for virus detection in the clinical setting, including cost, diagnostic accuracy, repeatability, and sensitivity/specificity for virus detection. In addition, the clinical implication of novel viruses in the human respiratory tract is not yet defined. Therefore, the accurate interpretation of Virochip in the clinical setting remains a formidable task. For example, where specimens are polymicrobial or viral material are present at low levels, clinical and epidemiological information might be required to draw clinically meaningful conclusions.

4. Interaction between respiratory viruses and bacteria

In a 25-year retrospective review from the Danish CF clinic, the first isolation of *P. aeruginosa* was most likely between October and March [16] coinciding with the peak of the *RSV* season. However, there are a number of other possible viral agents that would broadly fit the winter season, most notably *influenza, rhinovirus* and *metapneumovirus;* therefore, these findings must be interpreted with caution.

An increase in immunoglobulin A (IgA) antibodies to the O-antigen of *P. aeruginosa* is noted in 62% of viral infections [60]. This suggests a possible 'microbial synergism' between bacterial infections and infections with respiratory viruses in CF.

The first bacterial isolation of a given organism in CF has also been shown to often follow a viral infection. In the 17-month prospective study reported by Collinson et al. [26], 5 of the 6 first isolations of *P. aeruginosa* were made during the symptomatic phase of an upper respiratory tract infection or three weeks thereafter. In contrast, only one of the 6 initial infections with *P. aeruginosa* was identified during the asymptomatic period. Similarly, *H. influenzae* was recovered for the first time from 3 children within 3 weeks of an upper respiratory tract infection and the one new *S. aureus* infection was identified immediately following a viral infection.

Armstrong and colleagues have reported that 50% of CF respiratory exacerbations requiring hospitalisation are associated with isolation of a respiratory virus [21]. In their prospective study of repeated BAL in infants over a 5-year period, a respiratory virus was identified in 52% of infants hospitalised for a respiratory exacerbation, most commonly *RSV*; 11 of the 31 hospitalised infants (35%) acquired *P. aeruginosa* in the subsequent 12-60 month follow-up, compared to 3 of 49 (6%) non-hospitalised infants (Relative risk 5.8). This indicates that RSV infection was identified immediately following a viral infection.

Respiratory viruses can disrupt the airway epithelium and precipitate bacterial adherence. *Influenza A* infection has been shown to cause epithelial shedding to basement membrane with submucosal oedema and neutrophil infiltrate [61], while both influenza and adenovirus have a cytopathic effect on cultured nasal epithelium leading to destruction of the cell monolayer [62]. This epithelial damage results in an increase in the permeability of the mucosal layer [63, 64] and possibly facilitating bacterial adherence. Bacteria can also utilise viral glycoproteins and other virus-induced receptors on host cell membrane as bacterial receptors in order to adhere to virus-infected cells [65, 66].

Kim et al. [67] found that invariant natural killer T cells induce a type of macrophage activation driving the secretion of interleukin-13 leading to the production of globlet cell metaplasia and airway hyperactivity following infection with Sendai virus. The term 'invariant' stems from the fact that all invariant natural killer T cells in humans and mice use a unique T cell receptor that is essential for interaction with CD1d. CD1d molecules present lipid antigens to T lymphocytes rather than peptide antigens as in the case of major histocompatibility complex (MHC) class I and II molecules. Historically, MHC class II dependent CD4 and T lymphocytes, through their response to stimulation by environmental allergens, are keys to the pathogenesis of human asthma. The findings by the authors lead to the notion of the use of anti-interleukin-13 therapy as a potential therapy in patients.

Viral infections might predispose to secondary bacterial infections by impairing mucociliary function and triggering host inflammatory receptors [68, 69]. This phenomenon has been demonstrated both in vivo and in vitro [70, 71]. Avadhanula et al. [72] showed that different respiratory viruses use different mechanisms to enhance the adherence of bacteria to respiratory epithelial cells. In particular, *RSV* and *PIV type 3* up-regulate intercellular adhesion molecule-1 (ICAM-1), carcinoembryonic adhesion molecule 1 (CEACAM1) and platelet activating factor receptor (PAFr) but not mucin on the surfaces of A549, BEAS-2B and NHBE but not SAE cell lines. Much of the increased bacterial adhesion following *RSV* infection could be blocked by antibodies directed against these receptors. A549 and BEAS-2B are transformed cell lines derived from type II alveolar and normal bronchial cells, respectively. NHBE and SAE cells are primary epithelial cells obtained from bronchi and distal bronchial tree and are likely to include a heterogeneous population of cells.

Mechanisms independent of the expression of conventional receptors for bacteria, such as binding to viral proteins, could be responsible for enhanced adhesion [73]. Immunofluorescence microscopy demonstrates that bacteria binding to *RSV*-infected A549 cells adhere not only to these cells expressing viral antigens but also to uninfected epithelial cells. These data suggest that the ability to augment bacterial adhesion may result from a factor served by infected cells that exert a paracrine effect on adjacent epithelium. Cytokines or other inflammatory molecules are potential good candidates for such a mediator.

Rhinovirus has been shown to potentiate bacterial infections by inhibiting the secretion of TNF alpha and interleukin-8 by macrophages in vitro following co-infection with gram negative bacterial products, lipopolysaccharide (LPS), and gram positive bacterial products, lipoteichoic acid (LTA) [74]. This rhinovirus-dependent impairment of the macrophage immune response was not mediated by autocrine production of the anti-inflammatory cytokines interleukin-10 and PGE2, or by down-regulation of the cell surface receptor for LTA and LPS. In addition, the authors also show that rhinovirus inhibit the phagocytosis of bacterial products by macrophages. These findings support the notion that *rhinovirus* exposure resulted in a reduced ability to innate and adaptive immune responses against bacterial products, hence promoting the occurrence of bacterial and viral co-infections.

The lower respiratory tract is protected by local mucociliary mechanisms that involve the integration of the ciliated epithelium, periciliary fluid and mucus. Mucus acts as a physical and chemical barrier onto which particles and organisms adhere. Cilia lining the respiratory tract propel the overlying mucus to the oropharynx where it is either swallowed or expectorated. *Influenza* viral infection has been shown to precipitate the loss of cilial beat, and shedding of the columnar epithelial cells generally within 48 hours of infection [75]. Pittet et al. [76] showed that a prior *influenza* infection of tracheal cells in vivo does not increase the initial number of *pneumococci* found during the first hour of infection, but it does significantly reduce mucociliary velocity, and thereby reduces *pneumococcal* clearance during the first 2 hours after *pneumococcal* infection at both 3 and 6 days after an *influenza* infection. The defects in *pneumococcal* clearance were greatest at 6 days after *influenza* infection. Changes to the tracheal epithelium induced by *influenza* virus may increase susceptibility to a secondary *S. pneumoniae* infection by increasing *pneumococcal* adherence to the tracheal epithelium and/or decreasing the clearance of *S. pneumoniae* via the mucociliary escalator of the trachea, and thus increasing the risk of secondary bacterial infection.

De Vrankrijker et al. [77] showed that mice that were co-infected with *RSV* and *P. aeruginosa* had a 2,000 times higher colony-forming units (CFU) count of *P. aeruginosa* in the lung homogenates compared to mice that were infected with *P. aeruginosa* alone. Co-infected mice also had more severe lung function changes. These results suggest that *RSV* can facilitate the initiation of acute *P. aeruginosa* infection.

Another study also showed that *H. influenzae* and *S. pneumoniae* bind to both free *RSV* virions and epithelial cells transfected with cell-membrane-bound G protein, but not to secreted G protein. Pre-incubation with specific anti-G antibody significantly reduces bacterial adhesion to G protein-transfected cells [78].

Stark et al. [79] showed that mice that were exposed to *RSV* had significantly decreased *S. pneumonia, S. aureus* or *P. aeruginosa* clearance 1 to 7 days after *RSV* exposure. Mice that were exposed to both *RSV* and bacteria had a higher production of neutrophil-induced peroxide but less production of myeloperoxidase compared to mice that were exposed to *S. pneumoniae* alone. This suggests that functional changes in the recruited neutrophils may contribute to the decreased bacterial clearance.

More recently, Chattoraj et al. [15] demonstrated that acute infection of primary CF airway epithelial cells with rhinovirus liberates planktonic bacteria from biofilm. Superinfection with *rhinovirus* stimulates robust chemokine responses from CF airway epithelial cells that were pre-treated with mucoid *P. aeruginosa*. The authors also showed that these chemokine responses lead to a liberation of bacteria from mucoid *P. aeruginosa* biofilm and transmigration of planktonic bacteria from the apical to the basolateral surface of mucociliary-differentiated CF airway epithelial cells. Planktonic bacteria, which are more pro-inflammatory than their biofilm counterparts, stimulate increased chemokine responses in CF airway epithelial cells which, in turn, may contribute to the pathogenesis of CF exacerbations and subsequent prolonged intravenous antibiotic use and hospitalisation.

Contrary to the above reports, Chin et al. [32] performed a prospective study over a 2-year period on 35 adult CF patients. *P. aeruginosa* sputum density was analysed during stable, exacerbation and post-exacerbation assessments. PCR was used to detect respiratory viruses during exacerbations. The sputum density of *P. aeruginosa* in patients with or without a viral infection was compared using quantitative culture or by PCR. Twenty-two patients experienced 30 exacerbations during the study period; 50% were associated with a viral infection. There was no change in sputum density of *P. aeruginosa* from the stable to exacerbation state. Virus-associated exacerbations did not result in significant increases in *P. aeruginosa* sputum density compared to non-viral exacerbations.

Contrary to the above findings, Asner et al. [44] found the mean total bacterial density in sputum samples in virus-positive patients being two logs lower than that found in virus-negative patients ($p=0.299$). However, this could be explained by the fact that the median age of the virus-positive group was significantly lower than the virus-negative group. Virus-positive and virus-negative patients had similar IL-8, neutrophil percentage and neutrophil elastase levels.

Similarly, Kieninger et al. [80] performed a comprehensive investigation of the inflammatory response of CF airway epithelial cells on virus infection. Strong cytokine production was found in all cells studied, with the magnitude and type of inflammation differing depending on cell type and virus used. There was no exaggerated inflammatory response in CF, either during cytokine production or at the transcriptional level. Instead, there was a trend towards lower cytokine production in CF airway epithelial cells after virus infection, which was associated with increased cell death. The lower inflammatory response in CF can also be explained by additional pathophysiological mechanisms, such as interactions between anti-viral and pro-inflammatory pathways, which are likely to be involved [81]. It could also be speculated that because of chronic activation of pro-inflammatory pathways, CF airway epithelial cells are not able to respond sufficiently to further stimuli, such as virus infections. This might, in turn, lead to a lack of recruitment of effector immune cells resulting in longer duration and more severe respiratory symptoms.

TLRs are key mediators of type I interferon (IFN) during viral infections by recognizing various viral components. TLR7 and TLR9 have become apparent as universally important in inducing type I IFN during infection with most viruses, particularly by plasmacytoid dendritic cells [82]. New intracellular viral pattern recognition receptors leading to type I IFN production have been identified. CFTR mutations have been shown to affect the epithelial induction of type I IFN expression by airway cells in response to *P. aeruginosa* infection [83]. This is achieved by abolishing this signalling pathway, an important component of the innate immune system that protects mucosal surfaces. Based on available evidence, chronic colonisation of *P. aeruginosa* in CF airways can be hypothesised to increase the predisposition of viral infections; however, more in-depth studies are required to elucidate this hypothesis.

Taken together, these findings suggest conflicting data regarding the inflammatory response of the CF airway epithelium on virus infection and to some extent the symbiotic relationship between viruses and bacteria. Nonetheless, respiratory viruses may lead to epithelial disruption, increase neutrophil influx, inhibition of macrophage phagocytosis, destruction of mucociliary escalator, down-regulation of cilia beat, liberation of pro-inflammatory planktonic *P. aeruginosa* from biofilm and increased neutrophil-induced peroxide release, indirectly facilitating bacterial infection of the airway.

5. Prevention and treatment for respiratory viruses

The diversity of viral serotypes in causing infection has made vaccine preparation very difficult. Frequent mutations of viral proteins of RNA viruses (e.g. genetic drift and shift of *influenza*) have further hampered the prevention of the illness.

In the UK, it has been reported that 2,150 deaths during the 2011/12 season was attributable to influenza [84], though some of the deaths may be attributed to *RSV*. *Influenza* vaccines are the only commercially available vaccines against common respiratory viruses. They have been used since the mid-1940s and they now have an established role in the prevention of *influenza A and B* infections. Inactivated *influenza* vaccine is effective even in young children including those younger than 2 years [85]. The waning of vaccine-induced immunity over time requires annual re-immunisation even if the vaccine antigens are unchanged.

Recent vaccines contain antigens of two *influenza A* subtypes, strains of the currently circulating *H3N2 and H1N1 (Swine flu)* subtypes, and one *influenza B* virus. The current recommendation for *influenza* vaccination in the UK is to offer it to those over the age of 65, those with chronic heart, respiratory (including CF) or renal diseases and those who are diabetic or immunosuppressed.

Our group [34] recently showed that *influenza* vaccination provides protection against *influenza* acquisition in patients with CF, with 1 of 41 patients vaccinated having a positive nasal swab for influenza compared to 4 of the 22 non-vaccinated patients (p=0.046). Although *influenza* vaccination does not appear to have any impact on respiratory exacerbation rates, it does have a role in preventing live infections. In our study, respiratory exacerbation rates in the preceding 10 months before the study between the vaccinated and non-vaccinated groups were similar, indicating that these were unlikely to be the reasons influencing the decision on immunisation. The decision may be secondary to a combination of patient/parent education, social background, awareness of vaccination and accessibility of vaccination.

Due to the lack of randomised controlled studies looking at the efficacy of *influenza* vaccine in CF, the Cochrane review recommends clinicians to make their own judgements on the benefits and risks of this therapy in this cohort of patients [86]. In addition to vaccine, neuraminidase inhibitors have been shown to have a role in preventing *influenza A and B* infections [87].

Rhinovirus has more than 100 serotypes; therefore, it will be unlikely that a unifying vaccine can be developed. VP4, one of the non-enveloped capsids, is highly conserved among all of the rhinoviruses; anti-VP4 antibodies have recently been generated and been shown to have the potential for future vaccine development [88].

The development of an *RSV vaccine* has been hampered by the experience with formalin-inactivated whole *RSV* vaccine in the 1960s, as it caused 80% of *RSV* vaccinees to become hospitalised compared with 5% of controls, as well as two fatalities [89]. Current major research work has focused on a prophylaxis using a humanised mouse monoclonal antibody, Palizivumab. In patients with CF, monthly Palizivumab injection significantly reduced the hospitalisation rate for acute respiratory illness during the *RSV* season compared to those who were not immunised ($p<0.05$). The former group also had fewer hospital days for acute respiratory illness [90]. However, the Cochrane database systematic reviews were not able to draw any firm conclusions on the safety and tolerability of RSV prophylaxis with Palivizumab in infants with cystic fibrosis up to 2 years of age due to a lack of randomised controlled studies [91]. Further studies are required to evaluate the safety and effectiveness of this treatment in CF patients.

There is currently no licensed *PIV* vaccine. The formalin-inactivated vaccine generated in the 1960s was not able to prevent *PIV* infection and was soon abandoned. Recently, recombinant bovine *PIV type 3* and human *PIV type 3* attenuated vaccines are being evaluated in animal models as vectors for the delivery of other viral antigens such as *RSV*-G and *RSV*-F proteins. This bivalent vaccine combination provides high level of resistance to challenges with *PIV type 3* and *RSV* in animal models [92].

The conventional methods of vaccination are via the intramuscular and subcutaneous routes. Mucosal immunisation has recently been introduced as it represents an attractive manner of delivering vaccines. It is fast, simple, non-invasive and can be carried out by unskilled individuals. The use of mucosal vaccination seems logical in that most of respiratory viral infections initially start at the mucosal sites and therefore induce local immunity. In the autumn/winter of 2014/15 the annual nasal spray flu vaccine (Fluenz Tetra) became available for children aged 2, 3 and 4 year as part of the UK NHS childhood vaccination programme. The nasal spray flu vaccine is also for children aged 2-18 years who are "at risk" from flu, such as children with long-term health conditions.

Amantadine has been the conventional anti-viral against *influenza*. However, it is strain-specific as it is only effective against *influenza A* and has common side effects such as insomnia, poor concentration and irritability. It is now largely being replaced by neuraminidase inhibitors such as Zanamivir and Oseltamivir, which are licensed for the treatment of *influenza A and*

B, including *avian flu H5N1* and *swine flu H1N1*. However, Amantadine still has a role in dealing with Oseltamivir-resistant H1N1 virus. In children and adults, early initiation of neuraminidase inhibitors within 48 hours of the onset of symptoms can reduce the duration of flulike symptoms by 0.5 to 2.5 days [93]. Early use of these medications can also reduce development of complications such as pneumonia [94]. The 2009 pandemic *H1N1* virus remains susceptible to neuraminidase inhibitors, and Oseltamivir has been used extensively for treatment related to this viral infection. Resistance to Oseltamivir has been reported with *H1N1* viral infection but this is mainly restricted to immunocompromised individuals [95]. Zanamivir has a poor oral bioavailability, and intranasal application has been shown to be effective in treating experimental *influenza* infection with the reduction in symptoms caused, virus shedding and development of otitis media [96]. Intravenous use of Peramivir or Zanamivir could be life-saving in critically ill patients with *influenza* infection [97, 98]. However, currently the Cochrane database of systematic reviews does not recommend the routine use of neuraminidase inhibitors in influenza infection in CF because of the absence of high level evidence for the effectiveness of these interventions [99].

Ribavarin, a synthetic guanosine nucleoside that has a broad spectrum of anti-viral activity, has been used for treatment of infections related to *RSV, metapneumovirus, and parainfluenza and influenza viruses* [100]. Potential benefits of ribavarin therapy include the inhibition of RSV-specific IgE production in nasal secretions, which has been associated with the development of hypoxaemia and wheezing [101] and it has improved pulmonary functions [102]. Controlled studies also show that the use of ribavarin is effective in reducing the clinical severity score, duration of mechanical ventilation, supplemental oxygen use and days of hospitalisation [103]. Aerosolised ribavarin has been used for the treatment of *RSV*-related bronchiolitis and pneumonia. Intravenous formulation could be used for treatment of severe pneumonia, caused by infection *RSV, metapneumovirus, or parainfluenza virus*, on the basis of experience in immunocompromised patients [104]. Bonney et al. have shown that *metapneumovirus* can be successfully treated with a combination of intravenous ribavarin and immunoglobulin [105].

Although *rhinovirus* is the major cause of colds, its vast amount of serotypes has made development of anti-virals against it problematic. A 90% of *rhinovirus* serotypes gain entry into epithelial cells using ICAM-1 cellular receptors, and blockade of these receptors in experimental studies has shown reduced infection severity [106], but further study is required before this treatment option becomes widely available. Macrolide antibiotics, Bafilomycin A1 and Erythromycin have been shown to inhibit ICAM-1 epithelial expression and hypotheses about their potential as anti-inflammatory agents have yet to be definitive, as clinical proof is either negative or inconclusive [107].

Recently, an anti-rhinoviral agent known as Plecoranil, which acts by inhibiting the uncoating of Picornaviruses [108], the RV 3C protease inhibitor, Ruprintrivir[109] and soluble ICAM-1, Tremacamra[106] have shown promising results in early-stage clinical trials, but each of these medications was derailed by a combination of cost, pharmacokinetics, toxicity, drug interactions, and limited efficacy [110].

A previous study suggests that the increased morbidity in CF patients after virus infection is not due to an exaggerated inflammatory response of the airway epithelium but rather linked to increased cell death. Thus, they provide a rationale for implementing therapies aimed at controlling viruses and their replication rather than primarily targeting inflammation. In this respect, a promising candidate is the macrolide-antibiotic azithromycin, which is increasingly used in CF patients as a beneficial immunomodulatory agent [111] and has recently been shown to possess anti-viral properties [57].

6. Conclusion

As we become increasingly knowledgeable about the impact of respiratory virus infections in the context of CF exacerbations, screening for respiratory viruses should be part of the routine investigations for any CF patients that present with exacerbation symptoms. Using the appropriate sampling method in conjunction with sensitive and specific diagnostic technology will enable us to make appropriate clinical decisions surrounding the use of anti-virals and antibiotics.

Gaining further understanding in the pathogenesis of virus-induced respiratory exacerbations in CF may allow the development of new therapeutic techniques. If viral infection does predispose to bacterial infection, then influencing the interaction between viruses and bacteria could be a next pathway to diminish respiratory morbidity in patients with CF. The development of novel therapies will be exciting and this may improve their quality of life and prolong the lifespan of patients with CF.

However, there are still a number of research dilemmas that remain unanswered:

1. What are the standardised definitions of CF pulmonary exacerbation and pulmonary exacerbation severity score?
2. What is the optimal way for viral sampling?
3. What is the role of Virochip in routine viral identification?
4. How do respiratory viruses influence bacterial activities in chronically infected airways?
5. What influences the rate of respiratory viral clearance in CF respiratory tract?
6. What are the roles of anti-virals in CF?
7. What are the anti-viral properties of Azithromycin in CF?

Further understanding in the pathogenesis of viral infection in CF would be beneficial as this may provide insight to the above unresolved mysteries. At the moment, *influenza* vaccination and the use of neuraminidase inhibitors remain the only evidence based practice, albeit weak for the management of viral infections in CF.

Author details

Dennis Wat

Address all correspondence to: Dennis.Wat@lhch.nhs.uk

Liverpool Heart and Chest Hospital, Liverpool, United Kingdom

References

[1] Farrell PM. The prevalence of cystic fibrosis in the European Union. Journal of cystic fibrosis : official journal of the European Cystic Fibrosis Society. 2008;7(5):450-3.

[2] 2005 U.S. Cystic Fibrosis Foundation Annual Data Report to the Center Directors.. 2006.

[3] Riordan JR, Rommens JM, Kerem B, Alon N, Rozmahel R, Grzelczak Z, et al. Identification of the cystic fibrosis gene: cloning and characterization of complementary DNA. Science. 1989;245(4922):1066-73.

[4] Vawter GF, Shwachman H. Cystic fibrosis in adults: an autopsy study. Pathol Annu. 1979;14 Pt 2:357-82.

[5] Oppenheimer EH, Esterly JR. Pathology of cystic fibrosis review of the literature and comparison with 146 autopsied cases. Perspect Pediatr Pathol. 1975;2:241-78.

[6] Saiman L, Siegel J. Infection control in cystic fibrosis. Clin Microbiol Rev. 2004;17(1): 57-71.

[7] Rajan S, Saiman L. Pulmonary infections in patients with cystic fibrosis. Semin Respir Infect. 2002;17(1):47-56.

[8] Mahadeva R, Webb K, Westerbeek RC, Carroll NR, Dodd ME, Bilton D, et al. Clinical outcome in relation to care in centres specialising in cystic fibrosis: cross sectional study. Bmj. 1998;316(7147):1771-5.

[9] UK Cystic Fibrosis Registry Annual Data Report 2013: Summary 2014.

[10] Flume PA, Liou TG, Borowitz DS, Li H, Yen K, Ordonez CL, et al. Ivacaftor in subjects with cystic fibrosis who are homozygous for the F508del-CFTR mutation. Chest. 2012;142(3):718-24.

[11] Sawicki GS, Rasouliyan L, Pasta DJ, Regelmann WE, Wagener JS, Waltz DA, et al. The impact of incident methicillin resistant Staphylococcus aureus detection on pulmonary function in cystic fibrosis. Pediatr Pulmonol. 2008;43(11):1117-23.

[12] Thomassen MJ, Demko CA, Klinger JD, Stern RC. Pseudomonas cepacia colonization among patients with cystic fibrosis. A new opportunist. Am Rev Respir Dis. 1985;131(5):791-6.

[13] Nixon GM, Armstrong DS, Carzino R, Carlin JB, Olinsky A, Robertson CF, et al. Clinical outcome after early Pseudomonas aeruginosa infection in cystic fibrosis. J Pediatr. 2001;138(5):699-704.

[14] Aaron SD, Ramotar K, Ferris W, Vandemheen K, Saginur R, Tullis E, et al. Adult cystic fibrosis exacerbations and new strains of Pseudomonas aeruginosa. Am J Respir Crit Care Med. 2004;169(7):811-5.

[15] Chattoraj SS, Ganesan S, Jones AM, Helm JM, Comstock AT, Bright-Thomas R, et al. Rhinovirus infection liberates planktonic bacteria from biofilm and increases chemokine responses in cystic fibrosis airway epithelial cells. Thorax. 2011;66(4):333-9.

[16] Johansen HK, Hoiby N. Seasonal onset of initial colonisation and chronic infection with Pseudomonas aeruginosa in patients with cystic fibrosis in Denmark. Thorax. 1992;47(2):109-11.

[17] de Almeida MB, Zerbinati RM, Tateno AF, Oliveira CM, Romao RM, Rodrigues JC, et al. Rhinovirus C and respiratory exacerbations in children with cystic fibrosis. Emerging infectious diseases. 2010;16(6):996-9.

[18] Etherington C, Naseer R, Conway SP, Whitaker P, Denton M, Peckham DG. The role of respiratory viruses in adult patients with cystic fibrosis receiving intravenous antibiotics for a pulmonary exacerbation. Journal of cystic fibrosis : official journal of the European Cystic Fibrosis Society. 2014;13(1):49-55.

[19] Wat D, Doull I. Respiratory virus infections in cystic fibrosis. Paediatric respiratory reviews. 2003;4(3):172-7.

[20] Petersen NT, Hoiby N, Mordhorst CH, Lind K, Flensborg EW, Bruun B. Respiratory infections in cystic fibrosis patients caused by virus, chlamydia and mycoplasma--possible synergism with Pseudomonas aeruginosa. Acta paediatrica Scandinavica. 1981;70(5):623-8.

[21] Armstrong D, Grimwood K, Carlin JB, Carzino R, Hull J, Olinsky A, et al. Severe viral respiratory infections in infants with cystic fibrosis. Pediatric pulmonology. 1998;26(6):371-9.

[22] Hiatt PW, Grace SC, Kozinetz CA, Raboudi SH, Treece DG, Taber LH, et al. Effects of viral lower respiratory tract infection on lung function in infants with cystic fibrosis. Pediatrics. 1999;103(3):619-26.

[23] Pribble CG, Black PG, Bosso JA, Turner RB. Clinical manifestations of exacerbations of cystic fibrosis associated with nonbacterial infections. The Journal of pediatrics. 1990;117(2 Pt 1):200-4.

[24] Ramsey BW, Gore EJ, Smith AL, Cooney MK, Redding GJ, Foy H. The effect of respiratory viral infections on patients with cystic fibrosis. American journal of diseases of children. 1989;143(6):662-8.

[25] Wang EE, Prober CG, Manson B, Corey M, Levison H. Association of respiratory viral infections with pulmonary deterioration in patients with cystic fibrosis. The New England journal of medicine. 1984;311(26):1653-8.

[26] Collinson J, Nicholson KG, Cancio E, Ashman J, Ireland DC, Hammersley V, et al. Effects of upper respiratory tract infections in patients with cystic fibrosis. Thorax. 1996;51(11):1115-22.

[27] Smyth AR, Smyth RL, Tong CY, Hart CA, Heaf DP. Effect of respiratory virus infections including rhinovirus on clinical status in cystic fibrosis. Archives of disease in childhood. 1995;73(2):117-20.

[28] Olesen HV, Nielsen LP, Schiotz PO. Viral and atypical bacterial infections in the outpatient pediatric cystic fibrosis clinic. Pediatric pulmonology. 2006;41(12):1197-204.

[29] Influenza virus vaccine live intranasal--MedImmune vaccines: CAIV-T, influenza vaccine live intranasal. Drugs in R&D. 2003;4(5):312-9.

[30] Thompson WW, Shay DK, Weintraub E, Brammer L, Bridges CB, Cox NJ, et al. Influenza-associated hospitalizations in the United States. JAMA. 2004;292(11):1333-40.

[31] Ortiz JR, Neuzil KM, Victor JC, Wald A, Aitken ML, Goss CH. Influenza-associated cystic fibrosis pulmonary exacerbations. Chest. 2010;137(4):852-60.

[32] Chin M, De Zoysa M, Slinger R, Gaudet E, Vandemheen KL, Chan F, et al. Acute effects of viral respiratory tract infections on sputum bacterial density during CF pulmonary exacerbations. Journal of cystic fibrosis : official journal of the European Cystic Fibrosis Society. 2014.

[33] Punch G, Syrmis MW, Rose BR, Harbour C, Bye PT, Nissen MD, et al. Method for detection of respiratory viruses in the sputa of patients with cystic fibrosis. Eur J Clin Microbiol Infect Dis. 2005;24(1):54-7.

[34] Wat D, Gelder C, Hibbitts S, Bowler I, Pierrepoint M, Evans R, et al. Is there a role for influenza vaccination in cystic fibrosis? J Cyst Fibros. 2008;7(1):85-8.

[35] Flight WG, Bright-Thomas RJ, Tilston P, Mutton KJ, Guiver M, Morris J, et al. Incidence and clinical impact of respiratory viruses in adults with cystic fibrosis. Thorax. 2014;69(3):247-53.

[36] Wat D, Gelder C, Hibbitts S, Cafferty F, Bowler I, Pierrepoint M, et al. The role of respiratory viruses in cystic fibrosis. Journal of cystic fibrosis : official journal of the European Cystic Fibrosis Society. 2008;7(4):320-8.

[37] Abman SH, Ogle JW, Harbeck RJ, Butler-Simon N, Hammond KB, Accurso FJ. Early bacteriologic, immunologic, and clinical courses of young infants with cystic fibrosis identified by neonatal screening. J Pediatr. 1991;119(2):211-7.

[38] Brasfield D, Hicks G, Soong S, Tiller RE. The chest roentgenogram in cystic fibrosis: a new scoring system. Pediatrics. 1979;63(1):24-9.

[39] Conway SP, Simmonds EJ, Littlewood JM. Acute severe deterioration in cystic fibrosis associated with influenza A virus infection. Thorax. 1992;47(2):112-4.

[40] Shwachman H, Kulczycki LL. Long-term study of one hundred five patients with cystic fibrosis; studies made over a five- to fourteen-year period. AMA J Dis Child. 1958;96(1):6-15.

[41] Chrispin AR, Norman AP. The systematic evaluation of the chest radiograph in cystic fibrosis. Pediatr Radiol. 1974;2(2):101-5.

[42] Punch G, Syrmis MW, Rose BR, Harbour C, Bye PT, Nissen MD, et al. Method for detection of respiratory viruses in the sputa of patients with cystic fibrosis. European journal of clinical microbiology & infectious diseases : official publication of the European Society of Clinical Microbiology. 2005;24(1):54-7.

[43] Esposito S, Dacco V, Daleno C, Gambazza S, Montinaro V, Bisogno A, et al. Human rhinovirus infection in children with cystic fibrosis. Japanese journal of infectious diseases. 2014;67(5):399-401.

[44] Asner S, Waters V, Solomon M, Yau Y, Richardson SE, Grasemann H, et al. Role of respiratory viruses in pulmonary exacerbations in children with cystic fibrosis. Journal of cystic fibrosis : official journal of the European Cystic Fibrosis Society. 2012;11(5):433-9.

[45] Nokso-Koivisto J, Kinnari TJ, Lindahl P, Hovi T, Pitkaranta A. Human picornavirus and coronavirus RNA in nasopharynx of children without concurrent respiratory symptoms. Journal of medical virology. 2002;66(3):417-20.

[46] Nash EF, Whitmill R, Barker B, Rashid R, Whitehouse JL, Honeybourne D. Clinical outcomes of pandemic (H1N1) 2009 influenza (swine flu) in adults with cystic fibrosis. Thorax. 2011;66(3):259.

[47] Colombo C, Battezzati PM, Lucidi V, Magazzu G, Motta V, Alicandro G, et al. Influenza A/H1N1 in patients with cystic fibrosis in Italy: a multicentre cohort study. Thorax. 2011;66(3):260-1.

[48] Hoek RA, Paats MS, Pas SD, Bakker M, Hoogsteden HC, Boucher CA, et al. Incidence of viral respiratory pathogens causing exacerbations in adult cystic fibrosis patients. Scandinavian journal of infectious diseases. 2013;45(1):65-9.

[49] Kurt-Jones EA, Popova L, Kwinn L, Haynes LM, Jones LP, Tripp RA, et al. Pattern recognition receptors TLR4 and CD14 mediate response to respiratory syncytial virus. Nat Immunol. 2000;1(5):398-401.

[50] Haynes LM, Moore DD, Kurt-Jones EA, Finberg RW, Anderson LJ, Tripp RA. Involvement of toll-like receptor 4 in innate immunity to respiratory syncytial virus. J Virol. 2001;75(22):10730-7.

[51] Qureshi ST, Medzhitov R. Toll-like receptors and their role in experimental models of microbial infection. Genes Immun. 2003;4(2):87-94.

[52] Seki M, Higashiyama Y, Tomono K, Yanagihara K, Ohno H, Kaneko Y, et al. Acute infection with influenza virus enhances suspectibility to fatal pneumonia following Streptococcus pneumoniae infection in mice with chronic pulmonary colonisation with Psudomonas aeruginosa. Clin Exp Immunol. 2004;137(1):35-40.

[53] Zheng S, De B, Choudhary S, Comhair S, Goggans T, Slee R, et al. Impaired innate host defense causes suspectibility to respiratory virus infections in cystic fibrosis. Immunity. 2003;18(5):619-30.

[54] Zheng S, Xu W, Bose S, Banerjee A, Haque S, Erzurum S. Impaired nitirc oxide synthase-2 signaling pathway in cystic fibrosis airway epithelium. Am J Physiol Lung Cell Mol Physiol. 2004;287(2):L374-81.

[55] Xu W, Zheng S, Goggans TM, Kiser P, Quinones-Mateu ME, Janocha AJ, et al. Cystic fibrosis and normal human airway epithelial cell response to influenza a viral infection. J Interferon Cytokine Res. 2006;26(9):609-27.

[56] Sutanto EN, Kicic A, Foo CJ, Stevens PT, Mullane D, Knight DA, et al. Innate inflammatory responses of pediatric cystic fibrosis airway epithelial cells: effects of nonviral and viral stimulation. Am J Respir Cell Mol Biol. 2011;44(6):761-7.

[57] Gielen V, Johnston SL, Edwards MR. Azithromycin induces anti-viral responses in bronchial epithelial cells. The European respiratory journal. 2010;36(3):646-54.

[58] Schogler A, Kopf BS, Edwards MR, Johnston SL, Casaulta C, Kieninger E, et al. Novel antiviral properties of azithromycin in cystic fibrosis airway epithelial cells. The European respiratory journal. 2015;45(2):428-39.

[59] Chiu CY, Rouskin S, Koshy A, Urisman A, Fischer K, Yagi S, et al. Microarray detection of human parainfluenzavirus 4 infection associated with respiratory failure in an immunocompetent adult. Clin Infect Dis. 2006;43(8):e71-6.

[60] Przyklenk B, Bauernfeind A, Bertele RM. Viral infections in the respiratory tract in patients with cystic fibrosis. Serodign Immunother Infect Dis. 1988(2):217-25.

[61] Walsh JJ, Dietlein LF, Low FN, Burch GE, Mogabgab WJ. Bronchotracheal response in human influenza. Type A, Asian strain, as studied by light and electron microscopic examination of bronchoscopic biopsies. Arch Intern Med. 1961;108:376-88.

[62] Winther B, Gwaltney J, Hendley J. Respiratory virus infection of monolayer cultures of human nasal epithelial cells. Am Rev Respir Dis. 1990;141(4 Pt 1):839-45.

[63] Ohrui T, Yamaya M, Sekizawa K, Yamada N, Suzuki T, Terajima M, et al. Effects of rhinovirus infection on hydrogen peroxide- induced alterations of barrier function in the cultured human tracheal epithelium. Am J Respir Crit Care Med. 1998;158(1): 241-8.

[64] Igarashi Y, Skoner DP, Doyle WJ, White MV, Fireman P, Kaliner MA. Analysis of nasal secretions during experimental rhinovirus upper respiratory infections. J Allergy Clin Immunol. 1993;92(5):722-31.

[65] Sanford BA, Shelokov A, Ramsay MA. Bacterial adherence to virus-infected cells: a cell culture model of bacterial superinfection. J Infect Dis. 1978;137(2):176-81.

[66] Raza MW, Essery SD, Weir DM, Ogilvie MM, Elton RA, Blackwell CC. Infection with respiratory syncytial virus and water-soluble components of cigarette smoke alter production of tumour necrosis factor alpha and nitric oxide by human blood monocytes. FEMS Immunol Med Microbiol. 1999;24(4):387-94.

[67] Kim EY, Battaile JT, Patel AC, You Y, Agapov E, Grayson MH, et al. Persistent activation of an innate immune response translates respiratory viral infection into chronic lung disease. Nat Med. 2008;14(6):633-40.

[68] Murphy TF, Sethi S. Bacterial infection in chronic obstructive pulmonary disease. Am Rev Respir Dis. 1992;146(4):1067-83.

[69] Wilson R, Cole PJ. The effect of bacterial products on ciliary function. Am Rev Respir Dis. 1988;138(6 Pt 2):S49-53.

[70] Jiang Z, Nagata N, Molina E, Bakaletz LO, Hawkins H, Patel JA. Fimbria-mediated enhanced attachment of nontypeable Haemophilus influenzae to respiratory syncytial virus-infected respiratory epithelial cells. Infect Immun. 1999;67(1):187-92.

[71] White AJ, Gompertz S, Stockley RA. Chronic obstructive pulmonary disease. 6: The aetiology of exacerbations of chronic obstructive pulmonary disease. Thorax. 2003;58(1):73-80.

[72] Avadhanula V, Rodriguez CA, Devincenzo JP, Wang Y, Webby RJ, Ulett GC, et al. Respiratory viruses augment the adhesion of bacterial pathogens to respiratory epithelium in a viral species- and cell type-dependent manner. J Virol. 2006;80(4): 1629-36.

[73] Hament JM, Kimpen JL, Fleer A, Wolfs TF. Respiratory viral infection predisposing for bacterial disease: a concise review. FEMS Immunol Med Microbiol. 1999;26(3-4): 189-95.

[74] Oliver BG, Lim S, Wark P, Laza-Stanca V, King N, Black JL, et al. Rhinovirus exposure impairs immune responses to bacterial products in human alveolar macrophages. Thorax. 2008;63(6):519-25.

[75] Thompson CI, Barclay WS, Zambon MC, Pickles RJ. Infection of human airway epithelium by human and avian strains of influenza a virus. J Virol. 2006;80(16):8060-8.

[76] Pittet LA, Hall-Stoodley L, Rutkowski MR, Harmsen AG. Influenza virus infection decreases tracheal mucociliary velocity and clearance of Streptococcus pneumoniae. Am J Respir Cell Mol Biol.42(4):450-60.

[77] de Vrankrijker AM, Wolfs TF, Ciofu O, Hoiby N, van der Ent CK, Poulsen SS, et al. Respiratory syncytial virus infection facilitates acute colonization of Pseudomonas aeruginosa in mice. J Med Virol. 2009;81(12):2096-103.

[78] Avadhanula V, Wang Y, Portner A, Adderson E. Nontypeable Haemophilus influenzae and Streptococcus pneumoniae bind respiratory syncytial virus glycoprotein. J Med Microbiol. 2007;56(Pt 9):1133-7.

[79] Stark JM, Stark MA, Colasurdo GN, LeVine AM. Decreased bacterial clearance from the lungs of mice following primary respiratory syncytial virus infection. J Med Virol. 2006;78(6):829-38.

[80] Kieninger E, Vareille M, Kopf BS, Blank F, Alves MP, Gisler FM, et al. Lack of an exaggerated inflammatory response on virus infection in cystic fibrosis. The European respiratory journal. 2012;39(2):297-304.

[81] Subrata LS, Bizzintino J, Mamessier E, Bosco A, McKenna KL, Wikstrom ME, et al. Interactions between innate antiviral and atopic immunoinflammatory pathways precipitate and sustain asthma exacerbations in children. Journal of immunology. 2009;183(4):2793-800.

[82] Perry AK, Chen G, Zheng D, Tang H, Cheng G. The host type I interferon response to viral and bacterial infections. Cell Res. 2005;15(6):407-22.

[83] Parker D, Cohen TS, Alhede M, Harfenist BS, Martin FJ, Prince A. Induction of type I interferon signaling by Pseudomonas aeruginosa is diminished in cystic fibrosis epithelial cells. Am J Respir Cell Mol Biol. 2012;46(1):6-13.

[84] Green HK, Andrews N, Fleming D, Zambon M, Pebody R. Mortality attributable to influenza in England and Wales prior to, during and after the 2009 pandemic. PloS one. 2013;8(12):e79360.

[85] Heinonen S, Silvennoinen H, Lehtinen P, Vainionpaa R, Ziegler T, Heikkinen T. Effectiveness of inactivated influenza vaccine in children aged 9 months to 3 years: an observational cohort study. Lancet Infect Dis. 2010;11(1):23-9.

[86] Dharmaraj P, Smyth RL. Vaccines for preventing influenza in people with cystic fibrosis. The Cochrane database of systematic reviews. 2014;3:Cd001753.

[87] Harper SA, Bradley JS, Englund JA, File TM, Gravenstein S, Hayden FG, et al. Seasonal influenza in adults and children--diagnosis, treatment, chemoprophylaxis, and institutional outbreak management: clinical practice guidelines of the Infectious Diseases Society of America. Clin Infect Dis. 2009;48(8):1003-32.

[88] Katpally U, Fu TM, Freed DC, Casimiro DR, Smith TJ. Antibodies to the buried N terminus of rhinovirus VP4 exhibit cross-serotypic neutralization. J Virol. 2009;83(14): 7040-8.

[89] Kim HW, Canchola JG, Brandt CD, Pyles G, Chanock RM, Jensen K, et al. Respiratory syncytial virus disease in infants despite prior administration of antigenic inactivated vaccine. Am J Epidemiol. 1969;89(4):422-34.

[90] Giebels K, Marcotte JE, Podoba J, Rousseau C, Denis MH, Fauvel V, et al. Prophylaxis against respiratory syncytial virus in young children with cystic fibrosis. Pediatr Pulmonol. 2008;43(2):169-74.

[91] Robinson KA, Odelola OA, Saldanha IJ. Palivizumab for prophylaxis against respiratory syncytial virus infection in children with cystic fibrosis. The Cochrane database of systematic reviews. 2014;5:Cd007743.

[92] Schmidt AC, McAuliffe JM, Murphy BR, Collins PL. Recombinant bovine/human parainfluenza virus type 3 (B/HPIV3) expressing the respiratory syncytial virus (RSV) G and F proteins can be used to achieve simultaneous mucosal immunization against RSV and HPIV3. J Virol. 2001;75(10):4594-603.

[93] Shun-Shin M, Thompson M, Heneghan C, Perera R, Harnden A, Mant D. Neuraminidase inhibitors for treatment and prophylaxis of influenza in children: systematic review and meta-analysis of randomised controlled trials. BMJ. 2009;339:b3172.

[94] Yu H, Liao Q, Yuan Y, Zhou L, Xiang N, Huai Y, et al. Effectiveness of oseltamivir on disease progression and viral RNA shedding in patients with mild pandemic 2009 influenza A H1N1: opportunistic retrospective study of medical charts in China. BMJ. 2010;341:c4779.

[95] Bautista E, Chotpitayasunondh T, Gao Z, Harper SA, Shaw M, Uyeki TM, et al. Clinical aspects of pandemic 2009 influenza A (H1N1) virus infection. N Engl J Med. 2010;362(18):1708-19.

[96] Hayden FG, Treanor JJ, Betts RF, Lobo M, Esinhart JD, Hussey EK. Safety and efficacy of the neuraminidase inhibitor GG167 in experimental human influenza. Jama. 1996;275(4):295-9.

[97] Birnkrant D, Cox E. The Emergency Use Authorization of peramivir for treatment of 2009 H1N1 influenza. N Engl J Med. 2009;361(23):2204-7.

[98] Harter G, Zimmermann O, Maier L, Schubert A, Mertens T, Kern P, et al. Intravenous zanamivir for patients with pneumonitis due to pandemic (H1N1) 2009 influenza virus. Clin Infect Dis. 2010;50(9):1249-51.

[99] Jagannath VA, Asokan GV, Fedorowicz Z, Lee TW. Neuraminidase inhibitors for the treatment of influenza infection in people with cystic fibrosis. The Cochrane database of systematic reviews. 2014;2:Cd008139.

[100] Yin M, Brust J, van Tieu H, Hammer S. Antiherpes, anti-hepatitis virus, and anti-respiratory virus agents. In: Richman D, Whiyley R, Hayden F, editors. Clinical virology, 3rd edition. Washington: ASM Press; 2009. p. 217-64.

[101] Rosner IK, Welliver RC, Edelson PJ, Geraci-Ciardullo K, Sun M. Effect of ribavirin therapy on respiratory syncytial virus-specific IgE and IgA responses after infection. J Infect Dis. 1987;155(5):1043-7.

[102] Hiatt PT, D Laber, L. Pulmonary function (PF) following treatment with ribavarin in infants hospitalised with RSV bronchiolitis. Am Rev Respir Dis. 1990;141:A624.

[103] Smith DW, Frankel LR, Mathers LH, Tang AT, Ariagno RL, Prober CG. A controlled trial of aerosolized ribavirin in infants receiving mechanical ventilation for severe respiratory syncytial virus infection. N Engl J Med. 1991;325(1):24-9.

[104] Hopkins P, McNeil K, Kermeen F, Musk M, McQueen E, Mackay I, et al. Human metapneumovirus in lung transplant recipients and comparison to respiratory syncytial virus. Am J Respir Crit Care Med. 2008;178(8):876-81.

[105] Bonney D, Razali H, Turner A, Will A. Successful treatment of human metapneumovirus pneumonia using combination therapy with intravenous ribavirin and immune globulin. Br J Haematol. 2009;145(5):667-9.

[106] Turner RB, Wecker MT, Pohl G, Witek TJ, McNally E, St George R, et al. Efficacy of tremacamra, a soluble intercellular adhesion molecule 1, for experimental rhinovirus infection: a randomized clinical trial. Jama. 1999;281(19):1797-804.

[107] Suzuki T, Yamaya M, Sekizawa K, Hosoda M, Yamada N, Ishizuka S, et al. Erythromycin inhibits rhinovirus infection in cultured human tracheal epithelial cells. Am J Respir Crit Care Med. 2002;165(8):1113-8.

[108] Ledford RM, Patel NR, Demenczuk TM, Watanyar A, Herbertz T, Collett MS, et al. VP1 sequencing of all human rhinovirus serotypes: insights into genus phylogeny and susceptibility to antiviral capsid-binding compounds. J Virol. 2004;78(7):3663-74.

[109] Hayden FG, Turner RB, Gwaltney JM, Chi-Burris K, Gersten M, Hsyu P, et al. Phase II, randomized, double-blind, placebo-controlled studies of ruprintrivir nasal spray 2-percent suspension for prevention and treatment of experimentally induced rhinovirus colds in healthy volunteers. Antimicrobial agents and chemotherapy. 2003;47(12):3907-16.

[110] Turner RB. New considerations in the treatment and prevention of rhinovirus infections. Pediatr Ann. 2005;34(1):53-7.

[111] Equi A, Balfour-Lynn IM, Bush A, Rosenthal M. Long term azithromycin in children with cystic fibrosis: a randomised, placebo-controlled crossover trial. Lancet. 2002;360(9338):978-84.

2

New Research on the Importance of Cystic Fibrosis Transmembrane Conductance Regulator Function for Optimal Neutrophil Activity

Michelle M. White, Fatma Gargoum, Niall Browne, Killian Hurley, Noel G. McElvaney and Emer P. Reeves

Abstract

Despite tremendous recent advances in our understanding of the molecular and cellular basis of cystic fibrosis (CF), there remains a paradox of why recruited neutrophils fail to eradicate bacterial infections in the airways of individuals with CF. The focus of this chapter is on new research authenticating the CF neutrophil as a key player in disease pathogenesis. Studies specifying intrinsic abnormalities due to a lack of cystic fibrosis transmembrane conductance regulator (CFTR) function, along with reports indicating reprogrammed cell activity secondary to chronic bacterial infection and inflammation, will be discussed.

Keywords: cystic fibrosis, cystic fibrosis transmembrane conductance regulator, neutrophil function

1. Introduction

Cystic fibrosis (CF) is a multi-system disease resulting from mutations in the gene encoding the cystic fibrosis transmembrane conductance regulator (CFTR). In excess of 1900 CF mutations have been identified thus far [1], leading to misfolding of the CFTR protein and defective chloride (Cl^-) transport across cell membranes. CF affects various organs including the pancreas, liver, and intestinal tract, but the most severe complications often occur in the lung. CF related symptoms, although variable among patients, are typically present early in life and increase in severity with age despite aggressive therapeutic intervention. CFTR absence or malfunction causes defective ion transport across the epithelium, reduction in pericillary liquid volume, and persistent mucus hypersecretion. As a consequence, mucus accumulates on the airway surface and leads to chronic bacterial infection, exacerbated airway inflammation, and lung injury. Pulmonary inflammation in the CF setting has been observed as early as infancy and there is evidence of structural lung disease present in children with CF as young as 10 weeks old, with 50%–70% of children presenting with bronchiectasis by 3–5 years [2-6]. Additional studies have shown neutrophil-dominated airway inflammation in children with CF [7, 8], and with increasing age elevated levels of proinflammatory mediators including interleukin (IL)-8 [9], tumour necrosis factor-alpha (TNF-alpha) [10], and leukotriene B_4 (LTB_4) [11] serve to escalate the chronic neutrophil presence in the pulmonary circulation. Indeed, key studies have demonstrated that neutrophil-released granule proteins, particularly neutrophil elastase (NE), play a crucial pathological role (Figure 1) [12, 13]. In the healthy lung, neutrophils represent approximately 1% of the inflammatory cells; however, they account for 60–70% of the total cell count in CF bronchial lavage fluid [14, 15] and ~25% of CF children were positive for free NE activity in airway samples at 3 months old [16].

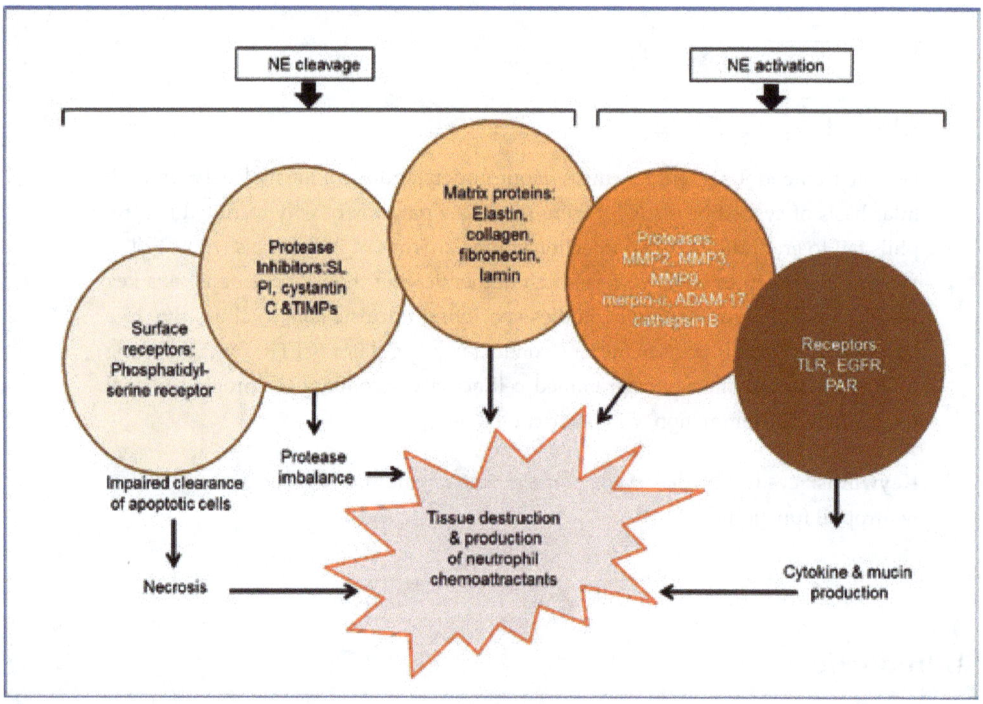

Figure 1. The potential effects of active NE in CF. Neutrophil elastase (NE) has the potential to cleave structural molecules and antiproteases causing an anti-protease imbalance and also activate enzymes and receptors that play a crucial pathological role in CF. Abbreviations used: NE, neutrophil elastase; SLPI, secretory leukocyte protease inhibitor; TIMPs, tissue inhibitors of metalloproteinases; MMP, metalloproteinase; TACE, tumour necrosis factor-alpha-converting enzyme; TLRs, toll-like receptors; EGFR, epidermal growth factor receptor; PAR, protease activated receptors.

Despite advances in our understanding of the molecular and cellular basis of CF, there persists an enigma as to why recruited neutrophils fail to eradicate bacterial infections in the lung. Support for the hypothesis that a genetic defect gives rise to dysregulated neutrophil responses in CF is shown by a study demonstrating upregulation of genes coding for both chemokines and proteins involved in signal transduction in CF [17]. A recent study has demonstrated that CXC chemokine receptors 1/2 (CXCR1/CXCR2) haplotypes in CF modulate antibacterial neutrophil functions against *P. aeruginosa* [18]. In addition, CF circulating neutrophils display an altered toll-like receptor (TLR) expression when compared to blood neutrophils from healthy subjects, including reduced expression of TLR2 [19, 20]. A recently published study identified IFRD1 (interferon-related developmental regulator 1), a histone-deacetylase-dependent transcriptional co-regulator expressed during terminal neutrophil differentiation, as a genetic modifier of CF disease severity. Neutrophils isolated from IFRD1 deficient mice exhibited impaired oxidative burst, bacterial clearance, and cytokine production leading to excessive bacterial burden and chronic infection of the lung [21]. Furthermore, levels of IFRD in bronchial epithelial cells with the *ΔF508* mutation were significantly reduced but could be rescued by treatment with glutathione suggesting down-regulation of IFRD1 expression in response to oxidative stress [22].

The focus of this chapter is on new research authenticating the CF neutrophil as a key player in disease pathogenesis. Studies published in the previous 10 years specifying intrinsic abnormalities due to a lack of CFTR function, along with reports indicating reprogrammed cell activity secondary to chronic bacterial infection and inflammation will be discussed. Our review of the literature was carried out using the MEDLINE database (from 2005 to the year 2015), Google Scholar, and The Cochrane Library databases using several appropriate generic terms.

2. The debate on CFTR expression by neutrophils

The year 2015 marks the 26th anniversary of the identification and isolation of the *CFTR* gene from epithelial cells [23]. This initial discovery was vital in the development of CFTR-targeted pharmacotherapy and resulted in an explosion of research aimed at identifying the expression of *CFTR* mRNA transcripts and protein levels in epithelial cells and non-epithelial cells alike. Although CF is a pleiotropic disease that affects multiple organs, disease progression is most pronounced in the airways and therefore researchers initially studied the expression of *CFTR* in epithelial cells found within the lungs. In this regard, Yoshimura and colleagues (1991) demonstrated the expression of *CFTR* mRNA transcripts in human bronchial epithelial cells [24], and Trapnall *et al.* demonstrated equal expression of *CFTR* mRNA transcripts from isolated respiratory tract epithelial cells from healthy controls and homozygous and heterozygous *ΔF508* patients with CF [25]. The level of research at this stage indicated that the expression of the *CFTR* was epithelial cell specific, yet the conclusions drawn from a further study by Yoshimura suggested that the *CFTR*-gene had characteristics of a house-keeping gene, suggesting that it may be present in other cell types [26]. This latter manuscript prompted researchers to examine *CFTR* mRNA transcripts in other cell types and in late 1991, Yoshimura demonstrated the expression of low levels of *CFTR* mRNA transcripts in non-epithelial cells, including T-lymphocytes, neutrophils, monocytes, and alveolar macrophages, all of human origin [26]. This was the first record of *CFTR* gene expression in a multitude of immune cell types, and the authors suggested an important role for CFTR Cl^- transport. In agreement, it was later demonstrated that alveolar macrophages from *CFTR* deficient mice retained the ability to phagocytose and generate an oxidative burst, but exhibited defective killing of internalized bacteria due to impaired acidification of the phagosome. Of interest, in this later study CFTR protein was not detected in either murine or human neutrophils [27] and further studies have shown CFTR independent phagosomal acidification in macrophages [28, 29]. Nevertheless, the expression of *CFTR* mRNA transcripts in human macrophages was confirmed by Del Porto, who published that the bactericidal capabilities of macrophages was CFTR dependent, indicating an important functional role for the CFTR protein in these immune cells [30].

Up to this point, no connection between abnormal neutrophil function and the expression of CFTR protein in human neutrophils had been made, and whether or not neutrophils express functional CFTR was still the topic of great debate among leading scientists and clinicians [5, 8, 13, 14], with relevance for the development of CFTR-targeting pharmacotherapy. This is emanating from worldwide laboratories equally committed to the pursuit of knowledge on the cause for impaired neutrophil activity in CF and also the potential consequence of the loss of functional CFTR Cl^- channels. Indeed, there is still great controversy as to the true nature of dysregulated neutrophil activity in CF and, for example, in 2010, McKeon and colleagues could only detect low levels of *CFTR* mRNA transcripts in human neutrophils by either reverse transcriptase polymerase chain reaction (RT-PCR) or real time PCR methods of amplification [31]. The authors could not detect CFTR protein expression in membrane or cytosolic fractions, or cell lysates from human neutrophils by Western blot analysis, suggesting that human neutrophils do not express CFTR protein and that the dysregulated neutrophil function in CF was due to the inflammatory status of the individual [31]. Similarly, a study by Morris *et al.*, (2005) who investigated altered phagocytosis of neutrophils in CF due to cell priming, did not detect CFTR protein in human neutrophils by Western blot analysis [32].

Over the years, a number of reasons for not detecting CFTR protein in neutrophil cell fractions by Western blot analysis have been put forward and include the susceptibility of CFTR protein to degradation, a lack of reliable anti-CFTR antibodies, and also boiling of cell fractions prior to electrophoresis. As these issues were addressed researchers have detected CFTR protein in human neutrophils and have established functional roles for membrane associated CFTR. In line with this concept, in 2006, Painter and colleagues demonstrated the presence of CFTR protein in human neutrophil membrane phagolysosomes by confocal microscopy, and also verified the expression of *CFTR* at a mRNA level, and at a protein level by Western blot analysis [33]. Interestingly, in this same study results demonstrated the expression of CFTR protein by Western blot analysis in a human myeloid cell line (HL-60 cells) differentiated into neutrophil-like cells [33]. This is in contrast to the study by Yoshimura *et al.*, who could not detect *CFTR* mRNA transcripts in HL-60 cells [24]. Further studies have identified *CFTR* mRNA transcripts in differentiated HL-60 cells and demonstrated CFTR protein localisation to the phagocytic vacuole, strengthening the similarities between HL-60 cells and human neutrophils [34].

Furthermore, expression of CFTR protein was confirmed by Pohl *et al.* (2014) in healthy control neutrophils and levels were severely impaired in neutrophils isolated from people with CF carrying the *ΔF508* or *G551D* mutation. By flow cytometry, this latter study also demonstrated that the percentage of CFTR positive cells significantly increased post phorbol ester stimulation [35], indicating upregulation of CFTR to the plasma membrane post activation. Interestingly, bacterial lipopolysaccharide (LPS)-stimulated murine neutrophils also demonstrated increased CFTR protein expression when compared to unstimulated cells, suggesting a role for CFTR in bacterial mediated neutrophil cell activation [36].

3. The role of CFTR in neutrophils: oxygen dependent and independent mechanisms of microbial killing

3.1. Oxygen dependent killing

The focus of this chapter will now turn to studies that have reported impaired neutrophil activity due to a lack of CFTR function. Of major relevance to bacterial killing in CF, reported defective killing of microbes due to conditions that prevail within the vacuole of phagocytosing neutrophils will be discussed. The process of neutrophil mediated bacterial clearance can be divided into two main processes: those that are oxygen independent and those that are oxygen dependent. With regards to oxidative mechanisms of microbial killing, the first indications that oxygen plays a role in the functionality of neutrophils was first discovered by Baldridge and Gerard [37]. By exposing canine neutrophils to bacteria they observed a significant increase in oxygen consumption [37], and later it was revealed that this increase in oxygen consumption was independent of mitochondrial respiration [38]. Following discovery of the respiratory burst, it was discovered that neutrophils from patients with chronic granulomatous disease (CGD) failed to mount a respiratory burst during phagocytosis and these individuals are characterised by an abnormality of neutrophil function and recurrent life-threatening infections [39, 40]. CGD provides the most definitive evidence for the physiological and clinical importance of the respiratory burst, or alternatively referred to as the NADPH oxidase (nicotinamide adenine dinucleotide phosphate oxidase). Indeed, patients with CGD have played a vital role in understanding the structure and mechanism of the NADPH oxidase (Figure 2). The burst of oxygen consumption upon phagocytosis and the absence of this process in CGD leading to impaired bacterial killing was understood to indicate that the oxygen consumed was converted to antimicrobial oxidants. By exposing neutrophils to opsonised bacteria, Cohen and colleagues demonstrated that 99% of oxygen consumed was converted to superoxide (O_2^-) [41] and the requirement of O_2^- as a precursor to hydrogen peroxide (H_2O_2) was confirmed [42]. It is not known what concentration of H_2O_2 is attained within the vacuole, with measurement from 0.01μM [42] to 100mM estimated, depending on the amount of phagocytosis and the intracellular pH [43]. These oxidants produced by neutrophils may also contribute to lung tissue damage and the shield against oxidant-modulated injury is the extracellular anti-oxidant glutathione; but this is significantly decreased in CF epithelial lining fluid [44-47]. Of major relevance is that CFTR has been linked to extracellular glutathione transport [48] and in paediatric reports of extremely high levels of protein oxidation have been detected in airway samples [49].

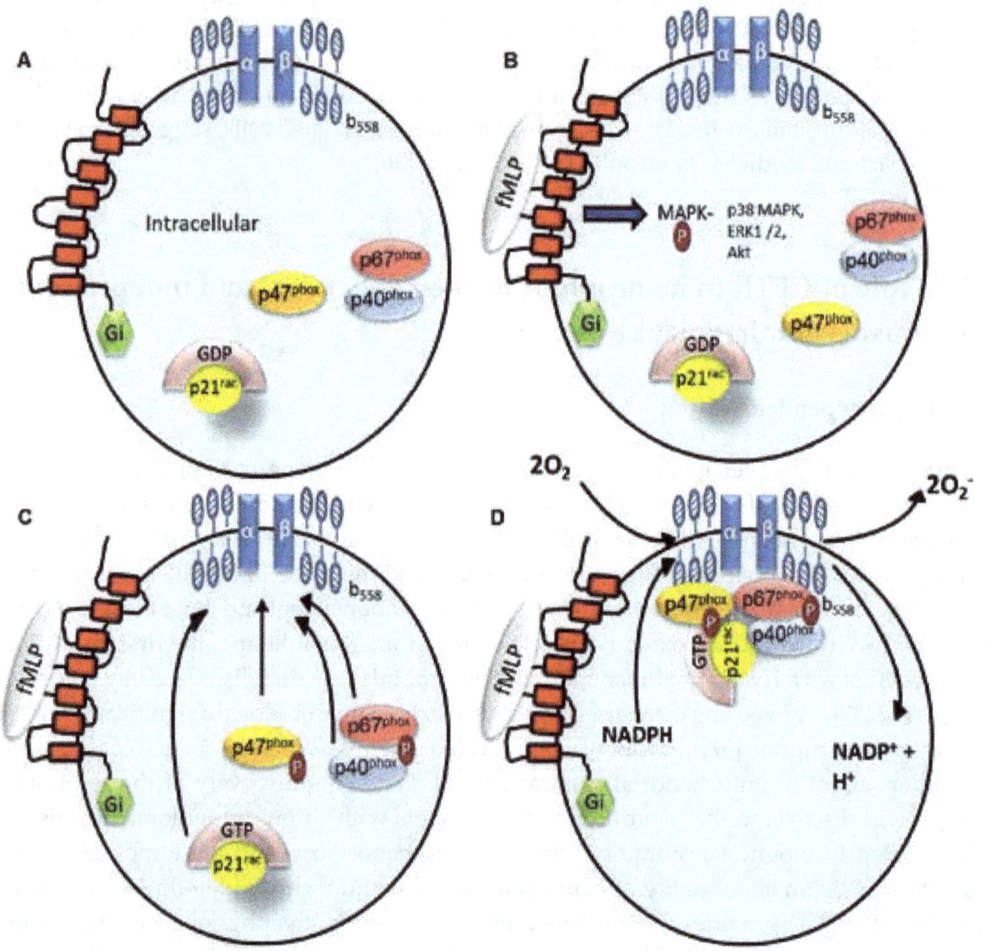

The neutrophil respiratory burst, or NADPH oxidase, generates superoxide (O_2^-) as the initial oxygen-derived reactive species in response to bacteria or a variety of soluble stimuli (fMLP). A) The enzyme complex is latent in quiescent unstimulated neutrophils and approximately 20% flavocytochrome b_{558} is found in the plasma membrane pool, and 80% in the specific granules. The active site of this enzyme is located in an integral membrane cytochrome, b_{558}, which consists of the two subunits $gp91^{phox}$ and $p21^{phox}$ (α and β subunits, respectively). B) Stimulation of the neutrophil by fMLP induces activation and phosphorylation (P) of a number of kinases including Akt. C) $p21^{rac}$ is converted into the active guanosine triphosphate GTP-bound form and the phosphorylation of the cytosolic components ($p67^{phox}$, $p47^{phox}$, and $p40^{phox}$) occurs. D) These subunits then translocate to the plasma membrane where they interact with cytochrome b_{558} to initiate reactive oxygen species production.

Figure 2. Schematic illustration of the NADPH oxidase of resting and fMLP activated cells.

H_2O_2 generated during the oxidative burst has limited bactericidal properties and the best-defined function of H_2O_2 in the antimicrobial activities of neutrophils comes from the function of H_2O_2 as a substrate for myeloperoxidase (MPO) in the presence of halides (chloride (Cl^-)). Neutrophil MPO was initially called verdoperoxidase, and later its name subsequently changed to MPO. It is present in exceptionally high concentrations in neutrophils, with levels estimated to be no less than 5% of the dry weight of the cell. MPO is synthesized and packaged into azurophilic, also referred to as primary granules of neutrophils, during the promyelocyte stage of granulocyte development and is present in mature resting granulocytes.

Mature MPO is a 150 kDa tetramer composed of two glycosylated 59–64 kDa heavy subunits and two unglycosylated 14 kDa light subunits as a pair of protomers linked together by a disulphide bond. When the phagosome containing microorganisms fuses with cytoplasmic granules, MPO, along with the other components of the granules, is released into the vacuole. A role for MPO as a component of the antimicrobial armoury of neutrophils was proposed with the finding that MPO was strongly microbial when combined with H_2O_2 and a halide [50, 51]. MPO and H_2O_2 form an enzyme-substrate complex, which oxidises ions to the toxic agent hypohalous acid. Any of the halide ions (I^-, Br^-, Cl^-) can be oxidised with iodide and bromide being more effective than Cl^- on a molar basis [51]. It is more likely however that the neutrophil uses Cl^- because it is present in high concentration in biological fluids, resulting in the formation of hypochlorous acid (HOCl). There are three proposed means of Cl^- transport to the phagosome: extracellular Cl^- intake during phagocytosis of a pathogen, stored Cl^- within granules released into the phagosome upon vesicle fusion, and passive or active transport of Cl^- from the cytosol to the phagosome [52]. Only active or passive transport has been suggested to provide a constant supply of Cl^- (Figure 3) [53] and two Cl^- ion channels (ClCs), ClC-3and CFTR have been implicated in the transport of Cl^- within the neutrophil and the phagosome [33, 54]. The influx of protons to the phagosomal lumen by V-ATPase has been demonstrated to facilitate the transport of Cl^- ions into the phagosome by ClCs including the CFTR [55] (Figure 3).

It is generally believed that HOCl is the most bactericidal oxidant known to be produced by the neutrophil. Levels of HOCl produced are based on calculations made after phorbol ester stimulation, which results in the secretion of O_2^- across the membrane to the surrounding supernatant and levels achieved are estimated at 80μM.

Levels produced in the phagocytic vacuole have been estimated using chlorinated fluorescein as a specific marker for HOCl production and by use of this technique it was calculated that 11% of oxygen consumed was converted to HOCl, resulting in 28μM within the phagosome [56]. HOCl is an extremely strong non-radical oxidant and bacterial targets include adenosine triphosphate (ATP)-generating systems [57], disruption of basement membranes or cell membranes, and fragmentation of proteins [58]. Chloramines are generated indirectly through the reaction of HOCl with amines, but are less reactive than HOCl but much more stable, and are therefore called "long lived oxidants." Because of the high intracellular concentration of the β-amino acid taurine, *N*-chlorotaurine is the major compound of low molecular weight long lived oxidants produced by neutrophils [59, 60]. Of major relevance to bacterial killing in CF it was reported that CF neutrophils had impaired chlorination of internalised bacteria within the phagosome when compared to healthy control neutrophils [33]. The authors highlighted the role of CFTR in facilitating Cl^- flux into the phagosome of neutrophils which was impaired in CF cells. This CFTR dysfunction resulted in limited availability of phagosomal Cl^- required for the generation of HOCl, resulting in reduced intravacuolar killing of *Pseudo-*

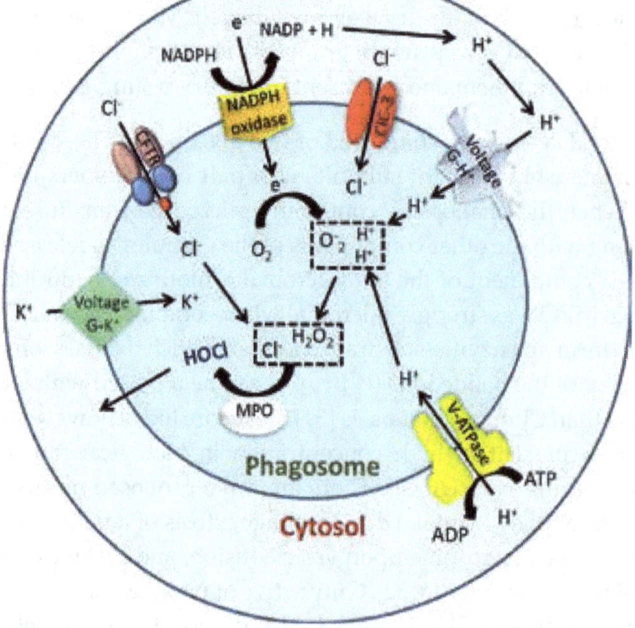

Upon activation of the NADPH oxidase, the cytochrome takes electrons from NADPH and passes them, via FAD and haem, to O_2 in the following reaction: NADPH + $2O_2$ → $NADP^+ + H^+ + 2O_2^-$. NADPH oxidase generates an electron current which is compensated through voltage gated ion influx of protons (Voltage G-H^+) and potassium (Voltage G-K^+). Cl^- transport is facilitated by CFTR and also other channels including ClC-3. The influx of H^+ to the phagosomal lumen by V-ATPase facilitates Cl^- transport into the phagosome by ClCs including the CFTR. O_2^- is a mild oxidant and reductant with restricted biological activity. H_2O_2 is a slow acting oxidising agent and HOCl is a strong non-radical oxidant.

Figure 3. Suggested mechanism of Cl^- and ion transport within the neutrophil phagosome.

monas aeruginosa, the archetype infecting organism in CF [33, 34, 53, 61]. Moreover, new data has shown that mutant CFTR fails to target to the neutrophil vacuole resulting in impaired intraphagosomal HOCl production and neutrophil microbial killing [62].

Having described the importance of MPO mediated halogenation for adequate microbial killing, there is also a need to mention that MPO deficiency occurs with a high prevalence and patients are not clinically afflicted by serious bacterial infections [63], with infections by *Candida* species being the main difficulty. Although more slowly than healthy cells, neutrophils deficient in MPO can kill bacteria *in vitro* [64], a result incompatible with the concept that HOCl is the major mediator of neutrophil bactericidal function in man. MPO deficient cells illustrate a prolonged respiratory burst resulting in increased levels of H_2O_2 and this coupled with non-oxidative methods of bacterial killing has been proposed to compensate for MPO deficiency. Furthermore, despite the fact that neutrophils of CGD patients do not produce O_2^- and H_2O_2, studies have shown that neutrophils from CGD patients are capable of killing significant numbers of phagocytosed bacteria and yeast [65, 66] and the presence of oxygen-independent microbial mechanisms in neutrophils is demonstrated by the ability of these cells to kill bacteria in the absence of oxygen [67].

3.2. Oxygen independent microbial killing

The presence of an oxygen independent microbial mechanism in neutrophils is demonstrated by the ability of these cells to kill bacteria under anaerobic conditions. Hirsch and colleagues reported that neutrophil lysates killed bacteria and that this effect was due to a substance they called phagocytin [68]. The component responsible for bacterial killing was localized to the cytoplasmic granules which are released into the phagocytic vacuole [69]. Neutrophil-derived microbial molecules are packaged within four distinct subgroups of granules (Figure 4) and are released either into the phagocytic vacuole or to the outside of the cell upon activation. Granule biogenesis follows the granulocyte differentiation pathway. The azurophilic (also referred to as primary) granules first emerge at the stage of the promyelocytes [70] and contain MPO, the serine proteases neutrophil elastase (NE), cathepsin G and proteinase 3, defensins and bacterial permeability-increasing protein [71], and are considered as the true microbial compartment mobilized upon phagocytosis. Later in differentiation, at the metamyelocyte stage, specific granules containing lactoferrin [72], 18 kDa human cathelicidin antimicrobial protein (hCAP-18], and lysozyme emerge [73], followed by a third population termed the gelatinase granules which predominantly contain gelatinase (matric metalloprotease (MMP)-9 and MMP-2), lysozyme, and leukolysin [74, 75]. A forth type of granule, called the secretory vesicles, appears at the stage of the mature neutrophil. Movement of the cytoplasmic granules following ingestion of bacteria was first observed by Robineaux and Frederic [76], and by use of chicken leukocytes with their large dense granules, Hirsch observed by phase contrast microscopy, degranulation and release of the granule contents directly into the phagocytic vacuole, by fusion of the granule membrane with the invaginated cell membrane [77]. As for any form of intracellular vesicle transport, degranulation is a tightly regulated process. Small GTPases of the Ras superfamily are known key regulators of cellular events including vesicle transport, cell division, control of cytoskeletal rearrangements, and nuclear assembly. Secondary and tertiary granules are tethered through a small GTPase Rab27a and its effector protein Munc13-4 [78] which interacts with the soluble N-ethylmaleimide association protein receptor (SNARE), a protein complex composed of vesicle-associated membrane proteins (VAMPs) on the vesicle surface and SNAP23 and STX4 on the plasma membrane [79-81]. Once the granule is docked the granule membrane fuses with the plasma membrane enabling release of granule contents. The small GTPase Rac2 has been shown necessary for the release of primary granules [82] but of interest, a sub-population of Rab27a positive primary granules was also found [83] with different Rab27a effectors Slp1 and Munc13-4 reported necessary for primary and tertiary granules release, respectively [84].

Although the neutrophil possesses an armoury of anti-microbial proteins and peptides, individual components have been shown to exert microbial effects. For example, NE has long been regarded as the major antibacterial protein and mice made homozygous for a disrupted NE gene have demonstrated impaired resistance to *Klebsiella pneumonia* and *Escherichia coli* sepsis [85]. A target for NE is the bacterial outer-membrane protein OmpA [86]. NE degradation of OmpA results in cell death as a result of loss of bacterial integrity by localized weakening of the cell wall followed by osmotic lysis [86]. The amino acid composition of cathepsin G shares 37% sequence homology with NE and plays a role in neutrophil responses against a

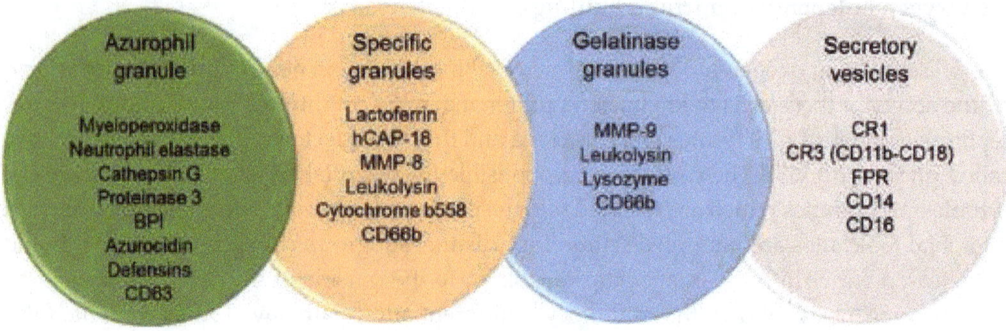

Figure 4. Granule and vesicle contents of the neutrophil. The most abundant organelles within the cytoplasm are the granules, which are membrane-bound organelles containing an array of antimicrobial proteins. Three major types have been identified, azurophilic, specific, and gelatinase-containing granules. A forth type of granule, called the secretory vesicles, are endocytic in nature and act as an internal reservoir of membrane/cytokine receptors.

variety of bacteria. Purified cathepsin G has been shown to inhibit the growth of several organisms including *Staphylococcus aureus, E. coli, P. aeruginosa,* and *Neisseria gonorrhoea* [87, 88]. Moreover, Tkalcevic and colleagues performed *in vivo* studies of mice deficient in cathepsin G, NE, or both and demonstrated the importance of cathepsin G in the successful clearance of *Aspergillus fumigatus*. Wild type mice almost completely cleared the fungal pathogen, while the single mutants showed an intermediate phenotype between the wild type and double mutants, thus establishing a critical role for both elastase and cathepsin G in the control of fungal infection *in vivo* [89].

Examples of proteins stored in specific (secondary) and gelatinase (tertiary) granules include human lactoferrin and MMPs. Lactoferrin is a major component of the specific granules and is active against a variety of pathogens [90]. This protein binds to bacteria through its highly positively charged *N*-terminus and displays antimicrobial properties against Gram-positive and Gram-negative bacteria by limiting the availability of environmental iron. However, since iron-saturated lactoferrin is also capable of killing certain bacteria, mechanisms other than iron depletion are involved. Further studies have indicated that peptides obtained after enzymatic hydrolysis of lactoferrin are much more effective in killing bacteria than is the intact protein. It is likely that the *N*-terminal cationic domain of human lactoferrin plays an essential role in the bactericidal activity and has been shown to be highly effective against infections with antibiotic-resistant *S. aureus* [91]. MMP-9 is stored in an inactive preform that requires activation by a serine protease such as NE. Its main function is the degradation of type V collagen in the extracellular matrix to aid migration to the site of infection [92]. The importance of MMP-9 in host defence was illustrated by a higher frequency of peritoneal sepsis in MMP-9 knockout mice due to impaired migration of neutrophils to the site of infection [93].

In spite of their original role in host defence, NE and proteinase 3 have been strongly implicated in the pulmonary pathology of CF. Indeed it has been shown that NE is the main mediator of proteolysis (Figure 1) but can also cause up-regulation of expression of other proteases including MMPs and cathepsins and as a result it has been proposed that neutralisation of NE activity is central to reducing the overall protease burden [94]. In line with this thought, NE has the ability to degrade structural proteins in the lung including elastin, collagen, and fibronectin and to promote IL-8 production by bronchial epithelial cells [95], to degrade antimicrobial peptides [96], and to degrade antiproteases including alpha-1 antitrypsin, SLPI [97], and elafin [98] leading to a protease/antiprotease imbalance [99]. Moreover, it has been shown that the process of primary granule release by CF neutrophils appears altered, as greater levels of NE [100] and MPO [101] were recorded in the extracellular fluids post stimulation with either CF airway samples, TNF-alpha and IL-8, or serum-opsonised particles. Of importance, altered cytosolic pH regulation in CF neutrophils has been demonstrated [102, 103], which could in turn influence the process of degranulation. In further support of increased primary granule release by CF neutrophils, MPO and NE levels have been reported to be present at significantly increased levels in airway samples from patients with CF compared to controls [49, 104]. Moreover, levels of NE degranulation were not significantly altered following intravenous antibiotic treatment of patients with CF, indicating continued dysregulation of neutrophil activity even with clinical improvement [105]. While the mechanism for excessive primary granule release by CF neutrophils has not been fully investigated [104, 106], new research on the cause of reduced secondary and tertiary granule release has recently been revealed [35]. Contrary to increased release of secondary and tertiary granules by neutrophils of individuals with airway disease linked to alpha-1 antitrypsin deficiency (AATD) [107], evidence was presented indicating that abnormal CFTR function contributes to impaired neutrophil killing in CF due to inadequate Rab27a activation, which regulates the release of antimicrobial proteins from secondary and tertiary granules. In this study reduced degranulation of lactoferrin of secondary granules and MMP-9 of tertiary granules from patients with CF compared to healthy control cells was observed, an effect mirrored in healthy control cells post CFTR inhibition. Collectively results revealed that CFTR inhibition or dysfunction reduces cytosolic Mg^{2+} levels resulting in impaired Rab27a activity, ultimately reducing the CF neutrophils ability to kill bacterial pathogens [35].

4. The involvement of CFTR in neutrophil adherence leading to migration

Before describing the process leading to neutrophil adhesion, it is important to stress the complexity of studying neutrophil adhesion and migration. Blood neutrophils isolated from patients with CF are chronically exposed to pro-inflammatory cytokines, including LTB_4 and IL-8, and pathogenic particles including fMLP (formyl-methionyl-leucyl-phenylalanine) and LPS, resulting in these cells being in a constant primed state. Therefore, independent of the expression of CFTR protein, neutrophils in CF may illustrate enhanced cell adherence and migration. To circumvent this dilemma and to eliminate the potential for bias towards inflammatory versus altered neutrophil adhesion due to a lack of CFTR function, an approach taken by researchers is to include neutrophils isolated from inflammatory control patients. For example, in 1998, Russell and colleagues demonstrated that L-selectin shedding is altered in patients with CF resulting in increased neutrophil adhesion in response to IL-8 and fMLP [108]. This paper reported that non-CF bronchiectasis patients did not possess alterations in L-selectin shedding, suggesting that the defect in L-selectin shedding is CF specific and could be a result of defective CFTR rather than the inflammatory status of the individual [108]. Indeed, CFTR expression in human neutrophils has provoked the idea that altered neutrophil migration and adhesion in CF could be caused by an intrinsic defect. Counteracting this concept however, Pohl *et al.* (2014) did not demonstrate impaired neutrophil migration in healthy control cells exposed to the CFTR inhibitor, CFTR(inh)-172, suggesting that altered neutrophil migration in CF is not inherent.

Circulating neutrophils generally adhere and migrate in response to pro-inflammatory mediators including TNF-alpha and pathogenic components including N-formyl peptides produced by bacteria. Lipid mediators involved in neutrophil adhesion and chemotaxis include LTB_4 [109, 110], with significantly increased levels quantified in sputum of patients with CF [111]. The chemokine IL-8 is the main neutrophil chemo-attractant involved in CF lung neutrophil infiltration [112], and increased levels of IL-8 have been detected in bronchial lavage fluid and sputum of patients with CF [113]. IL-8 is produced by a number of cells, including fibroblasts [114], epithelial cells [115], and by neutrophils themselves [116]. Interestingly, neutrophils isolated from children with CF demonstrate increased migration to IL-8 [117], and also release significantly increased levels of the chemokine when compared to the blood neutrophils of the same donor, suggesting that the environment that the cell is found triggers disproportionate release of IL-8 [116].

Neutrophils migrate in a multistep process consisting of rolling, tight binding, diapedesis, and migration. Initially, E-selectin and P-selectin are upregulated on the epithelium cell surface, and reversibly bind to L-selectin found on the neutrophil cell surface. In turn, L-selectin is shed from the neutrophil membrane resulting in up-regulation of integrins LFA-1 (CD11a/CD18) and MAC-1 (CD11b/CD18) which can both bind to ICAM-1 on the epithelium. Research studies have demonstrated that activation of integrins is in part mediated by IL-8 [118], and this is particularly relevant in CF as studies involving infants and children have demonstrated increased expression of IL-8 and ICAM-1, possibly indicating intrinsic inflammatory changes at a very early stage in disease progression supporting cell adhesion [119, 120]. This latter study is reinforced by data indicating that CF neutrophils show higher migratory responsiveness to IL-8 [117] supporting elevated numbers of neutrophils migrating to the airways. Moreover, neutrophil activation results in increased cytosolic Ca^{2+} levels triggering activation of calpain, a calcium dependent protease. Calpain has been demonstrated to liberate adhesion molecules CD11b and CD18, facilitating cell adhesion through the tight binding of integrins to epithelium cell surfaces [121]. Of major importance, studies have shown that CF neutrophils possess increased calpain activity, affecting cleavage of the cholesterol transporter caveolin-1, thereby modulating cholesterol trafficking to the plasma membrane [122]. Interestingly, and of major relevance to CF, Solomkin *et al.* (2007) demonstrated that cholesterol depletion in human neutrophils results in increased cell adhesion [123].

5. The involvement of CFTR in neutrophil apoptosis

Timely and effective neutrophil programmed cell death is essential for the resolution of inflammation [124, 125] and abnormal neutrophil apoptosis is associated with decreased antimicrobial defences [126], incomplete microbial clearance, and sustained inflammation [127, 128]. Three different pathways are involved in the regulation of apoptosis and particular attention will be given to signalling pathways that are relevant to the neutrophil as it has been recognised that neutrophils have unique mechanisms of cell death due to their short half-life and phagocytic activity (Figure 5). Essential to the regulation and execution of apoptosis are the caspases, a family of cytosolic proteases or cysteine-dependent aspartate-directed proteases, involved in all three pathways. The first pathway described is the mitochondrial or intrinsic pathway. This pathway responds to physical and chemical stress signals, including growth factor withdrawal, DNA damage, and endoplasmic stress, and is transduced by members of the Bcl-2 family, which ultimately trigger the mitochondrial outer membrane permeabilisation (MOMP). As a result, several pro-apoptotic mitochondrial proteins, the most important being cytochrome C, are released into the cytosol. Subsequently cytochrome C, apoptotic protease activating factor-1 (Apaf-1) and caspase-9 form the apoptosome [129-131], this results in the activation of caspase-9 which thereafter activates caspase-3 and initiates the execution of apoptosis. In addition, caspase-8 can cleave Bid into truncated Bid (TBid), which ultimately triggers MOMP, thus providing a link from the intrinsic pathway to the extrinsic pathway.

The second pathway, the extrinsic or external death receptor pathway, is activated in response to extracellular signals such as FasL and TNF-alpha and is mediated by the binding of these members of the tumour necrosis factor family to death receptors on the cell surface (e.g., Fas, TNFR). The binding of the FasL and TNF-alpha to its cognate receptor results in the multimerisation of the death receptor and the formation of the death inducing signal complex (DISC), containing multiple adaptor molecules such as the Fas associated death domain (FADD) or TNF-R1-associated death domain (FADD) or TNF-R1-associtaed death domain (TRADD). The respective adaptor death domain then interacts with caspase-8 [132, 133], which in turn leads to the autolytic activation from pro-caspase-8 to caspase-8. After activation and release of its active subunit (p18), caspase-8 then activates caspase-3, which finally executes apoptosis by releasing caspase-activated DNase (CAD) from its inhibitor (ICAD) with DNA fragmentation as a consequence [134]. The third pathway is the ER stress pathway. This pathway is thought to involve the activation of caspases, increase in cytosolic calcium and pro-apoptotic transcription factors in response to stress signals such as hypoxia, accumulation of unfolded protein, and alteration in calcium homeostasis within the ER [135, 136].

In the neutrophil the enzymatic activity of active caspase-3, -7, and -9 can be selectively inhibited by X-linked inhibitor of apoptosis (XIAP), a member of the conserved inhibitor of apoptosis (IAP) family of proteins [137]. Moreover, there are a number of key distinguishing features of neutrophil apoptosis. Firstly, the prominent role of the Bcl-2 homologue, Mcl-1, as a survival protein is central to the neutrophil's ability to undergo rapid apoptosis and may therefore limit the neutrophil's lifespan [138].

Mcl-1 is an unusual bcl-2 protein and can be rapidly turned over in the proteasome giving it a short half-life (2h) in the cell and is in contrast to the essential pro-apoptotic bcl-2 homologues, which are known to persist in the cell beyond 12 h. A critical excess of pro- over anti-apoptotic homologues decides the fate of the neutrophil and this eventually leads to loss of mitochondrial membrane potential and the progression of apoptosis [139]. Secondly, the involvement of

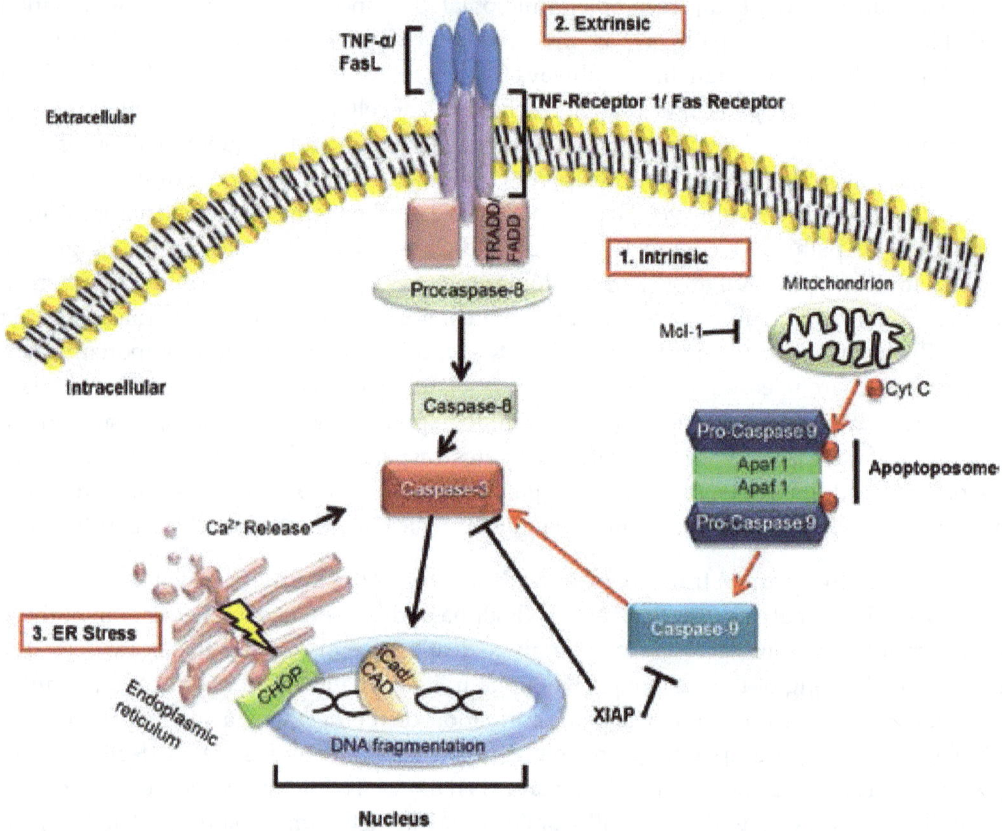

Figure 5. Summary schematic of apoptosis pathways in the neutrophil. [1] Intrinsic mitochondrial pathway (red): mitochondria release cytochrome c (Cyt C) in response to cellular stress. Together with apoptotic protease activating factor-1 (Apaf-1) and procaspase-9, Cyt C will form the apoptosome complex. This results in the proteolytic activation of the procaspase. Mature caspase-9 can then proteolytically activate caspase-3. [2] Extrinsic/ligand death-receptor pathway (black): death factors such as tumour necrosis factor alpha (TNF-alpha) and Fas ligand (FasL) trigger apoptosis by binding on death receptors such as tumour necrosis factor receptor 1 (TNFR1) and Fas. The death receptors recruit procaspase-8 by means of an adaptor protein, TNF-R1-associated death domain (TRADD), or Fas associated death domain protein (FADD). After cleavage the mature caspase-8 can then directly activate caspase-3. [3] Endoplasmic reticulum (ER) stress pathway (yellow bolt): the ER can also induce apoptosis as a reaction to ER stress by releasing intracytosolic calcium (Ca^{2+}) thereby activating effector caspases or through the expression of pro-apoptotic transcription factors such as CHOP. These different initiation pathways converge further downstream into activation of caspase-3. The effector caspase-3 cleaves ICAD (inhibitor of CAD) and releases it from CAD (caspase-activated DNase). CAD translocates from the cytoplasm to the nucleus and can now act as active endonuclease and fragment DNA. Inhibitors of apoptosis such as myeloid leukaemia cell differentiation protein (Mcl-1) and X-linked inhibitor of apoptosis (XIAP) act upstream against pro-apoptotic Bcl-2 family members at the mitochondria and downstream, directly inhibit caspases, respectively.

reactive oxygen species (ROS) is very specific to neutrophil apoptosis. The observation that neutrophils isolated from CGD patients which are known to be NADPH oxidase defective display a significant delayed spontaneous cell death relative to that of neutrophils from healthy donors is important [140]. This suggests that activation of the NADPH oxidase, with consequent production of ROS, is involved in spontaneous apoptosis and in regulating the programmed cell death of neutrophils during phagocytosis.

In contrast to the reported accelerated apoptosis in neutrophils from patients with airways disease associated with AATD [141], prolonged neutrophil survival has been reported in people with CF independent of infectious state and mutation type [142]. In support of this concept, Moriceau *et al.* (2010) illustrated that neutrophils isolated from heterozygous asymptomatic parents of people with CF exhibited delayed apoptosis [143, 144]. Moreover, the expression of the apoptosis-inducing membrane receptor Fas and its ligand have been reported reduced on CF neutrophils [145] while in addition, NE can degrade the phosphatidylserine receptor on macrophages, further delaying the removal of apoptotic neutrophils in CF [146].

6. The effect of CFTR mutation targeted therapy on neutrophil function

There can be no doubt that our grasp and understanding of the complex physiology of CFTR protein function has progressed majorly and permitted the development of exciting new treatments designed to target the basic defects of CF. Along with this, continuing improvements in clinical care have allowed improved outcomes for patients with CF including reduced morbidity and preserved lung function. As CFTR has been shown to be an integral membrane channel on neutrophils, the influence of new CFTR therapeutics on neutrophil function is an area of intense interest.

Class I mutations are thought to affect 5% of the CF population in Western society and in this class of *CFTR* mutations, there is complete absence of stable CFTR protein (due to non-sense mutations from premature stop codons) and thus replacement of the defective *CFTR* gene or changes in how the protein is made is required. However, the focus relating to the research surrounding gene addition therapy is its potential use in all class mutations in CF, with the ultimate aim of functional gene insertion and normalized *CFTR* expression. Studies on gene addition therapy have been developed to replace the mutant *CFTR* gene, and in this respect a phase II trial with non-viral lipid vector for DNA instillation has commenced. The study investigators have recommended monthly inhaled therapy for one-year duration (NCT 01621867). Further developments involve a lentiviral vector for gene therapy in this patient population [147] and the collective results of gene therapy on neutrophil function will be an exciting area of research in the future.

A second area of immense interest is the therapeutic use of aminoglycosides (e.g., gentamycin) and ataluren to cause read through of premature stop codons thereby allowing translation to continue to the end of transcription [148, 149]. Ataluren (PTC 124) is under investigation for its use and role in targeting premature stop codons. This compound has the potential to allow processing of premature stop codons, resulting in the production of normal length and functional CFTR, with insertion at the cell surface. Its beneficial effects have been proven with analysis of nasal chloride transport. The phase III trial in 238 patients with CF failed to achieve its primary end point (improvement in FEV_1) at 48 weeks, except in a small subgroup of patients not on concomitant nebulised aminoglycoside treatment [150].

Class II (e.g., *ΔF508*) and III *CFTR* mutations (e.g., *G551D*) have seen the advent of CFTR corrector and potentiator therapies. Corrector agents facilitate appropriate protein folding and targeting to the cell membrane. The correctors lumacaftor (VX 809) or VX 661 are designed to promote increased quantities of ΔF508 CFTR at the cell membrane surface. VX 809 has shown good results *in vitro* but it is likely that adequate correction of ΔF508 CFTR will need multi-compound drug therapy [147, 151]. The potentiator ivacaftor (VX 770) was originally developed to augment the activity and efficiency of the abnormal CFTR protein (Figure 6).

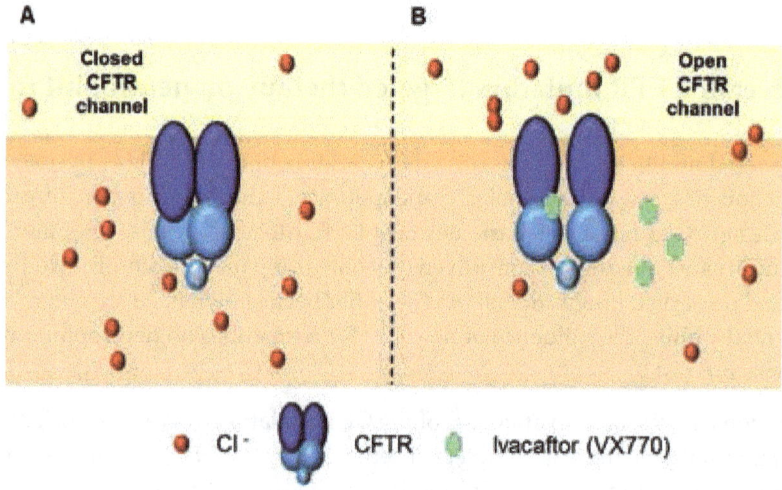

Figure 6. CFTR function in human epithelia. Panel (A) illustrates defective CFTR Cl^- transport due to the *G551D* mutation. Image (B) illustrates corrected function post VX-770 (ivacaftor) treatment.

Use of this therapy involved a well-designed randomized, double blind, placebo-controlled trial. The study subjects had at least one *G551D CFTR* mutation and were randomly assigned to ivacaftor 150 mg twice daily or placebo for 48 weeks. The treatment group showed a sustained improvement from baseline in FEV1 by 10% compared with the placebo group. They were also 55% less likely to suffer a pulmonary exacerbation compared with their placebo counter parts, had higher health scores, gained weight and normalization of their sweat chloride levels. These benefits were sustained for the duration of the trial and the frequency of adverse events in the two groups was equivocal [152]. A shortcoming of the use of ivacaftor is that only 2–3% of individuals with CF have the *G551D* mutation and research is currently underway to ascertain whether ivacaftor may be employed for other mutations. A multi-centre, phase II trial on the use of the CFTR corrector lumacaftor together with the CFTR potentiator ivacaftor for the treatment of patients with CF with the *ΔF508 CFTR* mutation was performed. The primary outcome was change in sweat chloride concentration with combination therapy in the *ΔF508* subjects, however a minimal effect on sweat chloride level was observed [153]. It is postulated that the reason behind this was that the potentiator rendered the CFTR protein less stable and increased its removal from the cell membrane. However, currently there is a very motivated area of research into double or triple combination treatment for synergistic ΔF508 CFTR correction [154].

Of relevance to the circulating neutrophil and as *CFTR* mRNA transcripts have been reported in neutrophils at an expression level similar to those found in monocytes and alveolar macrophages [24, 33], the effect of CFTR corrector and potentiator therapies on neutrophil function is an anticipated area of research. In a study by Pohl *et al.* (2014), the mechanism leading to impaired degranulation by CF neutrophils was shown to involve altered ion homeostasis caused by defective CFTR function and significantly decreased levels of GTP-bound Rab27a. Of major importance, treatment of *G551D* patients with ivacaftor, normalized neutrophil cytosolic ion levels, and activation of Rab27a thereby leading to increased degranulation and pseudomonal killing. These results confirm that intrinsic alterations of circulating neutrophils from patients with CF are corrected by ivacaftor thus illustrating additional clinical benefits for CFTR modulator therapy. In line with this concept, neutrophils of ivacaftor-treated subjects demonstrated decreased cell surface CD63, a marker of primary granule release [155].

7. Conclusion

A plethora of studies on neutrophil function in CF have been performed and demonstrate alterations in cellular activities including impaired microbial uptake [156, 157], defective intracellular kinase activation [116], cellular inactivation [158], and increased oxidant formation [106, 159]. Furthermore, an additional area of intense research has focused on persistent mammalian target of rapamycin (mTOR) and cyclic AMP response element binding protein (CREB) pathway activation in CF airway neutrophils [160], with more recent data suggesting that neutrophils express augmented cell surface nutrient transporter expression and glucose uptake, consistent with metabolic adaptation [161]. As the CF neutrophil may shape the inflammatory response and influence patient outcome, further research investigating the CF neutrophil is required. In addition, a promising development in the treatment of airway inflammation involves the correction of CFTR dysfunction. If CFTR dysfunction is corrected at a very early age, it is possible that neutrophil induced inflammation involving impaired trafficking, delayed apoptosis, impaired degranulation, and bacterial killing may be significantly curtailed.

Acknowledgements

We would like to thank the U.S. Cystic Fibrosis Foundation and Science Foundation Ireland under the Research Frontiers Programme (11/RFP/BMT/3094) and the Program for Research in Third Level Institutes administered by the Higher Education Authority in Ireland for support.

Author details

Michelle M. White, Fatma Gargoum, Niall Browne, Killian Hurley, Noel G. McElvaney and Emer P. Reeves*

*Address all correspondence to: emerreeves@rcsi.ie

Respiratory Research Division, Department of Medicine, Royal College of Surgeons in Ireland, Education and Research Centre, Beaumont Hospital, Dublin, Ireland

References

[1] De Boeck K, Zolin A, Cuppens H, Olesen HV, Viviani L. The relative frequency of CFTR mutation classes in European patients with cystic fibrosis. J Cyst Fibros. 2014;13(4):403-9.

[2] Mott LS, Park J, Murray CP, Gangell CL, De Klerk NH, Robinson PJ, et al. Progression of early structural lung disease in young children with cystic fibrosis assessed using CT. Thorax. 2012;67(6):509-16.

[3] Sly PD, Brennan S, Gangell C, De Klerk N, Murray C, Mott L, et al. Lung disease at diagnosis in infants with cystic fibrosis detected by newborn screening. American Journal of Respiratory and Critical Care Medicine. 2009;180(2):146-52.

[4] Davis SD, Fordham LA, Brody AS, Noah TL, Retsch-Bogart GZ, Qaqish BF, et al. Computed tomography reflects lower airway inflammation and tracks changes in early cystic fibrosis. American Journal of Respiratory and Critical Care Medicine. 2007;175(9):943-50.

[5] Wainwright CE, Vidmar S, Armstrong DS, Byrnes CA, Carlin JB, Cheney J, et al. Effect of bronchoalveolar lavage-directed therapy on Pseudomonas aeruginosa infection and structural lung injury in children with cystic fibrosis: a randomized trial. JAMA : The Journal of the American Medical Association. 2011;306(2):163-71.

[6] Stick SM, Brennan S, Murray C, Douglas T, Von Ungern-Sternberg BS, Garratt LW, et al. Bronchiectasis in infants and preschool children diagnosed with cystic fibrosis after newborn screening. The Journal of Pediatrics. 2009;155(5):623-8 e1.

[7] Armstrong DS, Hook SM, Jamsen KM, Nixon GM, Carzino R, Carlin JB, et al. Lower airway inflammation in infants with cystic fibrosis detected by newborn screening. Pediatr Pulmonol. 2005;40(6):500-10.

[8] Rosenfeld M, Gibson RL, McNamara S, Emerson J, Burns JL, Castile R, et al. Early pulmonary infection, inflammation, and clinical outcomes in infants with cystic fibrosis. Pediatr Pulmonol. 2001;32(5):356-66.

[9] Reeves EP, Williamson M, Byrne B, Bergin DA, Smith SG, Greally P, et al. IL-8 dictates glycosaminoglycan binding and stability of IL-18 in cystic fibrosis. J Immunol. 2010;184(3):1642-52.

[10] Mitola S, Sorbello V, Ponte E, Copreni E, Mascia C, Bardessono M, et al. Tumor necrosis factor-alpha in airway secretions from cystic fibrosis patients upregulate endothelial adhesion molecules and induce airway epithelial cell apoptosis: implications for cystic fibrosis lung disease. International Journal of Immunopathology and Pharmacology. 2008;21(4):851-65.

[11] Colombo C, Faelli N, Tirelli AS, Fortunato F, Biffi A, Claut L, et al. Analysis of inflammatory and immune response biomarkers in sputum and exhaled breath condensate by a multi-parametric biochip array in cystic fibrosis. International Journal of Immunopathology and Pharmacology. 2011;24(2):423-32.

[12] Birrer P, McElvaney NG, Rudeberg A, Sommer CW, Liechti-Gallati S, Kraemer R, et al. Protease-antiprotease imbalance in the lungs of children with cystic fibrosis. Am J Respir Crit Care Med. 1994;150(1):207-13.

[13] McElvaney NG, Nakamura H, Birrer P, Hebert CA, Wong WL, Alphonso M, et al. Modulation of airway inflammation in cystic fibrosis. In vivo suppression of interleukin-8 levels on the respiratory epithelial surface by aerosolization of recombinant secretory leukoprotease inhibitor. J Clin Invest. 1992;90(4):1296-301.

[14] Hartl D, Griese M, Kappler M, Zissel G, Reinhardt D, Rebhan C, et al. Pulmonary T(H)2 response in Pseudomonas aeruginosa-infected patients with cystic fibrosis. J Allergy Clin Immunol. 2006;117(1):204-11.

[15] Reinhardt N, Chen CI, Loppow D, Schink T, Kleinau I, Jorres RA, et al. Cellular profiles of induced sputum in children with stable cystic fibrosis: comparison with BAL. Eur Respir J. 2003;22(3):497-502.

[16] Sly PD, Gangell CL, Chen L, Ware RS, Ranganathan S, Mott LS, et al. Risk factors for bronchiectasis in children with cystic fibrosis. N Engl J Med. 2013;368(21):1963-70.

[17] Adib-Conquy M, Pedron T, Petit-Bertron AF, Tabary O, Corvol H, Jacquot J, et al. Neutrophils in cystic fibrosis display a distinct gene expression pattern. Mol Med. 2008;14(1-2):36-44.

[18] Kormann MS, Hector A, Marcos V, Mays LE, Kappler M, Illig T, et al. CXCR1 and CXCR2 haplotypes synergistically modulate cystic fibrosis lung disease. Eur Respir J. 2012;39(6):1385-90.

[19] Jann NJ, Schmaler M, Ferracin F, Landmann R. TLR2 enhances NADPH oxidase activity and killing of Staphylococcus aureus by PMN. Immunol Lett. 2010;135(1-2): 17-23.

[20] Petit-Bertron AF, Tabary O, Corvol H, Jacquot J, Clement A, Cavaillon JM, et al. Circulating and airway neutrophils in cystic fibrosis display different TLR expression and responsiveness to interleukin-10. Cytokine. 2008;41(1):54-60.

[21] Gu Y, Harley IT, Henderson LB, Aronow BJ, Vietor I, Huber LA, et al. Identification of IFRD1 as a modifier gene for cystic fibrosis lung disease. Nature. 2009;458(7241): 1039-42.

[22] Blanchard E, Marie S, Riffault L, Bonora M, Tabary O, Clement A, et al. Reduced expression of Tis7/IFRD1 protein in murine and human cystic fibrosis airway epithelial cell models homozygous for the F508del-CFTR mutation. Biochem Biophys Res Commun. 2011;411(3):471-6.

[23] Riordan JR, Rommens JM, Kerem B, Alon N, Rozmahel R, Grzelczak Z, et al. Identification of the cystic fibrosis gene: cloning and characterization of complementary DNA. Science. 1989;245(4922):1066-73.

[24] Yoshimura K, Nakamura H, Trapnell BC, Chu CS, Dalemans W, Pavirani A, et al. Expression of the cystic fibrosis transmembrane conductance regulator gene in cells of non-epithelial origin. Nucleic Acids Res. 1991;19(19):5417-23.

[25] Trapnell BC, Chu CS, Paakko PK, Banks TC, Yoshimura K, Ferrans VJ, et al. Expression of the cystic fibrosis transmembrane conductance regulator gene in the respiratory tract of normal individuals and individuals with cystic fibrosis. Proc Natl Acad Sci USA. 1991;88(15):6565-9.

[26] Yoshimura K, Nakamura H, Trapnell BC, Dalemans W, Pavirani A, Lecocq JP, et al. The cystic fibrosis gene has a "housekeeping"-type promoter and is expressed at low levels in cells of epithelial origin. J Biol Chem. 1991;266(14):9140-4.

[27] Di A, Brown ME, Deriy LV, Li C, Szeto FL, Chen Y, et al. CFTR regulates phagosome acidification in macrophages and alters bactericidal activity. Nat Cell Biol. 2006;8(9): 933-44.

[28] Haggie PM, Verkman AS. Cystic fibrosis transmembrane conductance regulator-independent phagosomal acidification in macrophages. J Biol Chem. 2007;282(43): 31422-8.

[29] Steinberg BE, Huynh KK, Brodovitch A, Jabs S, Stauber T, Jentsch TJ, et al. A cation counterflux supports lysosomal acidification. J Cell Biol. 2010;189(7):1171-86.

[30] Del Porto P, Cifani N, Guarnieri S, Di Domenico EG, Mariggio MA, Spadaro F, et al. Dysfunctional CFTR alters the bactericidal activity of human macrophages against Pseudomonas aeruginosa. PLoS One. 2011;6(5):e19970.

[31] McKeon DJ, Cadwallader KA, Idris S, Cowburn AS, Pasteur MC, Barker H, et al. Cystic fibrosis neutrophils have normal intrinsic reactive oxygen species generation. Eur Respir J. 2010;35(6):1264-72.

[32] Morris MR, Doull IJ, Dewitt S, Hallett MB. Reduced iC3b-mediated phagocytotic capacity of pulmonary neutrophils in cystic fibrosis. Clin Exp Immunol. 2005;142(1): 68-75.

[33] Painter RG, Valentine VG, Lanson NA, Jr., Leidal K, Zhang Q, Lombard G, et al. CFTR Expression in human neutrophils and the phagolysosomal chlorination defect in cystic fibrosis. Biochemistry. 2006;45(34):10260-9.

[34] Painter RG, Marrero L, Lombard GA, Valentine VG, Nauseef WM, Wang G. CFTR-mediated halide transport in phagosomes of human neutrophils. J Leukoc Biol. 2010;87(5):933-42.

[35] Pohl K, Hayes E, Keenan J, Henry M, Meleady P, Molloy K, et al. A neutrophil intrinsic impairment affecting Rab27a and degranulation in cystic fibrosis is corrected by CFTR potentiator therapy. Blood. 2014;124(7):999-1009.

[36] Su X, Looney MR, Su HE, Lee JW, Song Y, Matthay MA. Role of CFTR expressed by neutrophils in modulating acute lung inflammation and injury in mice. Inflamm Res. 2011;60(7):619-32.

[37] Baldridge C, Gerard, RW. The extra respiratory burst of phagocytosis. Am J Phsiol. 1933;103:235-6.

[38] Sbarra AJ, Karnovsky ML. The biochemical basis of phagocytosis. I. Metabolic changes during the ingestion of particles by polymorphonuclear leukocytes. J Biol Chem. 1959;234(6):1355-62.

[39] Good RA, Quie PG, Windhorst DB, Page AR, Rodey GE, White J, et al. Fatal (chronic) granulomatous disease of childhood: a hereditary defect of leukocyte function. Semin Hematol. 1968;5(3):215-54.

[40] Holmes B, Page AR, Good RA. Studies of the metabolic activity of leukocytes from patients with a genetic abnormality of phagocytic function. J Clin Invest. 1967;46(9): 1422-32.

[41] Cohen MS, Metcalf JA, Root RK. Regulation of oxygen metabolism in human granulocytes: relationship between stimulus binding and oxidative response using plant lectins as probes. Blood. 1980;55(6):1003-10.

[42] Root RK, Metcalf JA. H2O2 release from human granulocytes during phagocytosis. Relationship to superoxide anion formation and cellular catabolism of H2O2: studies with normal and cytochalasin B-treated cells. J Clin Invest. 1977;60(6):1266-79.

[43] Iyer GYN IM, Quastel JH. Biochemical Aspects of Phagocytosis. Nature. 1961;192:535-41

[44] Galli F, Battistoni A, Gambari R, Pompella A, Bragonzi A, Pilolli F, et al. Oxidative stress and antioxidant therapy in cystic fibrosis. Biochim Biophys Acta. 2012;1822(5): 690-713.

[45] Griese M, Ramakers J, Krasselt A, Starosta V, Van Koningsbruggen S, Fischer R, et al. Improvement of alveolar glutathione and lung function but not oxidative state in cystic fibrosis. Am J Respir Crit Care Med. 2004;169(7):822-8.

[46] Roum JH, Borok Z, McElvaney NG, Grimes GJ, Bokser AD, Buhl R, et al. Glutathione aerosol suppresses lung epithelial surface inflammatory cell-derived oxidants in cystic fibrosis. J Appl Physiol (1985). 1999;87(1):438-43.

[47] Roum JH, Buhl R, McElvaney NG, Borok Z, Crystal RG. Systemic deficiency of glutathione in cystic fibrosis. J Appl Physiol (1985). 1993;75(6):2419-24.

[48] Linsdell P, Hanrahan JW. Glutathione permeability of CFTR. Am J Physiol. 1998;275(1 Pt 1):C323-6.

[49] Kettle AJ, Chan T, Osberg I, Senthilmohan R, Chapman AL, Mocatta TJ, et al. Myeloperoxidase and protein oxidation in the airways of young children with cystic fibrosis. Am J Respir Crit Care Med. 2004;170(12):1317-23.

[50] Klebanoff SJ. Iodination of bacteria: a bactericidal mechanism. J Exp Med. 1967;126(6):1063-78.

[51] Klebanoff SJ. Myeloperoxidase-halide-hydrogen peroxide antibacterial system. J Bacteriol. 1968;95(6):2131-8.

[52] Winterbourn CC, Hampton MB, Livesey JH, Kettle AJ. Modeling the reactions of superoxide and myeloperoxidase in the neutrophil phagosome: implications for microbial killing. J Biol Chem. 2006;281(52):39860-9.

[53] Bonvillain RW, Painter RG, Adams DE, Viswanathan A, Lanson NA, Jr., Wang G. RNA interference against CFTR affects HL60-derived neutrophil microbicidal function. Free Radic Biol Med. 2010;49(12):1872-80.

[54] Moreland JG, Davis AP, Bailey G, Nauseef WM, Lamb FS. Anion channels, including ClC-3, are required for normal neutrophil oxidative function, phagocytosis, and transendothelial migration. J Biol Chem. 2006;281(18):12277-88.

[55] Aiken ML, Painter RG, Zhou Y, Wang G. Chloride transport in functionally active phagosomes isolated from Human neutrophils. Free Radic Biol Med. 2012;53(12): 2308-17.

[56] Jiang Q, Griffin DA, Barofsky DF, Hurst JK. Intraphagosomal chlorination dynamics and yields determined using unique fluorescent bacterial mimics. Chemical Research in toxicology. 1997;10(10):1080-9.

[57] Barrette WC, Jr., Hannum DM, Wheeler WD, Hurst JK. General mechanism for the bacterial toxicity of hypochlorous acid: abolition of ATP production. Biochemistry. 1989;28(23):9172-8.

[58] Albrich JM, Gilbaugh JH, 3rd, Callahan KB, Hurst JK. Effects of the putative neutrophil-generated toxin, hypochlorous acid, on membrane permeability and transport systems of Escherichia coli. J Clin Invest. 1986;78(1):177-84.

[59] Gottardi W, Nagl M. Chlorine covers on living bacteria: the initial step in antimicrobial action of active chlorine compounds. J Antimicrob Chemother. 2005;55(4):475-82.

[60] Gottardi W, Nagl M. N-chlorotaurine, a natural antiseptic with outstanding tolerability. J Antimicrob Chemother. 2010;65(3):399-409.

[61] Painter RG, Bonvillain RW, Valentine VG, Lombard GA, LaPlace SG, Nauseef WM, et al. The role of chloride anion and CFTR in killing of Pseudomonas aeruginosa by normal and CF neutrophils. J Leukoc Biol. 2008;83(6):1345-53.

[62] Ng HP, Zhou Y, Song K, Hodges CA, Drumm ML, Wang G. Neutrophil-mediated phagocytic host defense defect in myeloid Cftr-inactivated mice. PLoS One. 2014;9(9):e106813.

[63] Parry MF, Root RK, Metcalf JA, Delaney KK, Kaplow LS, Richar WJ. Myeloperoxidase deficiency: prevalence and clinical significance. Annals of Internal Medicine. 1981;95(3):293-301.

[64] Lehrer RI, Hanifin J, Cline MJ. Defective bactericidal activity in myeloperoxidase-deficient human neutrophils. Nature. 1969;223(5201):78-9.

[65] Reeves EP, Lu H, Jacobs HL, Messina CG, Bolsover S, Gabella G, et al. Killing activity of neutrophils is mediated through activation of proteases by K+ flux. Nature. 2002;416(6878):291-7.

[66] Segal AW, Geisow M, Garcia R, Harper A, Miller R. The respiratory burst of phagocytic cells is associated with a rise in vacuolar pH. Nature. 1981;290(5805):406-9.

[67] Mandell GL. Bactericidal activity of aerobic and anaerobic polymorphonuclear neutrophils. Infect Immun. 1974;9(2):337-41.

[68] Hirsch JG. Phagocytin: a bactericidal substance from polymorphonuclear leucocytes. J Exp Med. 1956;103(5):589-611.

[69] Zucker-Franklin D, Hirsch JG. Electron microscope studies on the degranulation of rabbit peritoneal leukocytes during phagocytosis. J Exp Med. 1964;120:569-76.

[70] Fouret P, Du Bois RM, Bernaudin JF, Takahashi H, Ferrans VJ, Crystal RG. Expression of the neutrophil elastase gene during human bone marrow cell differentiation. J Exp Med. 1989;169(3):833-45.

[71] Lacy P. Mechanisms of degranulation in neutrophils. Allergy, asthma, and clinical immunology. Official Journal of the Canadian Society of Allergy and Clinical Immunology. 2006;2(3):98-108.

[72] Esaguy N, Aguas AP, Silva MT. High-resolution localization of lactoferrin in human neutrophils: labeling of secondary granules and cell heterogeneity. J Leukoc Biol. 1989;46(1):51-62.

[73] Wang YB. Antibacterial mechanisms of lysozyme on Streptococcus mutans. Zhonghua ya yi xue hui za zhi Chinese Dental Journal / Dental Association, Republic of China. 1990;9(3):87-97.

[74] Gaggar A, Li Y, Weathington N, Winkler M, Kong M, Jackson P, et al. Matrix metalloprotease-9 dysregulation in lower airway secretions of cystic fibrosis patients. Am J Physiol Lung Cell Mol Physiol. 2007;293(1):L96-L104.

[75] Nie J, Pei D. Direct activation of pro-matrix metalloproteinase-2 by leukolysin/membrane-type 6 matrix metalloproteinase/matrix metalloproteinase 25 at the asn(109)-Tyr bond. Cancer Res. 2003;63(20):6758-62.

[76] Robineaux J, Frederic J. [Contribution to the study of neutrophil granulations of the polynuclears by phase contrast microcinematography]. Comptes rendus des seances de la Societe de biologie et de ses filiales. 1955;149(5-6):486-9.

[77] Hirsch JG. Cinemicrophotographic observations on granule lysis in polymorphonuclear leucocytes during phagocytosis. J Exp Med. 1962;116:827-34.

[78] Neeft M, Wieffer M, De Jong AS, Negroiu G, Metz CH, Van Loon A, et al. Munc13-4 is an effector of rab27a and controls secretion of lysosomes in hematopoietic cells. Mol Biol Cell. 2005;16(2):731-41.

[79] Borregaard N, Sorensen OE, Theilgaard-Monch K. Neutrophil granules: a library of innate immunity proteins. Trends Immunol. 2007;28(8):340-5.

[80] Mollinedo F, Martin-Martin B, Calafat J, Nabokina SM, Lazo PA. Role of vesicle-associated membrane protein-2, through Q-soluble N-ethylmaleimide-sensitive factor attachment protein receptor/R-soluble N-ethylmaleimide-sensitive factor attachment protein receptor interaction, in the exocytosis of specific and tertiary granules of human neutrophils. J Immunol. 2003;170(2):1034-42.

[81] Stow JL, Manderson AP, Murray RZ. SNAREing immunity: the role of SNAREs in the immune system. Nat Rev Immunol. 2006;6(12):919-29.

[82] Abdel-Latif D, Steward M, Macdonald DL, Francis GA, Dinauer MC, Lacy P. Rac2 is critical for neutrophil primary granule exocytosis. Blood. 2004;104(3):832-9.

[83] Munafo DB, Johnson JL, Ellis BA, Rutschmann S, Beutler B, Catz SD. Rab27a is a key component of the secretory machinery of azurophilic granules in granulocytes. Biochem J. 2007;402(2):229-39.

[84] Brzezinska AA, Johnson JL, Munafo DB, Crozat K, Beutler B, Kiosses WB, et al. The Rab27a effectors JFC1/Slp1 and Munc13-4 regulate exocytosis of neutrophil granules. Traffic. 2008;9(12):2151-64.

[85] Belaaouaj A, McCarthy R, Baumann M, Gao Z, Ley TJ, Abraham SN, et al. Mice lacking neutrophil elastase reveal impaired host defense against gram negative bacterial sepsis. Nat Med. 1998;4(5):615-8.

[86] Belaaouaj A, Kim KS, Shapiro SD. Degradation of outer membrane protein A in Escherichia coli killing by neutrophil elastase. Science. 2000;289(5482):1185-8.

[87] Odeberg H, Olsson I. Antibacterial activity of cationic proteins from human granulocytes. J Clin Invest. 1975;56(5):1118-24.

[88] Shafer WM, Onunka VC, Martin LE. Antigonococcal activity of human neutrophil cathepsin G. Infect Immun. 1986;54(1):184-8.

[89] Tkalcevic J, Novelli M, Phylactides M, Iredale JP, Segal AW, Roes J. Impaired immunity and enhanced resistance to endotoxin in the absence of neutrophil elastase and cathepsin G. Immunity. 2000;12(2):201-10.

[90] Arnold RR, Brewer M, Gauthier JJ. Bactericidal activity of human lactoferrin: sensitivity of a variety of microorganisms. Infect Immun. 1980;28(3):893-8.

[91] Nibbering PH, Ravensbergen E, Welling MM, Van Berkel LA, Van Berkel PH, Pauwels EK, et al. Human lactoferrin and peptides derived from its N terminus are highly effective against infections with antibiotic-resistant bacteria. Infect Immun. 2001;69(3):1469-76.

[92] Delclaux C, Delacourt C, D'Ortho MP, Boyer V, Lafuma C, Harf A. Role of gelatinase B and elastase in human polymorphonuclear neutrophil migration across basement membrane. Am J Respir Cell Mol Biol. 1996;14(3):288-95.

[93] Renckens R, Roelofs JJ, Florquin S, De Vos AF, Lijnen HR, Van't Veer C, et al. Matrix metalloproteinase-9 deficiency impairs host defense against abdominal sepsis. J Immunol. 2006;176(6):3735-41.

[94] Geraghty P, Greene CM, O'Mahony M, O'Neill SJ, Taggart CC, McElvaney NG. Secretory leucocyte protease inhibitor inhibits interferon-gamma-induced cathepsin S expression. J Biol Chem. 2007;282(46):33389-95.

[95] Walsh DE, Greene CM, Carroll TP, Taggart CC, Gallagher PM, O'Neill SJ, et al. Interleukin-8 up-regulation by neutrophil elastase is mediated by MyD88/IRAK/TRAF-6 in human bronchial epithelium. J Biol Chem. 2001;276(38):35494-9.

[96] Bergsson G, Reeves EP, McNally P, Chotirmall SH, Greene CM, Greally P, et al. LL-37 complexation with glycosaminoglycans in cystic fibrosis lungs inhibits antimicrobial activity, which can be restored by hypertonic saline. J Immunol. 2009;183(1): 543-51.

[97] Weldon S, McNally P, McElvaney NG, Elborn JS, McAuley DF, Wartelle J, et al. Decreased levels of secretory leucoprotease inhibitor in the Pseudomonas-infected cyst-

ic fibrosis lung are due to neutrophil elastase degradation. J Immunol. 2009;183(12): 8148-56.

[98] Guyot N, Butler MW, McNally P, Weldon S, Greene CM, Levine RL, et al. Elafin, an elastase-specific inhibitor, is cleaved by its cognate enzyme neutrophil elastase in sputum from individuals with cystic fibrosis. J Biol Chem. 2008;283(47):32377-85.

[99] Birrer P, McElvaney NG, Rudeberg A, Sommer CW, Liechti-Gallati S, Kraemer R, et al. Protease-antiprotease imbalance in the lungs of children with cystic fibrosis. Am J Respir Crit Care Med. 1994;150(1):207-13.

[100] Taggart C, Coakley RJ, Greally P, Canny G, O'Neill SJ, McElvaney NG. Increased elastase release by CF neutrophils is mediated by tumor necrosis factor-alpha and interleukin-8. Am J Physiol Lung Cell Mol Physiol. 2000;278(1): L33-41.

[101] Koller DY, Urbanek R, Gotz M. Increased degranulation of eosinophil and neutrophil granulocytes in cystic fibrosis. Am J Respir Crit Care Med. 1995;152(2):629-33.

[102] Coakley RJ, Taggart C, Canny G, Greally P, O'Neill SJ, McElvaney NG. Altered intracellular pH regulation in neutrophils from patients with cystic fibrosis. Am J Physiol Lung Cell Mol Physiol. 2000;279(1):L66-74.

[103] Coakley RJ, Taggart C, McElvaney NG, O'Neill SJ. Cytosolic pH and the inflammatory microenvironment modulate cell death in human neutrophils after phagocytosis. Blood. 2002;100(9):3383-91.

[104] Taggart C, Coakley RJ, Greally P, Canny G, O'Neill SJ, McElvaney NG. Increased elastase release by CF neutrophils is mediated by tumor necrosis factor-alpha and interleukin-8. Am J Physiol Lung Cell Mol Physiol. 2000;278(1):L33-41.

[105] Brockbank S, Downey D, Elborn JS, Ennis M. Effect of cystic fibrosis exacerbations on neutrophil function. Int Immunopharmacol. 2005;5(3):601-8.

[106] Witko-Sarsat V, Allen RC, Paulais M, Nguyen AT, Bessou G, Lenoir G, et al. Disturbed myeloperoxidase-dependent activity of neutrophils in cystic fibrosis homozygotes and heterozygotes, and its correction by amiloride. J Immunol. 1996;157(6): 2728-35.

[107] Bergin DA, Reeves EP, Hurley K, Wolfe R, Jameel R, Fitzgerald S, et al. The circulating proteinase inhibitor alpha-1 antitrypsin regulates neutrophil degranulation and autoimmunity. Sci Transl Med. 2014;6(217):217ra1.

[108] Russell KJ, McRedmond J, Mukherji N, Costello C, Keatings V, Linnane S, et al. Neutrophil adhesion molecule surface expression and responsiveness in cystic fibrosis. Am J Respir Crit Care Med. 1998;157(3 Pt 1):756-61.

[109] Hoover RL, Karnovsky MJ, Austen KF, Corey EJ, Lewis RA. Leukotriene B4 action on endothelium mediates augmented neutrophil/endothelial adhesion. Proc Natl Acad Sci USA. 1984;81(7):2191-3.

[110] Palmblad J, Malmsten CL, Uden AM, Radmark O, Engstedt L, Samuelsson B. Leukotriene B4 is a potent and stereospecific stimulator of neutrophil chemotaxis and adherence. Blood. 1981;58(3):658-61.

[111] O'Driscoll BR, Cromwell O, Kay AB. Sputum leukotrienes in obstructive airways diseases. Clin Exp Immunol. 1984;55(2):397-404.

[112] Dai Y, Dean TP, Church MK, Warner JO, Shute JK. Desensitisation of neutrophil responses by systemic interleukin 8 in cystic fibrosis. Thorax. 1994;49(9):867-71.

[113] Dean TP, Dai Y, Shute JK, Church MK, Warner JO. Interleukin-8 concentrations are elevated in bronchoalveolar lavage, sputum, and sera of children with cystic fibrosis. Pediatr Res. 1993;34(2):159-61.

[114] Smith RS, Fedyk ER, Springer TA, Mukaida N, Iglewski BH, Phipps RP. IL-8 production in human lung fibroblasts and epithelial cells activated by the Pseudomonas autoinducer N-3-oxododecanoyl homoserine lactone is transcriptionally regulated by NF-kappa B and activator protein-2. J Immunol. 2001;167(1):366-74.

[115] DiMango E, Zar HJ, Bryan R, Prince A. Diverse Pseudomonas aeruginosa gene products stimulate respiratory epithelial cells to produce interleukin-8. J Clin Invest. 1995;96(5):2204-10.

[116] Corvol H, Fitting C, Chadelat K, Jacquot J, Tabary O, Boule M, et al. Distinct cytokine production by lung and blood neutrophils from children with cystic fibrosis. Am J Physiol Lung Cell Mol Physiol. 2003;284(6):L997-1003.

[117] Brennan S, Cooper D, Sly PD. Directed neutrophil migration to IL-8 is increased in cystic fibrosis: a study of the effect of erythromycin. Thorax. 2001;56(1):62-4.

[118] Takami M, Terry V, Petruzzelli L. Signaling pathways involved in IL-8-dependent activation of adhesion through Mac-1. J Immunol. 2002;168(9):4559-66.

[119] Khan TZ, Wagener JS, Bost T, Martinez J, Accurso FJ, Riches DW. Early pulmonary inflammation in infants with cystic fibrosis. Am J Respir Crit Care Med. 1995;151(4): 1075-82.

[120] Verhaeghe C, Delbecque K, De Leval L, Oury C, Bours V. Early inflammation in the airways of a cystic fibrosis foetus. J Cyst Fibros. 2007;6(4):304-8.

[121] Dewitt S, Hallett MB. Cytosolic free Ca(2+) changes and calpain activation are required for beta integrin-accelerated phagocytosis by human neutrophils. J Cell Biol. 2002;159(1):181-9.

[122] White M AB, Cox S, McElvaney NG, Reeves EP. A neutrophil inflammatory impairment affects cell structure in cystic fibrosis and is indirectly corrected by CFTR potentiator therapy. The 28th Annual North American Cystic Fibrosis Conference; September 2014; Georgia World Congress Center, Atlanta, Georgia, USA Ped Pulmonol; 2014. p. ISSN 8755-6863.

[123] Solomkin JS, Robinson CT, Cave CM, Ehmer B, Lentsch AB. Alterations in membrane cholesterol cause mobilization of lipid rafts from specific granules and prime human neutrophils for enhanced adherence-dependent oxidant production. Shock. 2007;28(3):334-8.

[124] Witko-Sarsat V, Pederzoli-Ribeil M, Hirsch E, Sozzani S, Cassatella MA. Regulating neutrophil apoptosis: new players enter the game. Trends Immunol. 2011;32(3): 117-24.

[125] El Kebir D, Filep JG. Modulation of neutrophil apoptosis and the resolution of inflammation through beta2 Integrins. Front Immunol. 2013;4:60.

[126] Kennedy AD, DeLeo FR. Neutrophil apoptosis and the resolution of infection. Immunolog Res. 2009;43(1-3):25-61.

[127] Savill JS, Wyllie AH, Henson JE, Walport MJ, Henson PM, Haslett C. Macrophage phagocytosis of aging neutrophils in inflammation. Programmed cell death in the neutrophil leads to its recognition by macrophages. J Clin Invest. 1989;83(3):865-75.

[128] Nathan C. Neutrophils and immunity: challenges and opportunities. Nature Rev Immunology. 2006;6(3):173-82.

[129] Li P, Nijhawan D, Budihardjo I, Srinivasula SM, Ahmad M, Alnemri ES, et al. Cytochrome c and dATP-dependent formation of Apaf-1/caspase-9 complex initiates an apoptotic protease cascade. Cell. 1997;91(4):479-89.

[130] Liu X, Kim CN, Yang J, Jemmerson R, Wang X. Induction of apoptotic program in cell-free extracts: requirement for dATP and cytochrome c. Cell. 1996;86(1):147-57.

[131] Zou H, Henzel WJ, Liu X, Lutschg A, Wang X. Apaf-1, a human protein homologous to C. elegans CED-4, participates in cytochrome c-dependent activation of caspase-3. Cell. 1997;90(3):405-13.

[132] Kuwana T, Smith JJ, Muzio M, Dixit V, Newmeyer DD, Kornbluth S. Apoptosis induction by caspase-8 is amplified through the mitochondrial release of cytochrome c. J Biol Chem. 1998;273(26):16589-94.

[133] Muzio M, Chinnaiyan AM, Kischkel FC, O'Rourke K, Shevchenko A, Ni J, et al. FLICE, a novel FADD-homologous ICE/CED-3-like protease, is recruited to the CD95 (Fas/APO-1) death--inducing signaling complex. Cell. 1996;85(6):817-27.

[134] Tang D, Kidd VJ. Cleavage of DFF-45/ICAD by multiple caspases is essential for its function during apoptosis. J Biol Chem. 1998;273(44):28549-52.

[135] Han J, Murthy R, Wood B, Song B, Wang S, Sun B, et al. ER stress signalling through eIF2alpha and CHOP, but not IRE1alpha, attenuates adipogenesis in mice. Diabetologia. 2013;56(4):911-24.

[136] Rao RV, Hermel E, Castro-Obregon S, Del Rio G, Ellerby LM, Ellerby HM, et al. Coupling endoplasmic reticulum stress to the cell death program. Mechanism of caspase activation. J Biol Chem. 2001;276(36):33869-74.

[137] Altieri DC. Survivin and IAP proteins in cell-death mechanisms. Biochem J. 2010;430(2):199-205.

[138] Edwards SW, Derouet M, Howse M, Moots RJ. Regulation of neutrophil apoptosis by Mcl-1. Biochem Soc Trans. 2004;32(Pt3):489-92.

[139] Kroemer G, Galluzzi L, Brenner C. Mitochondrial membrane permeabilization in cell death. Physiol Rev. 2007;87(1):99-163.

[140] Kasahara Y, Iwai K, Yachie A, Ohta K, Konno A, Seki H, et al. Involvement of reactive oxygen intermediates in spontaneous and CD95 (Fas/APO-1)-mediated apoptosis of neutrophils. Blood. 1997;89(5):1748-53.

[141] Hurley K, Lacey N, O'Dwyer CA, Bergin DA, McElvaney OJ, O'Brien ME, et al. Alpha-1 antitrypsin augmentation therapy corrects accelerated neutrophil apoptosis in deficient individuals. J Immunol. 2014;193(8):3978-91.

[142] McKeon DJ, Condliffe AM, Cowburn AS, Cadwallader KC, Farahi N, Bilton D, et al. Prolonged survival of neutrophils from patients with Delta F508 CFTR mutations. Thorax. 2008;63(7):660-1.

[143] Moriceau S, Kantari C, Mocek J, Davezac N, Gabillet J, Guerrera IC, et al. Coronin-1 is associated with neutrophil survival and is cleaved during apoptosis: potential implication in neutrophils from cystic fibrosis patients. J Immunol. 2009;182(11): 7254-63.

[144] Moriceau S, Lenoir G, Witko-Sarsat V. In cystic fibrosis homozygotes and heterozygotes, neutrophil apoptosis is delayed and modulated by diamide or roscovitine: evidence for an innate neutrophil disturbance. J Innate Immun. 2010;2(3):260-6.

[145] Downey DG, Brockbank S, Martin SL, Ennis M, Elborn JS. The effect of treatment of cystic fibrosis pulmonary exacerbations on airways and systemic inflammation. Pediatr Pulmonol. 2007;42(8):729-35.

[146] Vandivier RW, Fadok VA, Hoffmann PR, Bratton DL, Penvari C, Brown KK, et al. Elastase-mediated phosphatidylserine receptor cleavage impairs apoptotic cell clearance in cystic fibrosis and bronchiectasis. J Clin Invest. 2002;109(5):661-70.

[147] Boyle MP, De Boeck K. A new era in the treatment of cystic fibrosis: correction of the underlying CFTR defect. Lancet Respir Med. 2013;1(2):158-63.

[148] Kerem E, Hirawat S, Armoni S, Yaakov Y, Shoseyov D, Cohen M, et al. Effectiveness of PTC124 treatment of cystic fibrosis caused by nonsense mutations: a prospective phase II trial. Lancet. 2008;372(9640):719-27.

[149] Wilschanski M, Famini C, Blau H, Rivlin J, Augarten A, Avital A, et al. A pilot study of the effect of gentamicin on nasal potential difference measurements in cystic fibro-

sis patients carrying stop mutations. Am J Respir Crit Care Med. 2000;161(3 Pt 1): 860-5.

[150] Kerem E, Konstan MW, De Boeck K, Accurso FJ, Sermet-Gaudelus I, Wilschanski M, et al. Ataluren for the treatment of nonsense-mutation cystic fibrosis: a randomised, double-blind, placebo-controlled phase 3 trial. Lancet Respir Med. 2014;2(7):539-47.

[151] Amaral MD, Farinha CM. Rescuing mutant CFTR: a multi-task approach to a better outcome in treating cystic fibrosis. Curr Pharmaceut Design. 2013;19(19):3497-508.

[152] Ramsey BW, Davies J, McElvaney NG, Tullis E, Bell SC, Drevinek P, et al. A CFTR potentiator in patients with cystic fibrosis and the G551D mutation. N Engl J Med. 2011;365(18):1663-72.

[153] Boyle MP, Bell SC, Konstan MW, McColley SA, Rowe SM, Rietschel E, et al. A CFTR corrector (lumacaftor) and a CFTR potentiator (ivacaftor) for treatment of patients with cystic fibrosis who have a phe508del CFTR mutation: a phase 2 randomised controlled trial. Lancet Respir Med. 2014;2(7):527-38.

[154] Bell SC, De Boeck K, Amaral MD. New pharmacological approaches for cystic fibrosis: promises, progress, pitfalls. Pharmacol Therapeut. 2015;145:19-34.

[155] Bratcher PE, Rowe SM, Reeves G, Roberts T, Szul T, Harris WT, Tirouvanziam R, Gaggar A. Alterations in blood leukocytes of G551D-bearing cystic fibrosis patients undergoing treatment with ivacaftor. J Cyst Fibros. 2015 Mar 11. pii: S1569-1993(15)00050-8.

[156] Hartl D, Latzin P, Hordijk P, Marcos V, Rudolph C, Woischnik M, et al. Cleavage of CXCR1 on neutrophils disables bacterial killing in cystic fibrosis lung disease. Nat Med. 2007;13(12):1423-30.

[157] Alexis NE, Muhlebach MS, Peden DB, Noah TL. Attenuation of host defense function of lung phagocytes in young cystic fibrosis patients. J Cyst Fibros. 2006;5(1):17-25.

[158] Tirouvanziam R, Gernez Y, Conrad CK, Moss RB, Schrijver I, Dunn CE, et al. Profound functional and signaling changes in viable inflammatory neutrophils homing to cystic fibrosis airways. Proc Natl Acad Sci USA. 2008;105(11):4335-9.

[159] Witko-Sarsat V, Delacourt C, Rabier D, Bardet J, Nguyen AT, Descamps-Latscha B. Neutrophil-derived long-lived oxidants in cystic fibrosis sputum. Am J Respir Crit Care Med. 1995;152(6 Pt 1):1910-6.

[160] Makam M, Diaz D, Laval J, Gernez Y, Conrad CK, Dunn CE, et al. Activation of critical, host-induced, metabolic and stress pathways marks neutrophil entry into cystic fibrosis lungs. Proc Natl Acad Sci USA. 2009;106(14):5779-83.

[161] Laval J, Touhami J, Herzenberg LA, Conrad C, Taylor N, Battini JL, et al. Metabolic adaptation of neutrophils in cystic fibrosis airways involves distinct shifts in nutrient transporter expression. J Immunol. 2013;190(12):6043-50.

3

New Molecular Diagnosis Approaches —From the Identification of Mutations to their Characterization

Anne Bergougnoux, Magali Taulan-Cadars,
Mireille Claustres and Caroline Raynal

Abstract

Molecular diagnosis of cystic fibrosis is based on the detection of mutation in the *CFTR* gene, identified in 1989. During the past 20 years, thanks to evolutions of diagnostic techniques, our knowledge of mutation spectrum and pathophysiological mechanisms involved in the disease has significantly improved. Sanger sequencing and quantitative methods greatly contributed to the identification of the 2,000 sequence variations reported worldwide in *CFTR*. We are now entering the new technological age with the generalisation of Next Generation Sequencing (NGS) technologies in diagnostics laboratories. These high throughput approaches allow scanning for the entire *CFTR* locus, including deep intronic regions, and in parallel other candidate genes that possibly influence the clinical evolution of patients. However, this powerful technology poses new challenge in test interpretation. In this chapter, we review the current and new technologies used in molecular diagnostics of cystic fibrosis, particularly NGS approaches. We also present current and new bioinformatics tools available for the interpretation of variants and *in vitro*/*ex vivo* and *in vivo* techniques that can be used to improve the characterization of the functional impact of *CFTR* variations.

Keywords: Next generation sequencing, *CFTR*, sequence variations, interpretation, functional characterization

1. Introduction

The autosomal recessive mode of inheritance of Cystic Fibrosis (CF) was suggested by Andersen and Hodges in 1945 when they described this disease as a pathological entity.

Since the discovery of the *CFTR* gene (and the predicted protein cystic fibrosis transmembrane conductance regulator) in 1989 [1], close to 2, 000 variations have been identified on this locus. *CFTR* gene studies represent one of the most frequent genetic analyses routinely performed worldwide, either to confirm the clinical diagnosis of CF or CFTR-related disorders (CFTR-RDs), or to offer carrier testing, prenatal or pre-implantation genetic diagnosis.

The most common severe mutation, p.Phe508del, is found in approximately 70% of CF alleles of European descent (therefore it is present in 49% of homozygous and 42% of compound heterozygous CF patients), with significant variations depending on ethnicities [2]. There is a clear decreasing northwest to southwest gradient in p.Phe508del frequency across Europe. Only four other mutations represent more than 1% of CF cases: p.Gly542*, p.Gly551Asp, p.Asn1303Lys, and p.Trp1282*. All other mutations are rare and many are private, only detected within a single family.

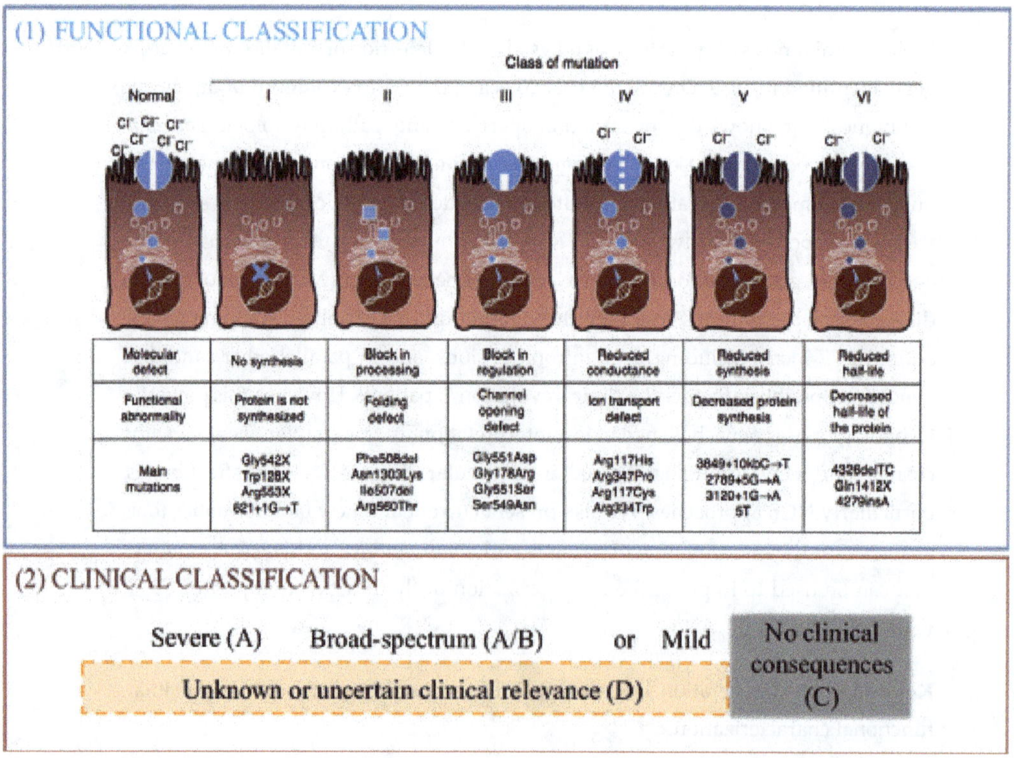

Figure 1. Two models for the classification of CFTR variants: (1) Functional: five classes of defective CFTR protein [3, 4, 5]; and (2) Clinical: four classes based on phenotypic expression in patients [6].

Therefore, a good knowledge of CFTR diseases and their molecular pathology is required when choosing tools and strategy and when interpreting results. Organization of regional or national networks of specialist clinical and molecular genetic laboratories is needed. Two models for the classification of sequence alterations have been proposed (Figure 1): (1) depending on their molecular impact on the CFTR chloride channel, which requires *in vitro/in vivo* functional assays, now less used due to the difficulty in accurately classifying the new reported variants [3, 4] or (2) by their clinical consequences on patients based on detailed and prospective clinical evaluation of patients associated with molecular findings [5].

However, even if the most severe mutations were studied *in vitro*, mild mutations or variants of unknown (clinical) significance (VUCs or VUS) were barely analysed. Thus, only one third of *CFTR* variations are functionally classified. Finally, in CF, as in other genetic diseases, new molecular diagnosis techniques such as Next Generation Sequencing (NGS) allow the analysis of the whole *CFTR* locus (including deep intronic regions) but increase the number of VUCS reported on patients.

Therefore, geneticists and clinicians have to combine CFTR epidemiological databases, functional *in vitro/in vivo* analysis and exhaustive clinical data to perform pertinent genotype/phenotype correlations in patients in order to provide appropriate genetic counselling to families.

2. Technical aspects of molecular diagnosis

The *CFTR* genetic testing strategy depends on the clinical and familial context and is classically performed step by step, as recommended [7]. As shown in Figure 2, tests are carried out in various situations, including confirmation of a clinical diagnosis, prenatal diagnosis (familial context or foetal suspicion of CF) and carrier screening.

A wide range of techniques is still used to identify *CFTR* gene sequence variations (presented in Table 1) and there is no gold standard or preferred method for routine testing. However, laboratories should be aware of the limitations of their chosen method (e.g. some mutations are not identified). Moreover, assay performance should always be verified before diagnostic use, even though commercial kits are CE-marked *in vitro* diagnostic devices (IVDD). In the perspective of accreditation (expected in France in 2020 for hospital diagnostic laboratories), all methods used in molecular biology should be validated before diagnostic use, notably by comparison with a reference method (Sanger sequencing for Single Nucleotide Variations and quantitative PCR for Copy Number Variations detection). This technical validation should be undertaken for NGS in the step 1 and 2 diagnosis.

Undetected *CFTR* mutations may lie within the introns or regulatory regions, which are not routinely explored but that will be soon analysed by NGS. Comparison between NGS and reference methods for the identification of *CFTR* variants on these unexplored regions will be a challenge.

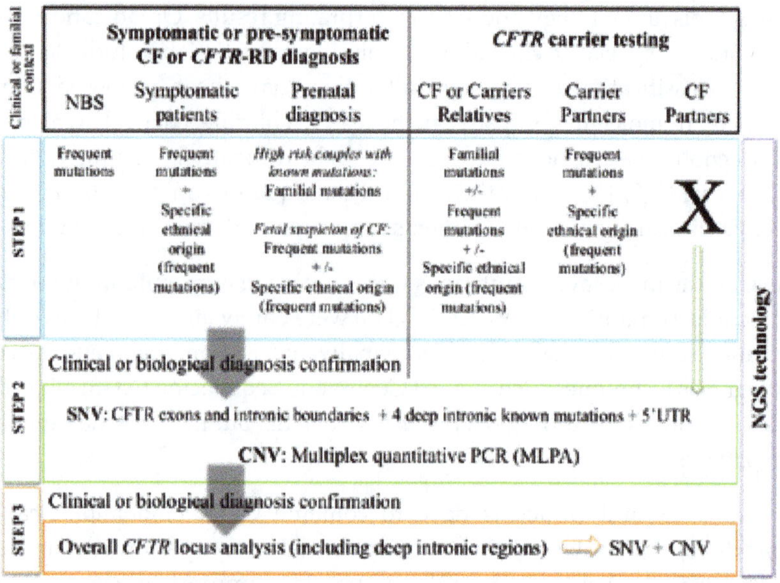

Figure 2. CF molecular diagnosis: a step-by-step strategy (modified from [7]). *NBS*: newborn screening; *SNV*: Single Nucleotide Variation; *CNV*: Copy Number Variation; *MLPA*: Multiplex Ligation-dependent Probe Amplification.

2.1. Current techniques to detect *CFTR* variants

2.1.1. Screening techniques (Step 1)

These approaches consist of genotyping a panel of frequent CF mutations using commercial kits (Table 1) that classically cover more than 80% of CF known mutations in European populations. Additional search for mutations specific to certain regions or ethnicities (frequency higher than 1% of CF alleles in the targeted population) completes the analyses.

Data on disease and carrier frequencies or mutation frequencies in various populations are available in the WHO report [8] and should be accurately known and used by laboratories.

For many patients carrying CF-causing mutations included in commercial panels, *CFTR* molecular analysis generally stops at this step. There is no need for additional studies, except the confirmation of mutations by a second method, as recommended by international guidelines for genetics diagnosis.

2.1.2. Scanning techniques (Step 2)

The high heterogeneity of *CFTR* mutations in CF and CFTR-RD populations makes the complete molecular screening of the 27 exons and parts of the regulatory regions (5'UTR, 3'UTR and partial intronic regions) essential.

Therefore, the analysis of the *CFTR* locus can be performed as follows:

- To detect SNV: scanning the 27 exons of the *CFTR* gene, intronic boundaries and four intronic regions with reported deep intronic mutations [9-12] and a part of the promoter. As an example, one can use Sanger sequencing with Single Condition Amplification Primers (SCAP) technique [13].
- To detect CNV (large *CFTR* rearrangements): scanning of exon by multiplex fluorescent quantitative PCR (Multiplex Ligation-dependent Probe Amplification or MLPA) or array-CGH [14].

These robust methods allow the detection of more than 97% of *CFTR* mutations involved in CF.

2.1.3. *Advantages and limits*

Classical screening or scanning methods used to detect mutations (in step 1 and 2) have high specificity and sensitivity (Table 1). Older techniques such as RFLP (restriction fragment length polymorphism), DGGE (denaturing gradient gel electrophoresis) or DHPLC (denaturing high performance liquid chromatography) were widely used in the past 20 years but were difficult to set up and showed inconstant performance. They have been progressively replaced by easy-to-use commercial kits, more appropriate for larger sample series. These kits allow PCR multiplexing and thus enable the detection of the most common CF mutations in one reaction. Sanger sequencing and quantitative PCR are the most effective to identify unknown mutations. However, all these classical methods are labour-intensive and time-consuming.

<table>
<tr><th>Method name</th><th>Mutations detected</th><th>Advantages</th><th>Limits</th></tr>
<tr><td colspan="4">Screening (step 1)</td></tr>
<tr><td>Reverse dot blot hybridization</td><td>Up to 20 mutations per multiplex</td><td rowspan="4">Appropriate for large series
High specificity
Cost effective</td><td>Partial hybridization if SNP on probe</td></tr>
<tr><td>ARMS (amplification refractory mutation system)</td><td>Up to 50 mutations</td><td>Primer Design difficult
Need of high agarose gel quality</td></tr>
<tr><td>OLA (Oligonucleotide ligation assay)</td><td>32 mutations (Abbott kit)</td><td>Partial hybridization if SNP on probe</td></tr>
<tr><td>NGS</td><td>139 to 166 CFTR variants</td><td>Need of sufficient coverage
In development (Illumina)</td></tr>
<tr><td colspan="4">Scanning (Step 2)</td></tr>
<tr><td>HRM (High Resolution Melting curve analysis)</td><td>Heterozygous variants</td><td>Appropriate for large series (e.g. epidemiological studies)</td><td>Exon by exon
Need of positive cases
Not adapted for homozygous variants</td></tr>
<tr><td>Sanger Sequencing</td><td>All sequenced bases</td><td>Close to 100% sensitivity</td><td>Expensive method
Can not detect CNV</td></tr>
<tr><td>Quantitative fluorescent multiplex PCR</td><td>Deletions, duplications, insertions</td><td>Simple and rapid</td><td>False positive if SNP on probe
Performance dependent on DNA quality</td></tr>
<tr><td>NGS (used for step 3)</td><td>All sequenced bases</td><td>Appropriate for large series
Cost effective</td><td>Need of sufficient coverage
In development (Illumina)</td></tr>
</table>

Table 1. Overview, advantages and limits of screening and scanning techniques used in molecular genetics diagnosis (adapted from [7])

2.2. Next Generation Sequencing (NGS)

2.2.1. Principle of NGS technologies

The development of Next Generation Sequencing (NGS) or Massively Parallel Sequencing (MPS) technologies with an immense capacity (up to 1 Terabase (Tb) of data per run with the HiSeq2500 system, Illumina) is a major technical progress in the field of human genetics. Since 2004, three principal NGS platforms have been commercially available, including (i) 454 GS FLX & GS junior from Roche (ii) Genome Analyzer, HiSeq & MiSeq from Illumina and (iii) SOLiD & Ion Torrent PGM from Life Technologies-Applied Biosystems (AB) [15]. These technologies differ in terms of sample library preparation workflow, enabling sequencing on any of the current NGS sequencers (e.g. Illumina, Life technologies, Roche). Since late 2004, three principal NGS firms developed sequencers commercially available (listed in Table 2).

454 pyrosequencing is a sequencing-by-synthesis method that measures the release of inorganic pyrophosphate upon incorporation of nucleotides, by converting it into luciferase chemiluminescent signals using a series of enzymatic reactions. Ion Torrent semiconductor technology is also based on a sequencing-by-synthesis approach but measures pH changes (instead of light) induced by the release of hydrogen ions as nucleotides are incorporated. SOLiD technology is a ligation-based sequencing system. DNA ligase is used to identify the nucleotide present at a given position in a DNA sequence; each base is read twice, which increases accuracy, even for homopolymeric regions. Base detection uses a mixture of labelled oligonucleotides, which queries the input strand with ligase. In Illumina system, clonal amplification is performed using a process termed 'bridge amplification' followed by two basic steps, initial priming and extending of the single-stranded, single-molecule template and bridge amplification of the immobilized template with immediately adjacent primers to form clusters. For sequencing, only dye-labelled terminators are added; then the sequence at that position is determined for all clusters; next, the dye is cleaved and another round of dye-labelled terminators is added.

Platform	GAII, HiSeq & MiSeq	Ion Torrent	SOLiD	GS FLX & GS Junior
Methodology	Sequencing by synthesis (Reversible termination)	Sequencing by synthesis	Sequencing by Ligation	Sequencing by synthesis (Pyrosequencing)
Loading	Adaptors on template DNA bind high density primers across surface of slide	Adaptors on template DNA bind primers on beads, one molecule per bead	Adaptors on template DNA bind primers on beads, one molecule per bead	Adaptors on template DNA bind primers on beads, one molecule per bead
Clonal amplification	Bridge PCR: Surface array on flow cell	Emulsion PCR: clusters on beads	Emulsion PCR: clusters on beads	Emulsion PCR: clusters on beads
Parallelisation	Random array on flow cell	Beads loaded on a chip	Beads bonded to high density glass slide	Beads loaded onto high density plate
Detection	Fluorescence	H^+ ions (sensitive pH meter)	Fluorescence	Light (luciferase)

Table 2. Overview of the main NGS technologies

2.2.1.1. *Target enrichment*

Targeted re-sequencing isolates genomic regions of interest in a sample library, allowing to focus efficiently and cost-effectively on a small subset of the genome, such as an exome, a particular chromosome, a set of genes or a region of interest such as a whole gene. Two main strategies can be envisioned: capture [16, 17] or amplification relevant genomic DNA [18-20] as shown in Table 3.

Strategy	Capture/hybridisation-based method			Amplicon-based method		
Methods	HaloPlex	SureSelect (Agilent) /SeqCap (NimbleGen)	Nextera (Illumina)	Microdoplet (RainDance Technologies)	Multiplex PCR (AmpliSeq, Life Technology & TrueSeq, Illumina)	Long-Range PCR Qiagen & "home" design
Main steps	Restriction enzyme digestion	Sonication/ nebulisation	Tagmentation with transposon	Sonication	PCR amplification	PCR amplification
	Probe hybridisation	PCR amplification + probe hybridisation	PCR amplification + probe hybridisation			Sonication/ nebulisation
						Ligation of sequencing adaptors

Table 3. Main strategies proposed for target enrichment

2.2.1.2. *Advantages and limits*

The main advantages of the technology are related to its capability to process a large number of samples in parallel. NGS technologies are time saving and lower the costs per patient, of step 1 and particularly step 2 molecular analyses. But, they also have significant limitations such as high error rates, enrichment of rare variants and large proportion of missing values, as well as the fact that most current analytical methods are designed for population-based association studies. With second generation sequencing, it is necessary to clonally amplify the isolated targets in order to generate sufficient signal for detection during the sequencing run generating clusters of many thousands of identical DNA targets. In addition, each NGS platform generates different read lengths that range from short (e.g. 35 bases) to long reads (over 500 bases). For a number of applications, including targeted re-sequencing, ChIP-Seq and RNA-Seq, short reads are highly informative and adequate. Conversely, longer reads are more suitable for *de novo* genome assembly, mapping of high homology regions (related gene family and pseudogenes) and sequencing of repetitive DNA regions, such as introns. This is an important consideration since short read length can make accurate assembly and alignment computationally challenging.

For some clinical applications, as NGS produces massive amounts of data, their analysis and interpretation are time-consuming, not trivial and a real challenge even if specific portions of a genome is analysed.

2.2.1.3. Bioinformatics software to analyse NGS data

Then, generated data are analysed by bioinformatics tools. Quality criteria such as confidence or coverage are guarantees for optimal sensitivity and specificity of a sequencing run. Bioinformatics analyses are frequently performed by using software developed by sequencers' companies. The three steps include (1) base calling and quality score computation, (2) assembly and alignment and (3) variant calling and annotation. Laboratories developed their own 'in-house' pipeline mainly to apply filters allowing an easy focus on causing-mutations. Others use free web resources to realign files including BWA (http://bio-bwa.sourceforge.net) or to perform a new variant calling such as Samtools and GATK [21-23]. Others serve as Viewer such as Integrative Genomics Viewer (http://www.broadinstitute.org/igv/). Galaxy website is an integrative platform offering the possibility to view and process files generated by NGS. Many databases, useful for variant annotation and sometimes inserted in others programs or pipelines, are publicly available including the 1000 Genomes Project [24] and the dbSNP database [25] (further described in part 3.1.1).

Many tracks are currently studied (i.e. improvement of bioinformatics tools, comparison of NGS approaches between CF laboratories, development of databases including newly detected NGS variants, publication of guidelines and definition of a diagnosis report model) to make CF molecular diagnosis by NGS suitable for different clinical and familial cases.

2.2.2. Indications and choice of CFTR analysed regions

In the case of Mendelian diseases caused by mutations in a single gene, like *CFTR* in Cystic Fibrosis, NGS sequencing of entire genome or exome is still useless and expensive. Collaborations between companies specialized in molecular diagnosis and academic laboratories recently led to the establishment of new molecular diagnosis tools based on NGS. Combination of (i) the enrichment of regions of interest by hybrid capture, circularization or Polymerase Chain Reaction (PCR) and (ii) high throughput sequencing now allows time-efficient and economical way to perform analyses. Use of NGS technology as a first intention is currently set up in laboratories, which will soon question the CF diagnosis strategy as a tree. As shown in Figure 2, in our actual CF molecular diagnosis strategy, NGS technology can be used instead of 'classical' techniques for the detection of a panel of common mutations (step 1) or to analyse the '*CFTR* exome' (step 2). Technical manipulations are similar for both, but filters can be used to focus on regions that contain mutations. Multiplicom® and Illumina® propose a locus specific design to library preparation for molecular analysis of the '*CFTR* exome'. CE-marked kits for *in vitro* diagnostic (CE-IVD) and efficient bioinformatics tools are commercialized. The latter could be performed by in-house pipelines or subcontract on commercial firms (Sophia Genetics®). SNV and indels are correctly detected (high specificity and sensitivity) and CNV detection is now available for some amplicon-based methods.

Furthermore, in patients with definite CF clinical diagnosis (positive sweat test, CF clinical features) and who carry no or only one CF mutation, step 3 analysis could be ultimately proposed, in combination with the analysis of potential modifiers genes (see next section)

In literature, three studies reported NGS *CFTR* sequencing (Table 4) on CF patients, CF carriers or controls samples [18, 26, 27]. Abou Tayoun and colleagues [26] first proposed a proof-of-concept for a '*CFTR* exome' analysis by NGS on 79 samples. Target enrichment was performed by PCR amplification (AmpliSeq Panel, Life technologies) and Sequencing on Ion Torrent Platform (PGM®). Their sequencing offered minimal coverage of 100X (depending on the Ion 314 or 318 chip used). Two others studies realized sequencing of the whole *CFTR* locus (close to 250 kb) including deep intronic *CFTR* regions (Figure 2, Step 3). Trujillano *et al.* [27] reported the *CFTR* re-sequencing by hybridization capture on a custom NimbleGen SeqCap EZ Choise array using HiSeq2000 (Illumina®) in a set of 92 samples. They highlighted the precise characterization of breakpoints of seven genomic rearrangements in *CFTR*.

We proposed a complete *CFTR* gene sequencing of DNA samples from patients with a confirmed CF clinical diagnosis but with an incomplete genotype [18]. Although large unexplored intronic regions might contain few mutations (about 1%–3% of CF mutations), we identified a new pathogenic mutation, which creates a pseudo-exon (Table 4). Moreover, we compared hybridization capture and Long-Range PCR to target enrichment and used a small-scale NGS platform for sequencing (GS Junior Sequencer, 454 Life Sciences®). Some promising variants were then confirmed as deleterious by *in vitro*/*ex vivo* functional assays. However, for most detected intronic variants, classification will be a long and difficult way. This approach is currently under development for CF diagnosis.

	Abou Tayoun et al., 2013 [25]	Trujillano et al., 2014 [26]	Bonini et al., 2015 [17]	
Samples	57 subjects already genotyped – 22 cell lines: 24 CF, 46 CF carriers, 9 controls	92 subjects already genotyped: 45 CF, 27 CF carriers, 20 CFTR-RD	18 CF subjects in whom only one mutation had identified	
Study objectif	Proof of concept of CFTR assay by NGS	Resequencing mutations Validation technique	Identification of the second mutation Comparison of two target enrichment approaches	
Sequencing protocol				
Regions analyzed	All *CFTR* exons and 20bp of all intron/splice sites (10 343bp)	All *CFTR* locus (208kb → 181kb after masking repetitive DNA elements)	All *CFTR* locus (250kb) 2.1million probes (60-90pb)	36 overlapping fragments (7.3-14.5kb)
Target enrichment	Custom AmpliSeq panel (Life technologies)	Hybrid capture: Custom NimbleGen SeqCap EZ	Hybrid capture: Custom NimbleGen SeqCap EZ	Long-Range -PCR (LR-PCR) enrichment
Initial DNA quantity per sample	20ng		500ng	750ng
Library preparation	2 separate primer pools (2x36 amplicons), end-repair, ligation to adaptators, quantification of Library pooled bar-coded libraries Clonal PCR	Sonication (Covaris End-repair, A-tailing, ligation to index adaptators (TrueSeq protocol CR), PCR amplification, quantification of Library (bioanalyzer), in-solution hybridization	Nebulization; End-repair, ligation to adaptators, quantification of Library, Clonal emulsion PCR	Nebulization; LR-PCREnd-repair, phosphorylation, ligation to MID adaptators, quantification of Library, Clonal emulsion PCR
Sample Multiplexing and cost	5 to 35 samples	8 to 24 samples	No multiplexing	4 samples
NGS technology	200bp single reads Ion 314TM (10Mb) or Ion 318 (1Gb) Ion torrent Personal Genome Machine (PGM)	2x100bp paired-end reads HiSeq 2000 instrument (Illumina)	Single or Paired-end reads, up to 450 bp GS Junior Sequencer (454 Life Sciences)	

	Abou Tayoun et al., 2013 [25]	Trujillano et al., 2014 [26]	Bonini et al., 2015 [17]	
Mapping	Human genome	Human genome (GATK pipeline and picard-tools)	Human Genome (454 Roche GS Junior data analysis pipeline)	Chromosome 7 (454 Roche GS Junior data analysis pipeline)
Minimal coverage		Mean: 231X 99,7% covered by minimum 5 reads	40X	
CFTR Sequencing statistics				
Specificity	97% (22 on 23 mutations)	100%	ND	
Sensitivity	100% (23 on 23 mutations)	100% (122 on 122 variants)	ND	
Reproducibility	100% (56 on 56 variants in 3 independent runs)	100% (8 on 8 variants)	ND	
Bioinformatics tools				
CNV	Depth-Of-Coverage tool from the Genome Analysis ToolKit (GATK) --> Log2 ratios < -0.7: deletion	Pindel; Conifer; PeSV-Fisher 5 large deletions, 1 duplication and 1 genomic rearrangement	ND	
SNV	7 variants per sample on average	115 SNV + 28 InDels on average per sample	197 variants on average per sample (118 in introns)	
Variant identification and calling	Not notified	Variant prediction tools: GATK Unified Genotyper, samtools mpileup, SHORE	Reference Mapper Mutalyzer SeqNext (JSI medical systems)	
Variant filter	Min coverage: 20 reads Threshold: 25% reads Both strands	GATK Variant filtration (MQ<30.0; QUAL<25.0; QD<4.0; DP<5; DP<2000; GQ<15) GATK Combine Variant	Threshold 30% of reads Heterozygous: Read support: 30-65% Homozygous >70%	
Databases	Variant frequency > 1% dbSNP Exome Variant Server CFMDB CFTR2	1000 Genomes project dbSNP Exome Variant Server CFMDB CFTR2	1000 Genomes project dbSNP	
In silico analysis	SIFT Mutation Taster	Annovar SIFT, PolyPhen2, PhyloP, Mutation Taster, phastCons UCSC Genome Browser	Annovar, HSF, MaxEnt, NNSplice, SIFT, Polyphen2, PhyloP, UCSC Genome Browser, Ensembl, MutationTaster	
Performance				
Diagnostic rate	ND	98.91%	88.9% (16 / 18)	
Particular cases	False positive c.2052del (2184delA) Sanger sequencing to determine the c. 1210-34TG(11-13)T(5-9) haplotype	In-house script to determine the c. 1210-34TG(11-13)T(5-9) haplotype	False positive c.2052del (2184delA) Sanger sequencing to determine the c. 1210-34TG(11-13);-12T(5-9) haplotype	
Advantages	Robust, specific, limited number of VUCs	Breakpoints of large genomic rearrangement accurately determined	LR-PCR more adapted for complete gene resequencing New intronic mutations identified	
Limits	SINE/LINE repeats (amplification and mapping) Homopolymer stretches (Sequencing)	GC rich genomic segments (target enrichment) Errors in index tags (sequencing)	SINE/LINE repeats (amplification and mapping) Homopolymer stretches (Sequencing) Uncaptured region in intron 3	

Table 4. Comparison of three NGS strategies for *CFTR* sequencing

2.3. Other loci

With the perspectives of high throughput molecular diagnosis in genetics laboratories, CF, CFTR-RDs and CF-like diseases could be simultaneously explored in patients using NGS. Various gene panels could be investigated according to patients' phenotypes. Therefore, NGS approaches could contribute to (i) identify and confirm the implication of modifiers genes and (ii) improve molecular diagnosis of atypical Cystic Fibrosis, CFTR-RDs or CF-like diseases. Several sequence changes located in the so-called 'modifier genes' have been associated with progression of lung disease in CF patients. A decrease of pulmonary function measured by FEV1 (the forced expired volume after 1 s of blowing out) was associated with SNVs in *EDNRA, ACER, IFRD1, IL8, MUC5AC* and *TGF-β1* genes. Haplotype 8.1 and variants in MBL2 gene were related to *Pseudomonas aeruginosa* colonization [28, 29]. SNVs in *SNAP23, PPP2R4, PPP2R1A and KRT19* were recently associated with a decrease of lung function. Interactions between CFTR and these altered proteins may modify CFTR trafficking and membrane stability and therefore modify phenotype of CF patients [30]. Moreover, changes in other modifier genes were suspected to have an effect on intestinal obstruction (*DCTN4, ADIPOR2* and *MSRA* genes), CF-associated diabetes (*TCF7L2* gene) or liver disease (*SERPIN1A1*) [31].

CFTR-Related disorders comprise congenital bilateral absence of vas deferens (CBAVD), pancreatitis, diffuse bronchiectasis and nasal polyposis. Classically, two *CFTR* mutations (a severe and a mild mutation or two mild mutations) are found in well-characterized CBAVD patients [32]. In addition, Sharma *et al*. reported 2 SNVs on *TGF-β1* and *ENDRA* genes associated with urogenital anomalies [33]. Chronic pancreatitis is caused by *CFTR* variations in some cases, and mutations in *CTRC, PRSS1, PRSS2* or *SPINK1* are also involved and must be analysed.

The implication of *CFTR* in diffuse bronchiectasis or nasal polyposis is more controversial [34]; variants in other genes were previously reported as possibly causative. However, the identification of mutations in other genes with sufficient significance remains difficult and needs large patient cohorts. In fact, in airway tract diseases, the influence of environment (pollutants, drugs/therapy and way of life) complicated the achievement of unbiased studies. Nevertheless, the hypothesis of oligogenism is supported by a study that reported mutations in ENaC channel genes (*SCNN1A, SCNN1B, SCNN1G*) or *SERPIN1A1* in CF-like patients (borderline sweat-test and suggestive CF clinical features without two *CFTR* mutations) [35].

Finally, a pleiotropic effect of *SLC26A9* on meconium ileus, pancreatic damage and lung disease has been identified [36], as well as *SLC9A3* for meconium ileus and lung disease and *SLC6A14* for meconium ileus and both lung disease and age at first *P. aeruginosa* infection [37]. Thus, the existence of pleiotropic effect of modifier genes on CF evolution may encourage the development of new therapeutic targets with multi-organ benefits.

3. Functional characterization of *CFTR* sequence variations

To provide appropriate diagnosis and prognosis to CF patients and also appropriate genetic counselling to families, the impact of variants identified by the techniques detailed above has to be functionally characterized.

Some variants such as frequent mutations (found in more than 1% of CF mutated alleles), nonsense or frameshift mutations are readily classified as pathogenic mutations. However, the frequent identification of rare sequence alterations of unknown pathogenicity (VUCS, VUS) substantially complicates test interpretation. Moreover, their number will increase with the diffusion of NGS technologies. To facilitate classification of these variants, CF laboratories have to combine several tools like central mutation databases or *CFTR* locus specific databases, *in silico* prediction tools and *ex vivo/in vivo* functional analyses [38, 39].

3.1. Epidemiological data and locus specific databases dedicated to *CFTR*

3.1.1. Core or central mutation databases

Their goal is to collect all sequence variations detected in all genes and to describe each mutation briefly. These databases are used to assess the frequency of a variation (minor allele frequency (MAF) lower or higher than 1%) in the general population (i.e. unaffected individuals). Since a MAF higher than 1% reflects a low probability for the variant to be pathogenic, such data may be highly informative for the interpretation of variants.

3.1.1.1. The National Center for Biotechnology Information (NCBI) short genetic variations database dbSNP

dbSNP [25] is the most comprehensive directory of single nucleotide variations. It catalogues short variations in nucleotide sequences from a wide range of organisms. Genetic Variations may be common, thus representing true polymorphisms, or they may be rare. Some of these rare human entries have additional information associated with them, including disease associations, genotype information and allele origin, as some variations are somatic rather than germ-line events. Genotypes and allele frequencies information for various populations from different studies, including data form the HapMap project, are also available.

3.1.1.2. Databases specifically collecting data from NGS projects

1000Genomes [24] aimed to find most genetic variants that have frequencies of at least 1% in samples from five populations: East Asian, South Asian, African, European and American ancestries. As in dbSNP, genotypes and allele frequencies information are available for a large number of variants [40].

Exome Variant Server [41] is a database that collects data of the NHLBI GO Exome Sequencing Project (ESP). This project aimed to discover novel genes and mechanisms contributing to various disorders by sequencing the protein coding regions of the human genome (i.e. exome) using NGS technology. As the *CFTR* gene is widely studied, this tool would not be of added value compared to dbSNP and 1000 Genomes.

3.1.2. Locus Specific Databases (LSDBs) dedicated to CFTR

LSDBs are now recognized as the best mode of collecting and curating lists of mutations related to human genetic diseases [42]. They compile in a single bioinformatics tool disease-causing and non-disease-causing sequence variations identified by genetics laboratories in families with a history of a given Mendelian disease. The most sophisticated ones integrate clinical and biological data, information on the geographic and/or ethnic origin, frequency of variations in the general population, mutation hot spots and all useful information for diagnosis, prognosis and the evaluation of genotype/phenotype relationships [43].

Here we choose to detail three LSDB dedicated to *CFTR* that provide complementary information for the interpretation and the characterization of variants identified in diagnostics practice.

3.1.2.1. Cystic fibrosis mutation database

The Cystic Fibrosis Mutation Database (CFMDB) [44] also called 'CFTR1' is an open access database dedicated to the collection of sequence variations in the *CFTR* gene for the international CF genetics research community. It was initiated by the Cystic Fibrosis Genetic Analysis Consortium (CFGAC) in 1989 and is maintained by the Cystic Fibrosis Centre at the Hospital for Sick Children in Toronto. CFMDB allows the direct submission of new variants by laboratories, by filling out an on- line standardized form with the possibility to detail phenotypic data, genotype (i.e. other variants identified in patient) or epidemiological data. The key point of this database is to collect the largest number of *CFTR* sequence variations identified in patients, relatives and partners. On the other side, because the submission procedure applies only to the initial report of each variant, CFMDB does not provide frequency data, available with the two other databases described below. Finally, contributors do not always follow HGVS recommendations and a same variant can be reported by several laboratories under different names, possibly leading to misinterpretation or misreporting in diagnosis reports.

3.1.2.2. Clinical and functional translation of CFTR database CFTR2

CFTR2 [45] is a website designed to provide information about specific CF mutations to patients, researchers and the general public. For each mutation included in the database, it provides information about whether a given mutation causes cystic fibrosis when combined with another CF-causing mutation and clinical and biological information (sweat chloride, lung function, pancreatic status and pseudomonas infection rates) in patients carrying the mutation. A specific section for health practitioners and scientists provides more in-depth and research-related information.

The goal of the CFTR2 project is to categorize all mutations seen in CF patients as disease-causing (always resulting in CF when combined with another CF-causing mutation), neutral or mutation of varying clinical consequences (CF and CFTR-RD). Mutations that have not been fully analysed are considered of unknown clinical significance.

The major advantages of CFTR2 are (i) the collection of detailed clinical characteristics on large cohorts of individuals [46] that provide useful information related to a given genotype, and (ii) results of functional testing that are key arguments for their final interpretation [47].

However, this database only collects clinical and genetic data of CF patients (from national registers) that can lead to a bias of phenotypic spectrum assessment of several mutations considered as CF-causing mutations while they were also reported in CFTR-RD patients in *trans* of other CF-causing mutations.

3.1.2.3. The French molecular database CFTR-France

CFTR-France [48] has been developed since 2012 with the aim to collect, store and process any category of variants identified in the *CFTR* gene, thanks to the collaboration of nine French laboratories with high expertise in the molecular analyses of this gene. Its specificity is to compile and annotate any category of variations (disease-causing, non-disease-causing and variants of unknown clinical significance) that have been identified by collaborators in patients affected with CF or CFTR-RD, in foetuses with abnormal ultrasonography (e.g. echogenic bowel), newborns with pending or inconclusive diagnosis and asymptomatic individuals carrying at least one sequence variation on each CFTR gene (i.e. carrying two variations in *trans*). The database includes the main clinical data of these individuals, genetic information from familial segregation studies and various variant annotations (frequency in patients and controls populations, sequence homology, predicted or experimentally assessed functional impact, etc.), allowing the analysis of genotype/phenotype relationships.

Thus, *CFTR*-France, by collecting all phenotypes, reflects the phenotypic spectrum of a large number of mutations. It also reports mutations in complex alleles with association frequencies (related to all individuals recorded in the database), and gives the up-to-date HGVS nomenclature of mutations.

Data collected in *CFTR*-France are provided by level 2 (specialised) and reference laboratories, so that patients analysed only by level 1 laboratories (searching for the most common mutations) are not included in the database.

Note: Access to *CFTR*-France is currently restricted to collaborators. A public access program is in progress for the medical and scientific community and for patients and families.

3.2. *In silico* prediction analyses

3.2.1. Variants located in exons and exon-intron boundaries

3.2.1.1. Prediction tools for the assessment of the impact on protein

Prediction methods of amino acid substitutions use protein sequence, structure and/or annotation. Disease-causing mutations that affect protein function tend to occur at evolutionarily conserved sites and/or at key positions in protein structure. Multiple sequence alignment of orthologous sequences reveal what positions have been conserved through evolution, and these positions are supposed to be important for protein function. Annotation can enhance prediction for variants located in structurally and functionally important domains, but this information is often sparse.

The issue of the efficiency of prediction tools in assessing possible pathogenicity of missense variants in the *CFTR* gene is of major interest, since they constitute the vast majority of VUS identified in patients. Diagnostics laboratories frequently use those tools and particularly in problematic situations. Unfortunately their performance has not been clearly established and results (i.e. score of pathogenicity) may be discordant for a given variant.

Predictions of the impact of non-synonymous substitutions in CFTR are mainly based on multiple sequence alignment of orthologous sequences. Indeed, even if a partial 3D model of the CFTR protein has been established [49, 50], prediction tools do not take into account these elements in the final 'score of pathogenicity'. It is classically recommended to use several prediction tools to obtain concordant predictions that could be considered for variant interpretation.

Table 5 summarizes bioinformatics programs classically used by diagnostics laboratories [51-53] and the new software SuSPect [54].

Method and Web site	Algorithm	Output
PolyPhen 2 [54]	Sequence conservation, structure to model position of amino acid substitution, and SWISS-PROT annotation	Score ranges from 0 to a positive number, where 0 is neutral, and a high positive number is damaging
SIFT [55]	Sequence homology: scores are calculated using position-specific scoring matrices with Dirichlet priors	Score ranges from 0 to 1, where 0 is damaging and 1 is neutral
Align GVGD [56]	Multiple sequence alignments to characterise the biochemical properties (composition, polarity and volume) of the observed amino acids at each position	The prediction classes form a spectrum (C0, C15, C25, C35, C45, C55, C65) with C65 most likely to interfere with function and C0 least likely.
SuSPect [57]	Sequence-, structure*- and systems biology-based features to predict the phenotypic effects of missense mutations. Algorithm trained using VariBench (contains information for experimentally verified effects) **Structure-based comparison with other ABC transporters*	Table of scores from 0-100, colour-coded according to predicted deleteriousness (blue=neutral, red=disease-causing). A score of 50 is recommended as a cut-off between neutral and disease-causing variants
Alamut© [58] Commercial software (Interactive Biosoftware)	Databases: RefSeq, dbSNP, Uniprot, InterPro, UCSC Genome Browser Database, PubMed, Ensembl. And Automated access to on-line prediction tools: PolyPhen2, SIFT, Align GVGD Access to splicing prediction tools (detailed in Section III.2.1.2.) **"Alamut Batch"** **High-throughput annotation software for NGS analysis**	Summarized report of the results of different prediction tools, according to their output format **Designed for intensive variant analysis workflows**

Table 5. Bioinformatics tools for the prediction of amino acid changes: websites, characteristics and output format [55-59]

A recent work has emphasised the importance of sequence alignments on the performance of prediction tools [60]. The authors constructed custom multiple sequence alignments called phenotype-optimized sequence ensembles (POSEs) that was tested on a training set of *CFTR* mutations.

A previous work already suggested that providing SIFT or PolyPhen-2 with custom alignments increased their performance relative to the default alignments employed by the algorithms [61]. This could explain that, if Alamut© is a highly interesting tool with its ease of use, some predictions obtained by using each tool separately with a custom algorithm could differ from Alamut© results (obtained with default alignments).

3.2.1.2. Prediction tools for the assessment of the impact on pre-mRNA splicing

Splicing mechanisms comprise exon recognition within large pre-mRNA molecules and the precise removal of flanking introns. Three elements constitute the core splicing signals: the intronic branch point, the acceptor site (or 3'splice site), including an inconstant upstream polypyrimidine tract (PPT), and the donor site (or 5' splice site). These core human splice site motifs contain only a part of the information that defines exons, whereas the rest corresponds to less conserved splicing regulatory elements. The latter are located within the exon or flanking introns, promoting or inhibiting exon recognition through exonic/intronic splicing enhancers (ESE or ISE) or silencers (ESS or ISS), respectively (Figure 3).

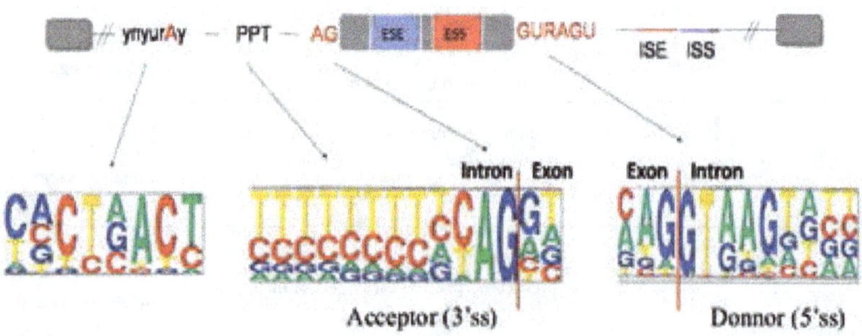

Figure 3. A schematic of key splicing motifs and regulatory elements. Adapted by Le Guédard-Méreuze S. from Wang and Burge, 2008 [62, 63].

Many bioinformatics tools have been developed to predict which splicing modification is the most probable for a given sequence variation — exon skipping, cryptic splice sites activation, use of *de novo* splice sites — or if the variant may be considered as neutral regarding its impact on splicing. Most algorithms were developed based on biostatistical and experimental analyses of information contained in the genomic sequence. They provide a score depending on the strength of the considered splice site. Indeed, the strength of splicing motifs is a key parameter to predict the impact of a sequence variation. Performance of these tools has been widely studied by comparing the results of predictions with experimental assays for various genes including *CFTR* [39, 63-66]. In 2012, Houdayer and collaborators performed a large-scale study of VUCS in BRCA genes in order to assess the performance of six prediction tools [67]. This work provided guidelines for the proper use of these tools and for the interpretation of prediction results.

Table 6 summarizes principle and main characteristics of the most 'popular' bioinformatics programs and ASSEDA, a recently developed program [68-73].

Method and Web site	Algorithm	Output
MaxEntScan [72]	Based on a Maximum Entropy Model (MEM): Modelling the sequences of short sequence motifs such as those involved in RNA splicing which simultaneously accounts for non-adjacent as well as adjacent dependencies between positions.	
Human Splicing Finder (HSF) [73] Associates weight matrix model (WMM) and Maximum Entropy Model (MEM)	**Consensus splice sites**	
	HSF (WMM): Quantification of the relative likelihood of candidate splice site sequence to show coincidence with consensus sequence	Numerical Score (0-100)
	MaxEnt (MEM): Statistical approach representing the least biased approximation for the distribution of sequence motifs, from available data (real and decoy splice sites). Incorporates local adjacent and non-adjacent position dependencies	Numerical Score (0-10)
	cis-regulatory elements	
	ESEfinder* RESCUE-ESE* Predicted PESE AND PESS Octamers from Zhang & Chasin *See Prediction tools for *cis*-regulatory elements	See Prediction tools for *cis*-regulatory elements
NNSplice [74]	Machine learning approach that recognizes sequence patterns once it is trained with sets of DNA sequences encompassing authentic and decoy splice sites. Based on a hidden Markov Model (HMM): Incorporates local adjacent position dependencies	Score between 0 and 1
Automated Splice Site and Exon Definition Analysis (ASSEDA) [75] *Restricted access: registration required*	Analyses splicing mutations according to changes in total exon information: information content of a spliced exon from the cumulative contributions of sequences recognized by the spliceosomal machinery and the distribution distances separating binding sites within the same exon.	$\Delta Ri_{,total}$ values (differences in probability of relative inclusion or exclusion of the wild type and mutated exon in mature mRNA)
Prediction tools for cis-regulatory elements		
ESEfinder [76]	Prediction of SR protein specific putative ESE, based on an in vitro SELEX approach dependent on addition of individual SR proteins	ESE motif score
RESCUE-ESE [77] (Relative enhancer and silencer classification by unanimous enrichment)	Statistical approach based upon different distribution of hexamers in exons and introns with different properties (e.g. weak and strong splice sites)	Z-score (Highlights extremely over- or under-represented hexamers)

Table 6. Main characteristics of several Splicing prediction tools [74-79]

It is important to note that consequences on splicing of exonic synonymous and non-synonymous *CFTR* variants must be assessed, as suggested by recent of experimental studies [39, 80].

3.2.2. *Deep intronic variants*

The examples of insertion of intronic sequences called pseudo-exons (or cryptic exons) in mature transcripts of various genes are becoming ever more numerous and their role in human diseases has been largely demonstrated. We saw in section 2.2 that NGS strategies currently allow scanning of *CFTR* deep intronic regions [18], resulting in a growing number of new identified deep intronic variants.

Bioinformatics tools described above, which assess the impact of variants on splicing, can also be used to evaluate deep intronic mutations. We tested these algorithms on mutations identified in CF patients after NGS sequencing of the entire *CFTR* locus and they showed satisfactory results [18]. Indeed, prediction tools allowed the selection of possible disease-causing mutations (i.e. predicted impact on splicing by inclusion of pseudo-exons) and predictions were confirmed by *in vitro* functional studies using minigene constructs (see section 3.3.1.1) and by direct analysis of aberrant transcripts from nasal epithelial cells of patients (see 3.3.2.1).

3.3. *In vitro/ex vivo* functional analyses

3.3.1. *Cell lines transfection experiments*

The type of cells used for transfection depends on the tissue that is studied and the clinical context. Pulmonary (BEAS-2B, A549, Calu-3) or intestinal/colic (CACO-2, T84) immortalized cells (by SV40 or carcinoma) contain an appropriate concentration of transcriptional and splicing factors for CFTR protein synthesis. Cells stably transfected with mutated *CFTR* can also be used (CFBe41o-, CFPAC-1). Stable expression is usually obtained by lentivirus transduction and transient transfection by chemical agent (Polyfect, interferin). In this case, the endogenous CF molecular and cellular context (inflammation) should also be considered.

3.3.1.1. *Splicing assessment*

Minigenes are autonomic cyclic entity containing promoter and exons and are produced by clonal amplification in bacteria [81, 82]. They contain a genomic segment from the gene of interest (here *CFTR*) that includes exon and flanking intronic regions (length can range from ten to thousands of nucleotides, an average of 300 bp) or only intronic regions in the case of evaluation of potential creation of a pseudo-exon. To determine whether a mutation is responsible for altered splicing, minigenes can also include *cis*-regulatory elements if affected (ESE, ESS, ISE or/and ISS) [83]. These regions of interest are framed by two invariable exons, which are part of the system. Every assay of transfection in cell lines compares the wild-type and mutated (through directed mutagenesis) constructs [84]. All *CFTR* exons are needed to produce a mature and functional protein. Thus, a modification of transcript in the *in vitro* system suggests that the assessed *CFTR* change has a deleterious effect on exon splicing. An ever-increasing number of mini-gene studies have been performed to assess the pathogenicity of *CFTR* variants [39, 60, 80, 84]. This strategy, despite its limitations, is of high interest in the overall strategy for the characterization of rare sequence variations.

3.3.1.2. Expression vectors for the quantification of mRNA, protein or CFTR-specific chloride conductance

Full-length *CFTR* cDNA is classically inserted in expression vector system (e.g. pcDNA3 or p-Tracer) upon a promoter that may be drug-activated (G418, tetracycline or doxycycline-activation). To assess point variants or small indels, directed mutagenesis is carried out (usually QuikChange Mutagenesis kits®, Agilent Technologies). To assess molecular consequences of large rearrangements concerning one or more exons, a truncated *CFTR* cDNA can be inserted in the expression vector [85-87]. Transient or stable transfection can be performed in eukaryotic cells (describe in III.3.1. section). 3-HA tag (in the fourth loop of *CFTR*) can be introduced to easily visualize protein expression. Then, measurement of mRNA expression and evaluation of function and localization of the CFTR protein can be performed for each alternative transcript construct, compared to wild-type.

Automated real-time RT-PCR allows the relative straightforward quantification of mRNA transcripts with specific primers and appropriate reference genes for normalization. mRNA level informs about future protein quality and quantity.

Protein assessment consists in the implementation of complementary experiments for protein quantification, evaluation of its maturation or its cellular localization. Main techniques are detailed below. The effect of variants on CFTR expression and maturation is assessed based on the detection of immature (core-glycosylated, B band, ~150-kD) and/or mature (additional glycosylation in the Golgi, C band ~170-190 kDa) CFTR forms by immunoblotting. Long-term pulse-chase experiments can provide additional information on the lifetime of CFTR on cellular compartments [88]. Immunocytochemical assays (Immunofluorescence (IF) based) can highlight the cellular localization of the CFTR protein. However, most difficulties noted in IF experiments relate to non-specific antibody staining and the effect of sample processing on characteristics of cell development. Moreover, confusion between cell surface (where CFTR is active) and subsurface (where it would not) may occur. Therefore, more sensitive and specific antibodies as well as co-localization assays with other cell surface markers (such as β-tubulin or WGA) are needed. Finally, this remains a qualitative or semi-quantitative method.

CFTR function and activity, i.e. CFTR-specific chloride conductance, can be determined by patch-clamp electrophysiology, halide selective electrode technique, radioisotope efflux assays and by fluorescence-based halide efflux measurement. The use of a CFTR-activating appropriate drug (such as forskolin, isobutylmethylxanthine (IBMX), isoproterenol, terbutaline, genistein, adenosine, etc.) or ATP followed by specific CFTR inhibitor CFTRinh-172 permits CFTR-dependant or independent chloride transport, respectively. To date, the easiest approach developed consists in Iodide efflux based on fluorescence measurement. YFP fluorescence is dependent on YFP expression levels and iodide concentration. Compared with conventional plate-bound CFTR functional assays, the flow cytometric approach can be used to study CFTR function in cell suspension. It may be further adjusted to study CFTR function in heterologous cell populations using cell surface markers and selection of cells that display high CFTR function. Technical limitations include the need to perform this assay in specialized centres (using expensive imaging equipment).

All these methods offer the possibility to evaluate the functional consequences of molecular abnormalities on CFTR and finally improve the classification of variants.

3.3.2. *Ex vivo CF patients' cells assays*

3.3.2.1. *Analyses on primary airway cells and tissues*

Characterization of *CFTR* molecular defect can partially be performed directly after biopsies of tissues that show sufficient CFTR expression. Nasal or lung airway epitheliums are optimal. These tissues are accessible by minimally invasive interventions and display an endogenous expression of CFTR transcripts and protein. Moreover, nasal and bronchial epitheliums show the same cellular composition (ciliated, goblet, columnar and immune cells) although ratios differ slightly [89]. Since quantification and detection of aberrant splicing and quantification or localization of proteins are possible in human tissues, information that they bring is crucial to assess the effect of variants and to propose a functional classification. However, this approach has its limitations and requires other functional assays to perform large-scale genotype–phenotype correlation studies. In addition, especially for nasal tissue, the low quantity of cells collected (out of 500.000 cells per brushing) only allows 'one-shot' tests and hinders mechanistic assays. Moreover, highly variable CFTR expression in heterogeneous cell types, in healthy individuals and in p.Phe508del homozygous patients has been described, varying from 0 to 100% [90]. Other genetic (see below) or environmental parameters could also modify CFTR expression levels.

3.3.2.2. *Ex vivo culture of primary airway cells*

Culture of primary cells from CF patients can be performed with brushed nasal or bronchial cells after biopsies. Wild-type endogenous CFTR protein is expressed at the apical membrane of polarized cells. Therefore, *in vitro* monolayer culture seems no longer adapted. Obtaining polarized cells is promoted by air–liquid interface culture (ALI), proposed since the 2000s, by an *ex vivo* system of collagen-coated porous membrane on which cells are platted after a phase of monolayer amplification or directly after nasal brushing. Basal adherent cells differentiate in all airways epithelial cell types, which organize into a pseudo-stratified epithelium [91].

This model offers the opportunity to perform functional assays described above to determine CFTR dysfunction. Molecular defect induced by a specific mutation can be qualitatively determined if the cell donor is homozygous for this mutation.

Technical limitations such as bacterial or fungi contaminations or absence of adherence complicate culture of cells obtained from CF patients. Moreover, further studies are needed to determine if extrapolation is possible between observations in primary cells directly after brushing and after several weeks in culture media, particularly for quantitative level assessment.

3.3.2.3. Intestinal current measurement (ICM)

ICM was developed as a research tool to assess CFTR function in the 1990s and has been used as a diagnostic test since the early 2000s [92, 93]. At least four superficial rectal biopsies per patient, obtained by suction, are needed and mounted on adequate tissue sliders. ICM consists in blocking epithelial sodium channels by amiloride and stimulates cAMP-mediated CFTR-depending chloride transport in a chloride-free solution with forskolin or IBMX. Cholinergic chloride transport and histaminic reaction were also evaluated and the sum of the response $\Delta Isc_{forskolin/IBMX+carbachol+histamine}$ appears to be the best parameter to evaluate CFTR function by ICM, but reference values and ranges have not been established. This combination of ionic responses discriminates patients with CF from healthy subjects but not CF patients with pancreatic insufficiency (PI) or sufficiency (PS). ICM can detect a loss of CFTR function above 80%, therefore CF carriers and CFTR-RD patients may not be identified by this method. Moreover, mild mutations could result in a false-negative ICM.

ICM is not altered by secondary damage on tissue and thus better reveals the primary CFTR dysfunction (compared with nasal potential difference, see below). A new functional CFTR assay using primary CF intestinal organoïds derived from patients and cultured *in vitro* may offer new tools to screen for therapy [94].

Finally, setup and maintenance of dedicated equipment by experienced and trained staff limits its use.

3.3.3. In vivo biomarkers assays of CFTR function

Sweat chloride Test (ST) and Nasal potential difference (NPD) measurement are used as diagnostic tests for CF. In atypical clinical context these *in vivo* tests can give additional arguments to further explore the *CFTR* locus (cf. Figure 2 that describes the molecular diagnostics step-by-step strategy). Furthermore, they provide complementary information for the interpretation of *CFTR* variations.

ST higher than 60 mmol/L is the 'gold standard' and discriminates between healthy and typical CF. Sweat electrolytes are higher in the most severely affected and are lower in those with mild mutation, who have partial rescue of channel function [95-97]. There are two major advantages for the use of sweat test in the evaluation of the *CFTR* mutation severity: (i) stability of the measure throughout life and (ii) non-invasive way of measurement which maintains skin integrity. Indeed, sweat electrolytes levels reflect the primary defect on the CFTR protein and do not highlight secondary consequences of its absence or dysfunction on affected organs. Furthermore, a new means for assessing the secretory function of CFTR has been recently developed based on β-adrenergic-mediated sweating. This method provides a unique evaluation of the purely secretory function of CFTR *in vivo*. It has been shown to be more sensitive in individuals carrying mutations that commonly exhibit normal or borderline sweat chloride rates, such as c.3718-2477C>T (legacy name: 3849+10kbC>T) [98].

The transepithelial NPD measurement estimates the net ion conductance across the nasal airway epithelium and indirectly measure CFTR activity. Sodium conductance is determined after amiloride perfusion (Na+). NPD parameters discriminate CF and CFTR-RD phenotypes and a correlation between NPD and disease severity has been shown [99], although there is an overlap in subjects with mild phenotype [97]. However, other sources of phenotypic variability (modifiers genes or environment) and technical limitations (i.e. maintenance of dedicated equipment and trained personnel) contribute to the inconsistencies of NPD across genotype-phenotype correlation studies. CFTR expression and NPD response can also be modified if nasal epithelium is affected by rhinosinusitis, polyposis or exposure to smoking [100]. However, despite the difficulty of setting up this technique, NPD assessment could be used as a complementary step to support CFTR dysfunction in inconclusive clinical cases and then to confirm the deleterious effect of *CFTR* variants identified in these patients.

4. Conclusion

New issues are emerging from the use of NGS technology in CF molecular diagnosis. On one hand, NGS approaches offer new possibilities by multiplexing samples and provide a wider coverage of the *CFTR* locus including deep intronic regions. NGS assay design can also include additional modifiers genes [31]. On the other hand, molecular diagnoses in emergency contexts challenge the possibility of sample multiplexing, and the increased number of VUCS will require complex functional analyses. However, as tools described above are constantly improving, the knowledge about *CFTR* variations is rapidly expanding, allowing geneticists and clinicians to provide patients with high quality information and adequate genetic counselling. Finally, the functional characterization of CFTR variations will provide rationale for a personalised medicine strategy driven by patients' genotype in the very near future.

Acknowledgements

We acknowledge all members of the technical team for CF molecular diagnosis: Jean-Pierre Altieri, Fanny Verneau and Lise Larrieu. We also thank the coordination team of the *CFTR*-France genetic database: Corinne Bareil and Corinne Thèze and all the collaborating members of this project. We are also grateful to the French Network of laboratories specialized in molecular diagnosis of CF (GenMucoFrance). Finally, we thank the French Association against CF (Vaincre la Mucoviscidose) for its constant support.

Author details

Anne Bergougnoux[1*], Magali Taulan-Cadars[2], Mireille Claustres[2] and Caroline Raynal[1]

*Address all correspondence to: anne.bergougnoux@inserm.fr

1 Laboratory of Molecular Genetics, Montpellier Hospital, France

2 Montpellier University, France

References

[1] Riordan JR, Rommens JM, Kerem B, Alon N, Rozmahel R, Grzelczak Z, Zielenski J, Lok S, Plavsic N, Chou JL, et al. Identification of the cystic fibrosis gene: cloning and characterization of complementary DNA. Science. 1989 Sep 8;245(4922):1066-73. Erratum in: Science 1989 Sep 29;245(4925):1437.

[2] Casals T, Ramos MD, Giménez J, Larriba S, Nunes V, Estivill X. High heterogeneity for cystic fibrosis in Spanish families: 75 mutations account for 90% of chromosomes. Hum Genet. 1997 Dec;101(3):365-70.

[3] Tsui LC. The spectrum of cystic fibrosis mutations. Trends Genet. 1992 Nov;8(11): 392-8.

[4] Welsh MJ, Smith AE. Molecular mechanisms of CFTR chloride channel dysfunction in cystic fibrosis. Cell. 1993 Jul 2;73(7):1251-4. Review.

[5] Quintana-Gallego E, Delgado-Pecellín I, Calero Acuña C. CFTR protein repair therapy in cystic fibrosis. Arch Bronconeumol. 2014 Apr;50(4):146-50. doi: 10.1016/j.arbres. 2013.07.013. [Article in English, Spanish].

[6] Castellani C, Cuppens H, Macek M Jr, Cassiman JJ, Kerem E, Durie P, Tullis E, Assael BM, Bombieri C, Brown A, Casals T, Claustres M, Cutting GR, Dequeker E, Dodge J, Doull I, Farrell P, Ferec C, Girodon E, Johannesson M, Kerem B, Knowles M, Munck A, Pignatti PF, Radojkovic D, Rizzotti P, Schwarz M, Stuhrmann M, Tzetis M, Zielenski J, Elborn JS. Consensus on the use and interpretation of cystic fibrosis mutation analysis in clinical practice. J Cyst Fibros. 2008 May;7(3):179-96. doi: 10.1016/ j.jcf.2008.03.009. Review.

[7] Dequeker E, Stuhrmann M, Morris MA, Casals T, Castellani C, Claustres M, Cuppens H, des Georges M, Ferec C, Macek M, Pignatti PF, Scheffer H, Schwartz M, Witt M, Schwarz M, Girodon E. Best practice guidelines for molecular genetic diagnosis of cystic fibrosis and CFTR-related disorders--updated European recommendations. Eur J Hum Genet. 2009 Jan;17(1):51-65. doi: 10.1038/ejhg.2008.136.

[8] World Health Organisation Report "The molecular genetic epidemiology of cystic fibrosis". Available on: http://www.who.int/genomics/publications/en/ HGN_WB_04.02_report.pdf [Accessed: 2015-02-07]

[9] Abeliovich D, Lavon IP, Lerer I, Cohen T, Springer C, Avital A, Cutting GR. Screening for five mutations detects 97% of cystic fibrosis (CF) chromosomes and predicts a

carrier frequency of 1:29 in the Jewish Ashkenazi population. Am J Hum Genet. 1992 Nov;51(5):951-6.

[10] Chillón M, Dörk T, Casals T, Giménez J, Fonknechten N, Will K, Ramos D, Nunes V, Estivill X. A novel donor splice site in intron 11 of the CFTR gene, created by mutation 1811+1.6kbA-->G, produces a new exon: high frequency in Spanish cystic fibrosis chromosomes and association with severe phenotype. Am J Hum Genet. 1995 Mar; 56(3):623-9.

[11] Costantino L, Claut L, Paracchini V, Coviello DA, Colombo C, Porcaro L, Capasso P, Zanardelli M, Pizzamiglio G, Degiorgio D, Seia M. A novel donor splice site characterized by CFTR mRNA analysis induces a new pseudo-exon in CF patients. J Cyst Fibros. 2010 Dec;9(6):411-8. doi: 10.1016/j.jcf.2010.08.009.

[12] Faà V, Incani F, Meloni A, Corda D, Masala M, Baffico AM, Seia M, Cao A, Rosatelli MC. Characterization of a disease-associated mutation affecting a putative splicing regulatory element in intron 6b of the cystic fibrosis transmembrane conductance regulator (CFTR) gene. J Biol Chem. 2009 Oct 30;284(44):30024-31. doi: 10.1074/jbc.M109.032623. Epub 2009 Sep 15.

[13] Bareil C, Guittard C, Altieri JP, Templin C, Claustres M, des Georges M. Comprehensive and rapid genotyping of mutations and haplotypes in congenital bilateral absence of the vas deferens and other cystic fibrosis transmembrane conductance regulator-related disorders. J Mol Diagn. 2007 Nov;9(5):582-8.

[14] Costantino L, Rusconi D, Claut L, Colombo C, Novara F, Paracchini V, Porcaro L, Capasso P, Zuffardi O, Seia M. A wide methodological approach to identify a large duplication in CFTR gene in a CF patient uncharacterised by sequencing analysis. J Cyst Fibros. 2011 Dec;10(6):412-7. doi: 10.1016/j.jcf.2011.06.007.

[15] Metzker ML. Sequencing technologies—the next generation Nat Rev Genet. 2010 Jan; 11:31-46.

[16] Bodi K, Perera AG, Adams PS, Bintzler D, Dewar K, Grove DS, Kieleczawa J, Lyons RH, Neubert TA, Noll AC, Singh S, Steen R, Zianni M. Comparison of commercially available target enrichment methods for next-generation sequencing. J Biomol Tech. 2013 Jul;24(2):73-86. doi: 10.7171/jbt.13-2402-002.

[17] Chilamakuri CS, Lorenz S, Madoui MA, Vodák D, Sun J, Hovig E, Myklebost O, Meza-Zepeda LA. Performance comparison of four exome capture systems for deep sequencing. BMC Genomics. 2014 Jun 9;15:449. doi: 10.1186/1471-2164-15-449.

[18] Bonini J, Varilh J, Raynal C, Thèze C, Beyne E, Audrezet MP, Ferec C, Bienvenu T, Girodon E, Tuffery-Giraud S, Des Georges M, Claustres M, Taulan-Cadars M. Small-scale high-throughput sequencing-based identification of new therapeutic tools in cystic fibrosis. Genet Med. 2015 Jan 8. doi: 10.1038/gim.2014.194.

[19] Tewhey R, et al. Microdroplet-based PCR enrichment for large-scale targeted sequencing. Nature Biotech. 2009;27:1025-31.

[20] Guo Y, Long J, He J, Li CI, Cai Q, Shu XO, Zheng W, Li C. Exome sequencing generates high quality data in non-target regions. BMC Genomics. 2012 May 20;13:194. doi: 10.1186/1471-2164-13-194.

[21] Li H, Handsaker B, Wysoker A, et al. The sequence alignment/map format and SAMtools. Bioinformatics. 2009;25:2078-9.

[22] McKenna A, Hanna M, Banks E, Sivachenko A, Cibulskis K, Kernytsky A, Garimella K, Altshuler D, Gabriel S, Daly M, DePristo MA. The genome analysis toolkit: a MapReduce framework for analyzing next-generation DNA sequencing data. Genome Res. 2010;20:1297-1303.

[23] Treangen TJ, Salzberg SL. Repetitive DNA and next-generation sequencing: computational challenges and solutions. Nat Rev Genet. 2011 Nov 29;13(1):36-46. doi: 10.1038/nrg3117.

[24] 1000 Genomes Project Database. Available on: http://www.1000genomes.org/ [Accessed: 2015-02-07]

[25] NCBI Short Genetic Variations Database. Available on: http://www.ncbi.nlm.nih.gov.gate2.inist.fr/projects/SNP/ [Accessed: 2015-02-07]

[26] Abou Tayoun AN, Tunkey CD, Pugh TJ, Ross T, Shah M, Lee CC, Harkins TT, Wells WA, Tafe LJ, Amos CI, Tsongalis GJ. A comprehensive assay for CFTR mutational analysis using next-generation sequencing. Clin Chem. 2013 Oct;59(10):1481-8. doi: 10.1373/clinchem.2013.206466.

[27] Trujillano D, Ramos MD, González J, Tornador C, Sotillo F, Escaramis G, Ossowski S, Armengol L, Casals T, Estivill X. Next generation diagnostics of cystic fibrosis and CFTR-related disorders by targeted multiplex high-coverage resequencing of CFTR. J Med Genet. 2013 Jul;50(7):455-62. doi: 10.1136/jmedgenet-2013-101602. Epub 2013 May 17.

[28] Guo X, Pace RG, Stonebraker JR, Commander CW, Dang AT, Drumm ML, Harris A, Zou F, Swallow DM, Wright FA, O'Neal WK, Knowles MR. Mucin variable number tandem repeat polymorphisms and severity of cystic fibrosis lung disease: significant association with MUC5AC. PLoS One. 2011;6(10):e25452. doi: 10.1371/journal.pone.0025452. Epub 2011 Oct 6.

[29] Guillot L, Beucher J, Tabary O, Le Rouzic P, Clement A, Corvol H. Lung disease modifier genes in cystic fibrosis. Int J Biochem Cell Biol. 2014 Jul;52:83-93. doi: 10.1016/j.biocel.2014.02.011.

[30] Gisler FM, von Kanel T, Kraemer R, Schaller A, Gallati S. Identification of SNPs in the cystic fibrosis interactome influencing pulmonary progression in cystic fibrosis. Eur J Hum Genet. 2013 Apr;21(4):397-403. doi: 10.1038/ejhg.2012.181.

[31] Cutting GR. Modifier genes in Mendelian disorders: the example of cystic fibrosis. Ann N Y Acad Sci. 2010 Dec;1214:57-69. doi: 10.1111/j.1749-6632.2010.05879.x. Review.

[32] Claustres M, Guittard C, Bozon D, Chevalier F, Verlingue C, Ferec C, Girodon E, Cazeneuve C, Bienvenu T, Lalau G, Dumur V, Feldmann D, Bieth E, Blayau M, Clavel C, Creveaux I, Malinge MC, Monnier N, Malzac P, Mittre H, Chomel JC, Bonnefont JP, Iron A, Chery M, Georges MD. Spectrum of CFTR mutations in cystic fibrosis and in congenital absence of the vas deferens in France. Hum Mutat. 2000;16(2):143-56.

[33] Sharma H, Mavuduru RS, Singh SK, Prasad R. Heterogeneous spectrum of mutations in CFTR gene from Indian patients with congenital absence of the vas deferens and their association with cystic fibrosis genetic modifiers. Mol Hum Reprod. 2014 Sep; 20(9):827-35. doi: 10.1093/molehr/gau047.

[34] Bergougnoux A, Viart V, Miro J, Bommart S, Molinari N, des Georges M, Claustres M, Chiron R, Taulan-Cadars M. Should diffuse bronchiectasis still be considered a CFTR-related disorder? J Cyst Fibros. 2015 pii: S1569-1993(15)00054-5.

[35] Ramos MD, Trujillano D, Olivar R, Sotillo F, Ossowski S, Manzanares J, Costa J, Gartner S, Oliva C, Quintana E, Gonzalez MI, Vazquez C, Estivill X, Casals T. Extensive sequence analysis of CFTR, SCNN1A, SCNN1B, SCNN1G and SERPINA1 suggests an oligogenic basis for cystic fibrosis-like phenotypes. Clin Genet. 2014 Jul;86(1):91-5. doi: 10.1111/cge.12234.32

[36] Bakouh N, Bienvenu T, Thomas A, Ehrenfeld J, Liote H, Roussel D, Duquesnoy P, Farman N, Viel M, Cherif-Zahar B, Amselem S, Taam RA, Edelman A, Planelles G, Sermet-Gaudelus I. Characterization of SLC26A9 in patients with CF-like lung disease. Hum Mutat. 2013 Oct;34(10):1404-14. doi: 10.1002/humu.22382.

[37] Li W, Soave D, Miller MR, Keenan K, Lin F, Gong J, Chiang T, Stephenson AL, Durie P, Rommens J, Sun L, Strug LJ. Unraveling the complex genetic model for cystic fibrosis: pleiotropic effects of modifier genes on early cystic fibrosis-related morbidities. Hum Genet. 2014 Feb;133(2):151-61. doi: 10.1007/s00439-013-1363-7.

[38] Practice guidelines for the Interpretation and Reporting of Unclassified Variants (UVs) in Clinical Molecular Genetics, 2007. Available on: http://cmgsweb.shared.hosting.zen.co.uk/ [Accessed: 2015-02-07]

[39] Raynal C, Baux D, Theze C, Bareil C, Taulan M, Roux AF, Claustres M, Tuffery-Giraud S, des Georges M. A classification model relative to splicing for variants of unknown clinical significance: application to the CFTR gene. Hum Mutat. 2013;34:774-874.

[40] 1000 Genomes Project Consortium, Abecasis GR, Altshuler D, Auton A, Brooks LD, Durbin RM, Gibbs RA, Hurles ME, McVean GA. A map of human genome variation from population-scale sequencing. Nature. 2010 Oct 28;467(7319):1061-73. doi: 10.1038/nature09534. Erratum in: Nature 2011 May 26;473(7348):544.

[41] NHLBI GO Exome Sequencing Project. Available on: http://evs.gs.washington.edu/EVS/ [Accessed: 2015-02-07]

[42] Claustres M, Horaitis O, Vanevski M, Cotton RG. Time for a unified system of mutation description and reporting: a review of locus-specific mutation databases. Genome Res. 2002;12:680-8.

[43] Cotton RGH, Auerbach AD, Beckmann JS, Blumenfeld OO, Brookes AJ, Brown AE, et al. Recommendations for locus-specific databases and their curation. Hum Mutat. 2008;29(1):2-5.

[44] Cystic Fibrosis Mutation Database (CFMDB). Available on: www.genet.sickkids.on.ca/cftr/ [Accessed: 2015-02-07]

[45] Clinical and Functional Translation of CFTR (CFTR2), US CF Foundation, Johns Hopkins University, The Hospital for Sick Children, John Hopkins, USA. Available on: http://www.cftr2.org/ [Accessed: 2015-02-07]

[46] Castellani C, CFTR2 Team. CFTR2: how will it help care? Paediatr Respir Rev. 2013 May;14(Suppl 1):2-5. doi: 10.1016/j.prrv.2013.01.006.

[47] Sosnay PR, Siklosi KR, Van Goor F, Kaniecki K, Yu H, Sharma N, Ramalho AS, Amaral MD, Dorfman R, Zielenski J, Masica DL, Karchin R, et al. Defining the disease liability of variants in the cystic fibrosis transmembrane conductance regulator gene. Nat Genet. 2013;45:1160-7.

[48] CFTR-France. Available on: https://cftr.iurc.montp.inserm.fr/CFTR/ (Restricted access) [Accessed: 2015-02-07]

[49] He L1, Aleksandrov AA, Serohijos AW, Hegedus T, Aleksandrov LA, Cui L, Dokholyan NV, Riordan JR. Multiple membrane-cytoplasmic domain contacts in the cystic fibrosis transmembrane conductance regulator (CFTR) mediate regulation of channel gating. J Biol Chem. 2008 Sep 26;283(39):26383-90. doi: 10.1074/jbc.M803894200.

[50] Mornon JP, Lehn P, Callebaut I. Atomic model of human cystic fibrosis transmembrane conductance regulator: membrane-spanning domains and coupling interfaces. Cell Mol Life Sci. 2008 Aug;65(16):2594-612. doi: 10.1007/s00018-008-8249-1.

[51] Adzhubei IA, Schmidt S, Peshkin L, Ramensky VE, Gerasimova A, Bork P, Kondrashov AS, Sunyaev SR. A method and server for predicting damaging missense mutations. Nat Methods. 2010 Apr;7(4):248-9. doi: 10.1038/nmeth0410-248.

[52] Ng PC, Henikoff S. SIFT: predicting amino acid changes that affect protein function. Nucleic Acids Res. 2003 Jul 1;31(13):3812-4.

[53] Tavtigian SV, Deffenbaugh AM, Yin L, Judkins T, Scholl T, Samollow PB, de Silva D, Zharkikh A, Thomas A. Comprehensive statistical study of 452 BRCA1 missense sub-

stitutions with classification of eight recurrent substitutions as neutral. J Med Genet. 2006;43(4):295-305.

[54] Yates CM, Filippis I, Kelley LA, Sternberg MJ. SuSPect: enhanced prediction of single amino acid variant (SAV) phenotype using network features. J Mol Biol. 2014 Jul 15;426(14):2692-701. doi: 10.1016/j.jmb.2014.04.026.

[55] PolyPhen 2. Available on: http://genetics.bwh.harvard.edu/pph2/ [Accessed: 2015-02-08]

[56] SIFT. Available on: http://sift.jcvi.org/www/SIFT_BLink_submit.html [Accessed: 2015-02-08]

[57] Align GVGD. Available on: http://agvgd.iarc.fr/agvgd_input.php [Accessed: 2015-02-08]

[58] SuSPect. Available on: www.sbg.bio.ic.ac.uk/suspect [Accessed: 2015-02-08]

[59] Alamut©. http://www.interactive-biosoftware.com/ (Commercial software, not available online)

[60] Masica DL, Sosnay PR, Cutting GR, Karchin R. Phenotype-optimized sequence ensembles substantially improve prediction of disease-causing mutation in cystic fibrosis. Hum Mutat. 2012 Aug;33(8):1267-74. doi: 10.1002/humu.22110.

[61] Hicks S, Wheeler DA, Plon SE, Kimmel M. Prediction of missense mutation functionality depends on both the algorithm and sequence alignment employed. Hum Mutat. 2011;32:661-8.

[62] Le Guédard-Méreuze S. Mutations in splicing cis-regulatory elements: role in human genetic diseases [thesis in French]. Université Montpellier 1, 2009.

[63] Spurdle AB, Couch FJ, Hogervorst FB, Radice P, Sinilnikova OM, IARC Unclassified Genetic Variants Working Group. Prediction and assessment of splicing alterations: implications for clinical testing. Hum Mutat. 2008 Nov;29(11):1304-13. doi: 10.1002/humu.20901.

[64] Vreeswijk MP, Kraan JN, van der Klift HM, Vink GR, Cornelisse CJ, Wijnen JT, Bakker E, van Asperen CJ, Devilee P. Intronic variants in BRCA1 and BRCA2 that affect RNA splicing can be reliably selected by splice-site prediction programs. Hum Mutat. 2009 Jan;30(1):107-14. doi: 10.1002/humu.20811.

[65] Sharma N, Sosnay PR, Ramalho AS, Douville C, Franca A, Gottschalk LB, Park J, Lee M, Vecchio-Pagan B, Raraigh KS, Amaral MD, Karchin R, Cutting GR. Experimental assessment of splicing variants using expression minigenes and comparison with in silico predictions. Hum Mutat. 2014 Oct;35(10):1249-59. doi: 10.1002/humu.22624.

[66] Houdayer C, Caux-Moncoutier V, Krieger S, Barrois M, Bonnet F, Bourdon V, Bronner M, Buisson M, Coulet F, Gaildrat P, Lefol C, Léone M, Mazoyer S, Muller D, Remenieras A, Révillion F, Rouleau E, Sokolowska J, Vert JP, Lidereau R, Soubrier F,

Sobol H, Sevenet N, Bressac-de Paillerets B, Hardouin A, Tosi M, Sinilnikova OM, Stoppa-Lyonnet D. Guidelines for splicing analysis in molecular diagnosis derived from a set of 327 combined in silico/in vitro studies on BRCA1 and BRCA2 variants. Hum Mutat. 2012 Aug;33(8):1228-38.doi: 10.1002/humu.22101.

[67] Yeo G, Burge CB. Maximum entropy modeling of short sequence motifs with applications to RNA splicing signals. J Comput Biol. 2004;11(2-3):377-94.

[68] Desmet FO, Hamroun D, Lalande M, Collod-Béroud G, Claustres M, Béroud C. Human Splicing Finder: an online bioinformatics tool to predict splicing signals. Nucleic Acids Res. 2009 May;37(9):e67. doi: 10.1093/nar/gkp215.

[69] Shapiro MB, Senapathy P. RNA splice junctions of different classes of eukaryotes: sequence statistics and functional implications in gene expression. Nucleic Acids Res. 1987 Sep 11;15(17):7155-74.

[70] Reese MG, Eeckman FH, Kulp D, Haussler D. Improved splice site detection in Genie. J Comput Biol. 1997 Fall;4(3):311-23.

[71] Mucaki EJ, Shirley BC, Rogan PK. Prediction of mutant mRNA splice isoforms by information theory-based exon definition. Hum Mutat. 2013 Apr;34(4):557-65. doi: 10.1002/humu.22277.

[72] Cartegni L, Wang J, Zhu Z, Zhang MQ, Krainer AR. ESEfinder: a web resource to identify exonic splicing enhancers. Nucleic Acids Res. 2003;31:3568-71.

[73] Fairbrother WG, Yeh RF, Sharp PA, Burge CB. Predictive identification of exonic splicing enhancers in human genes. Science. 2002;297:1007-13.

[74] MaxEntScan. Available on: http://genes.mit.edu/burgelab/maxent/Xmaxentscan_scoreseq.html [Accessed: 2015-02-08]

[75] Human Splicing Finder, version 2.4.1. Available on: http://www.umd.be/HSF/ [Accessed: 2015-02-08]

[76] NNSplice. Available on: http://www.fruitfly.org/seq_tools/splice.html [Accessed: 2015-02-08]

[77] Automated Splice Site and Exon Definition Analyses (ASSEDA). Available on: http://splice.uwo.ca/ (Restricted access: registration required) [Accessed: 2015-02-08]

[78] ESEfinder. Available on: http://rulai.cshl.edu/tools/ESE/ [Accessed: 2015-02-08]

[79] Relative enhancer and silencer classification by unanimous enrichment (RESCUE ESE). Available on: http://genes.mit.edu/burgelab/rescue-ese/ [Accessed: 2015-02-08]

[80] Aissat A, de Becdelievre A, Golmard L, Vasseur C, Costa C, Chaoui A, Martin N, Costes B, Goossens M, Girodon E, Fanen P, Hinzpeter, A. Combined computational-experimental analyses of CFTR exon strength uncover predictability of exon- skipping level. Hum Mutat. 2013;34:873-81.

[81] Burn TC, Connors TD, Klinger KW, Landes GM. Increased exon-trapping efficiency through modifications to the pSPL3 splicing vector. Gene. 1995;161(2):183-7.

[82] Cooper TA. Use of minigene systems to dissect alternative splicing elements. Methods. 2005 Dec;37(4):331-40.

[83] Singh G, Cooper TA. Minigene reporter for identification and analysis of cis elements and trans factors affecting pre-mRNA splicing. Biotechniques. 2006 Aug;41(2):177-81.

[84] Goina E, Fernandez-Alanis E, Pagani F. Approaches to study CFTR pre-mRNA splicing defects. Methods Mol Biol. 2011;741:155-69. doi: 10.1007/978-1-61779-117-8_11.

[85] Scott A, Petrykowska HM, Hefferon T, Gotea V, Elnitski L. Functional analysis of synonymous substitutions predicted to affect splicing of the CFTR gene. J Cyst Fibros. 2012 Dec;11(6):511-7. doi: 10.1016/j.jcf.2012.04.009.

[86] Taulan M, Guittard C, Theze C, Claustres M, Georges MD, A novel double 312 deletion underscores the importance of characterizing end points of the CFTR large 313 rearrangements. Eur J Hum Genet. 2009;17(12):1683-87.

[87] Taulan M, Viart V, Theze C, Guittard C, Altieri JP, Templin C, Mely L, Claustres M, des Georges M. Identification of a novel duplication CFTRdup2 and functional impact of large rearrangements identified in the CFTR gene. Gene. 2012 Jun 1;500(2): 194-8. doi: 10.1016/j.gene.2012.03.043.

[88] Aleksandrov AA, Kota P, Aleksandrov LA, He L, Jensen T, Cui L, Gentzsch M, Dokholyan NV, Riordan JR. Regulatory insertion removal restores maturation, stability and function of DeltaF508 CFTR. J Mol Biol. 2010 Aug 13;401(2):194-210. doi: 10.1016/ j.jmb.2010.06.019.

[89] Bergougnoux A, Claustres M, de Sario A. Nasal epithelial cells, a tool to study DNA methylation in airway diseases. Epigenomics. 2015 Feb;7(1):119-26. doi: 10.2217/epi. 14.65.

[90] van Meegen MA, Terheggen-Lagro SW, Koymans KJ, van der Ent CK, Beekman JM. Apical CFTR expression in human nasal epithelium correlates with lung disease in cystic fibrosis. PLoS One. 2013;8(3):e57617. doi: 10.1371/journal.pone.0057617.

[91] Hajj R, Baranek T, Le Naour R, Lesimple P, Puchelle E, Coraux C. Basal cells of the human adult airway surface epithelium retain transit-amplifying cell properties. Stem Cells. 2007 Jan;25(1):139-48.

[92] Hirtz S, Gonska T, Seydewitz HH, Thomas J, Greiner P, Kuehr J, Brandis M, Eichler I, Rocha H, Lopes AI, Barreto C, Ramalho A, Amaral MD, Kunzelmann K, Mall M. CFTR Cl- channel function in native human colon correlates with the genotype and phenotype in cystic fibrosis. Gastroenterology. 2004 Oct;127(4):1085-95.

[93] De Jonge HR, Ballmann M, Veeze H, Bronsveld I, Stanke F, Tümmler B, Sinaasappel M. Ex vivo CF diagnosis by intestinal current measurements (ICM) in small aperture, circulating Ussing chambers. J Cyst Fibros. 2004 Aug;3 Suppl 2:159-63.

[94] Dekkers JF, Wiegerinck CL, de Jonge HR, Bronsveld I, Janssens HM, de Winter-de Groot KM, Brandsma AM, de Jong NW, Bijvelds MJ, Scholte BJ, Nieuwenhuis EE, van den Brink S, Clevers H, van der Ent CK, Middendorp S, Beekman JM. A functional CFTR assay using primary cystic fibrosis intestinal organoids. Nat Med. 2013 Jul;19(7):939-45. doi: 10.1038/nm.3201.

[95] Farrell PM, Koscik RE. Sweat chloride concentrations in infants homozygous or heterozygous for F508 cystic fibrosis. Pediatrics. 1996 Apr;97(4):524-8.

[96] Davis PB, Schluchter MD, Konstan MW. Relation of sweat chloride concentration to severity of lung disease in cystic fibrosis. Pediatr Pulmonol. 2004 Sep;38(3):204-9.

[97] Wilschanski M, Dupuis A, Ellis L, Jarvi K, Zielenski J, Tullis E, Martin S, Corey M, Tsui LC, Durie P. Mutations in the cystic fibrosis transmembrane regulator gene and in vivo transepithelial potentials. Am J Respir Crit Care Med. 2006 Oct 1;174(7): 787-94. Epub 2006 Jul 13.

[98] Quinton P, Molyneux L, Ip W, Dupuis A, Avolio J, Tullis E, Conrad D, Shamsuddin AK, Durie P, Gonska T. β-adrenergic sweat secretion as a diagnostic test for cystic fibrosis. Am J Respir Crit Care Med. 2012 Oct 15;186(8):732-9. doi: 10.1164/rccm. 201205-0922OC.

[99] Ho LP, Samways JM, Porteous DJ, Dorin JR, Carothers A, Greening AP, Innes JA. Correlation between nasal potential difference measurements, genotype and clinical condition in patients with cystic fibrosis. Eur Respir J. 1997 Sep;10(9):2018-22.

[100] Bagheri-Hanson A, Nedwed S, Rueckes-Nilges C, Naehrlich L. Intestinal current measurement versus nasal potential difference measurements for diagnosis of cystic fibrosis: a case-control study. BMC Pulm Med. 2014 Oct 4;14:156. doi: 10.1186/1471-2466-14-156.

4

Cystic Fibrosis and Fertility

Rosaria Casciaro, Federico Cresta,
Federica Favilli and Laura Minicucci

Abstract

In the last 20 years, the prognosis of cystic fibrosis (CF) has slightly increased and nowadays more than 50% of CF patients are adults. An obvious consequence of this deep change is the increasing question about fertility in both males and females.

Almost 97% of male CF patients are infertile, having significant anatomical abnormalities of the reproductive tract, in most cases a congenital bilateral absence of the vas deferens (CBAVD); even if anatomical defect plays an important role, cystic fibrosis transmembrane conductance regulator (CFTR) is directly involved in many aspects of male reproduction, with well-known consequences in spermatozoa capacitation and bicarbonate secretion.

Actually, male CF patients can become parents with assisted fertilization techniques: intracytoplasmic sperm injection (ICSI), currently the most used fertilization treatment worldwide, has dramatically improved the assisted reproduction outcomes for men with obstructive azoospermia.

Most CF women have a normal reproductive tract and may be able to conceive spontaneously, but multifactorial fertility problems can affect them also: the main cause could be the difficult transport of sperm through the female reproductive tract, secondary to thick secretions, but also lung function and nutritional status at the time of conception significantly influence their fertility.

Keywords: Cystic fibrosis, CFTR, Congenital bilateral absence of the vas deferens, Fertility, In vitro fertilization, Pregnancy

1. Introduction

As the life expectancy of cystic fibrosis (CF) patients continues to increase, and more patients become adults with a chronic disease, researching the impact of this disorder on male and female infertility has become increasingly important.

Although most men with CF have significant anatomical abnormalities of the reproductive tract causing infertility, most women with CF have anatomically normal reproductive tracts and up to half of them may be able to conceive spontaneously.

Assisted reproductive technologies can help both infertile male and female patients with CF in achieving successful parenthood. In addition, for women more health characteristics including baseline pulmonary function have to be evaluated as predictors of health and pregnancy outcomes.

2. Fertility in men with cystic fibrosis

CF is a systemic illness that affects multiple organ systems, including lungs, endocrine and epithelial tissues, gastrointestinal system, pancreas, and reproductive tract. Because of the dramatic improvement made in prognosis in CF population in the last two decades, reproductive function has become one of the new red flags in the management of CF adult patients. Infertility in CF males has been extensively studied and found in most cases to be secondary to atrophy or malformation of the vas deferens, leading to an obstructive azoospermia (Figure 1).

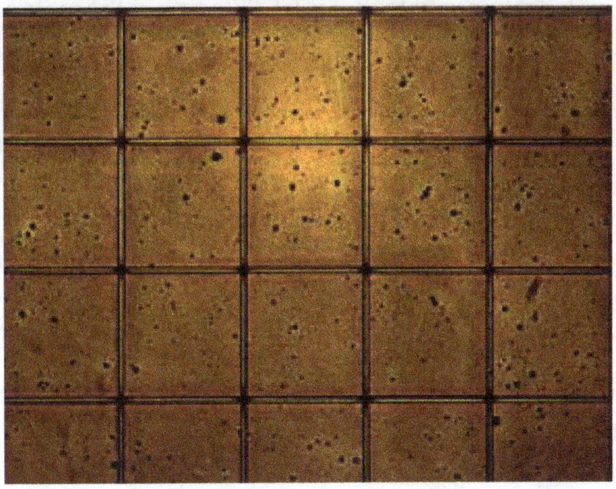

Figure 1. Spermiogram performed in our 34-year-old patient affected by CF documents azoospermia

2.1. Pathogenesis

Cystic fibrosis transmembrane conductance regulator (CFTR) is a gene located on chromosome 7 (7q31.2), encoding for a protein located in the apical membranes of epithelial cells; it was identified in 1989 and its role in the pathogenesis of CF is now well known. CF is a disease characterized by a defect in electrolyte and fluid transport in exocrine tissues; it could present several different clinical manifestations, including chronic lung disease, pancreas insufficiency, and infertility [1].

In literature, it is reported that almost 97% of male CF patients are infertile [2]: this infertility is primarily secondary to an obstructive azoospermia. The defective CFTR ion channel function causes an early obstruction of male genital tract, due to the dehydrated secretions: this mechanism drives to deep structural changes in reproductive tract, causing in most cases a congenital bilateral absence of the vas deferens (CBAVD). In early studies on CF adult patients with azoospermia, CBAVD was reported in all the population studied. At the light of these findings, Holscalaw et al. [3] speculated a unique genetic cause of CF and CBAVD. Usually, the proximal part of epididymis is present and this allows the sperm collection in CF patients to obtain spermatozoa.

Obstructive dysfunction is not the only cause of infertility in males with CF: further studies demonstrated that CFTR may also play a critical role in spermatogenesis and sperm maturation [4]; an increased CFTR mutation frequency in a population of men with reduced sperm quality is also reported [5]. Histological examination of CF testicular biopsies shows a wide range of spermatogenesis abnormalities, including a decreased count of mature spermatids and maturation arrest. These findings could be the expressions of CFTR abnormalities in seminiferous tubules or spermatozoa.

CFTR plays a role in many aspects of male reproduction, with well-known consequences in CBAVD and CF. It has not only ion channel functions but also it is a versatile signaling molecule and interacts with more than 180 other proteins. CFTR is expressed throughout the whole genital tract [6], but we do not know yet what is CFTR's role in the male accessory glands other than the epididymis.

A significant role in sperm function was also suggested by the involvement of CFTR in uterine HCO_3^- secretion and its effect on the fertilizing capacity of sperm [7]. CFTR is present in human sperm and it is involved in both sperm motility and capacitation phases. CF mice sperm has reduced sperm motility and capacitation with reduced fertility rate in vitro and in vivo [8]: these findings suggest a significant role of CFTR in sperm functions also.

2.2. CBAVD

CBAVD is a congenital condition in which vas deferens fails to develop properly, causing male infertility because of the total obstruction of reproductive tract. CBAVD accounts for approximately 1–2% of all infertility in males and is the result of genetic abnormalities [9]. More than half of the men with CBAVD (62–80%) carry a CFTR mutation and this condition is considered to be one of the most common CFTR-related diseases. Anatomical abnormalities include bilateral or unilateral absence of the vas deferens and seminal vesicles anomalies.

Subjects with CBAVD usually have no clinical symptoms of CF, but the finding of subclinical CF features is not uncommon (mild chloride elevation at sweat test, chronic sinusitis, nasal polyps) and actually many experts consider CBAVD as a mild CF form [9].

2.3. Other genital abnormalities

Genital abnormalities may develop early in CF, but in children these are less common than described in adults. In 2002, Blau et al. [10] described genital abnormalities in male children with CF, performing pelvic and scrotal ultrasonography in 12 CF boys aged 2–12 years. They found seminal vesicles hypoplasia, testicular microlithiasis, and abnormalities of the epididymal head, such as cysts, hypo-, or hyper-echogenicity. These findings are more frequent in pancreatic-insufficient than in pancreatic-sufficient CF patients. The reported experience represents a very small population of CF children, and larger longitudinal studies will be necessary to better define the onset and progression of urogenital abnormalities in CF males.

In CF adults, testes are usually symmetric and have a normal echogenicity, but mild inhomogeneity or striated appearance can be documented with ultrasounds. Focal inhomogeneities seem to be rare, as testicular nodules. Didymus cysts, epididymal cysts (also multiple) with sediments and/or calcifications are common. Usually, vas deferens is absent, but a structure attributable to spermatic cord could be revealed bilaterally or unilaterally in some cases, usually with a significant stenosis.

Several features can influence the anatomical genital phenotype in these patients (as genotype, clinical features, age), and further studies will be crucial to find risk factors and significant correlation for these abnormalities in CF.

2.4. Fertility management in men with CF

Over the last 20 years, the relevant improvement in survival of CF patients and the concomitant development of new assisted conception methods have significantly increased the opportunities for these patients to become parents. It is therefore very important to start an early and effective management of fertility issues in males with CF.

The clinical management of reproductive issues in males affected by CF has to begin during puberty with periodic evaluation of testicular volume/consistency and all the other virilization signs, indicating a congruous testosterone production. Hormonal levels (as LH, FSH, and testosterone serum concentration) are usually normal in male CF, indicating a regular spermatogenesis in most cases. It could be also useful as a deeper examination to detect the presence of vas deferens (usually palpable in the upper portion of scrotum), but the definitive diagnosis of CBAVD can be made with radiological exams.

There is not a considerable literature about the morphological study of the scrotum in adult CF patients, but trans-rectal ultrasounds could be considered a good instrument to evaluate abnormalities in shape, volume, and structure of testes, epididymis, and spermatic cord.

Also scrotal ultrasound with high-definition instruments is non-invasive and executable without any discomfort for the patient and could be useful in order to analyze the extra pelvic portion of the vas deferens (from the groin to the testicle) and all the scrotal structures.

The diagnosis of azoospermia could be simply supported and confirmed by semen analysis. In case of seminal vesicles abnormalities, semen analysis will also show an acid pH, due to lack of fructose concentrations in sperm, and often the volume of ejaculate is low: in these cases, the sperm is produced by the prostate, with no contribute from vesicles. Typically, men with the absence of the vas deferens have low-volume (often less than 0.5 ml) and acidic semen [11].

2.5. Assisted reproduction in men with CF

2.5.1. Counseling

CF men and their partners, who want to start assisted reproduction treatments, need an adequate genetic, medical, and psychological counseling. Genetic tests have to be performed in the patient (if not already done) and in the partner, in order to define the risk of generating an affected child. In case of incomplete genetic assessment or high risk of CF recurrence, prenatal or pre-implantation genetic diagnosis could also be recommended; it is important to consider ethic and legislative issues, because in some countries pre-implantation genetic tests are not allowed. All these procedures have relevant psychological, ethical, and sanitary costs, so alternative measures (as adoption or use of sperm donor) could be considered.

Another important issue is the prognosis of the potential father affected by CF. This delicate aspect asks the intervention of CF-clinician and psychologist, together with an experienced fertility specialist.

2.5.2. Sperm collection

Sperm retrieval is a procedure used to obtain sperm for fertility purposes. In general, it is necessary in case of azoospermia or if men are unable to ejaculate. In almost all cases, sperm retrieval must be utilized in combination with in vitro fertilization (IVF) and intracytoplasmic sperm injection (ICSI) for reasonable pregnancy rates to be obtained [12].

The sperm collection could be performed by aspiration from epididymis or directly from the testis. In CF the proximal part of the epididymis is usually present, so the procedure is usually quietly simple. The techniques of collection include:

- Percutaneous epididymal sperm aspiration (PESA) from the caput of the epididymis, usually simple to localize and good reservoir of sperm; aspiration is performed with fine needle after local anesthetization and is usually fast and well tolerated by the patient
- Microsurgical epididymal sperm aspiration (MESA)
- Percutaneous testicular aspiration (TESA) performed with local anesthetization (Figure 2) as for PESA
- Testicular surgical biopsy (Figure 3)
- Testicular sperm extraction (TESE), an in vivo microdissection of testicular tubules finalized to the identification of normal tubules (Figure 4), suitable for an effective sperm collection

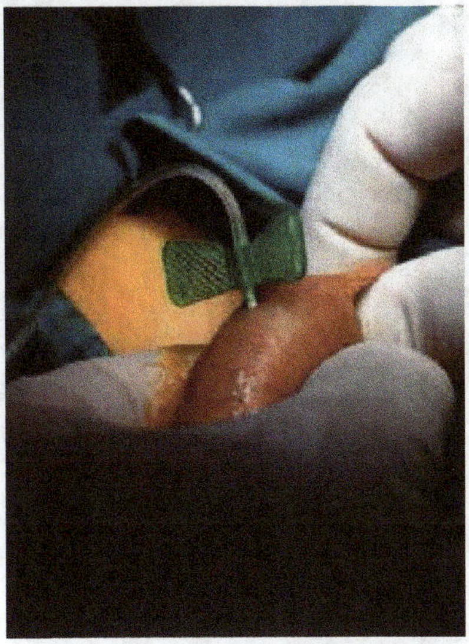

Figure 2. Percutaneous testicular aspiration (TESA) performed with local anesthetization

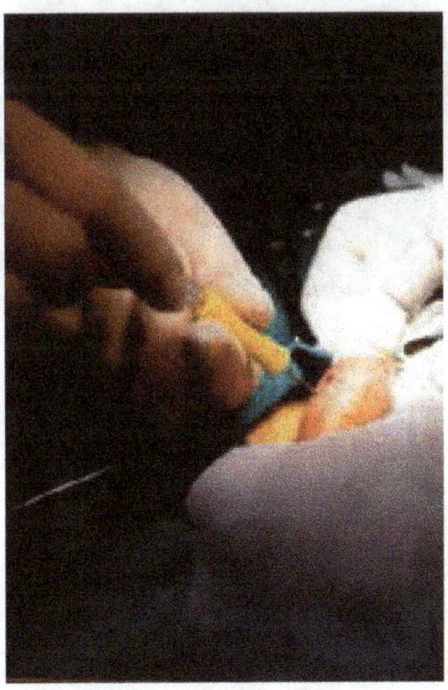

Figure 3. Percutaneous testicular biopsy

Cryopreservation of sperm is possible and represents a good chance for future use, but usually repeated epididymal aspiration is required. These procedures are usually performed on the same day of the partner's oocytes collection (Figure 5) to assure high counts of motile sperm in the time of fecundation.

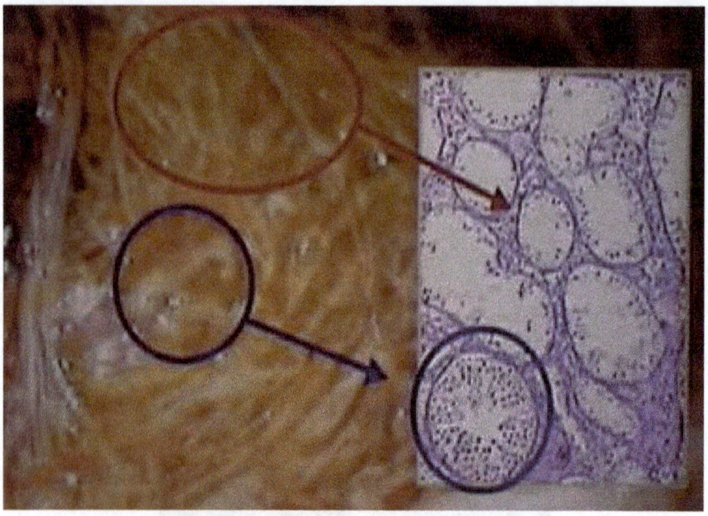

Figure 4. Microsurgical identification of tubules with spermatogenesis (TESE technique)

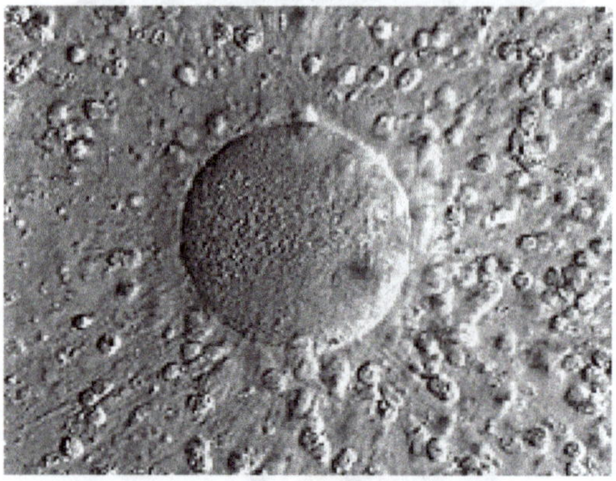

Figure 5. Oocytes culture

2.5.3. Assisted reproduction treatments

The first experience of in vitro fertilization with sperm obtained by epididymal aspiration was in 1985 [13]; in the next years, several experiences also in CBAVD patients have been reported [14]. In that period, the fertilization rates were low (less than 20%), with very poor birth rates.

A dramatic increase in assisted reproduction outcomes for men with obstructive azoospermia has been represented by ICSI, introduced first in the 1990s. The first large experience with ICSI in the United States was published by Sherins et al. in 1995 [15]. This technique is generally performed following an in vitro fertilization procedure to extract one to several oocytes from a woman. The procedure is done under a microscope, using multiple micromanipulation devices, in order to allow the direct injection of a single sperm in a human oocyte.

This technique is currently the most used fertilization treatment worldwide and it has deeply increased the chances of successful fertilizations and pregnancies; ICSI technique allows to have the same fertilization and pregnancy rates between CF males and men with no vas deferens obstructive disease (Figure 6).

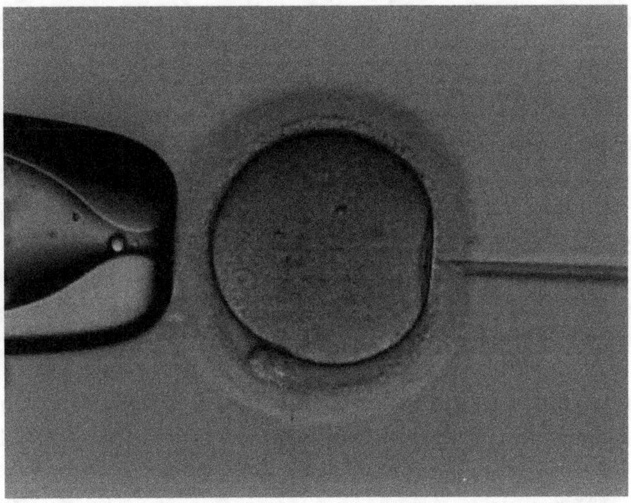

Figure 6. ICSI technique

3. Fertility in women with cystic fibrosis

Although most men with CF have significant anatomical abnormalities of the reproductive tract, most CF women have an anatomically normal reproductive tract and may be able to conceive spontaneously, but in literature it is reported that only slightly more than half of them have spontaneous pregnancies. The fertility problems in CF female are multifactorial: the main cause would be the difficult transport of sperm through the female reproductive tract, secondary to thick secretions; but certainly also the underlying medical conditions (especially lung function and nutritional status) have a major impact on fertility in these patients. The improved health and longevity of CF women naturally leads to an increased number of CF women who become or desire to become pregnant.

The first reported successful pregnancy in a CF woman was in 1960 [16], and in 1966 13 pregnancies in 10 different patients were reported [17]. These early reports were discouraging. However, with aggressive management of infections and significant improvement in pulmonary and nutritional interventions, pregnancies today are well tolerated in CF, especially in women with mild to moderate disease [18, 19]. The North American CF Registry reported in 2007 that 3–4% of CF women over 17 years old become pregnant each year [20].

3.1. Pathogenesis

Despite CF has long been associated with female infertility, the underlying causes remain unclear. Actually, we know that the majority of CF women have a normal fertility, but ovulation disturbance may occur in patients with advanced disease [21], also with amenorrhea in the most compromised subjects. Although most girls have normal menstrual cycles, there is a higher incidence of missed or irregular periods and amenorrhea. This is more likely in those with a reduced percentage of body fat and may occur in case of malnutrition or alimentary disorders.

Fertility problems may be related to lung disease severity, poor weight, and to an unsatisfying control of CF-related diabetes [22]. Historically, the predictors of poor pregnancy outcome for mother and/or fetus were a forced vital capacity (FVC) of less than 50% of the predicted value and poor nutritional status. In the past, an FVC of less than 50% of the predicted value was an absolute contraindication to pregnancy.

For several years, it has been postulated that the thickened cervical mucus present in CF women reproductive tract could lead to fertility disturbance. Normally, when the egg is released from the ovary, cervical and uterine mucus thins and allows easier passage of sperm into the uterus and fertilization. Increased thickness of this mucus in women with CF may theoretically act as a barrier to sperm penetration and could reduce fertility, but nowadays the majority of women with CF can become pregnant without any difficulty.

In 2008, Hodges et al. [23] studied the mouse model of CF, indicating that in CF mice the major cause of decreased fertility is the impaired sperm transport within female reproductive tract. In their experience, excess cervical mucus played a minor role, because instead of a physical barrier, the decreased fertilization seemed to be due to an inadequate fluid production in reproductive system, with a subsequent decrease in sperm number in the oviduct. CFTR could play not only an important role in female reproductive tract fluid control but also in sperm capacitation with its bicarbonate transport.

3.2. Impact of pregnancy on CF

The physiologic changes associated with pregnancy may contribute to increased morbidity and mortality risks for the mother in CF women. Volumetric increase of abdomen with the consequent upward displacement of diaphragm causes a decrease in functional residual volume, and the concomitant increase in resting minute ventilation can lead to a relevant breath disturbance. Also gas exchange has deep alterations in pregnant women, with an increased alveolar–arterial oxygen gradient, especially in supine position [24].

In a recent study [25], it is reported that adjusting for the FEV1 percent predicted, weight, height, and pulmonary exacerbation rate per year, pregnancy is not associated with an increased risk of death. Pregnancy did not appear to be harmful even in a subset of women with diabetes mellitus or with FEV1 less than 40% of predicted. Important predictors of pregnancy outcome for the fetus are the severity of maternal pulmonary impairment and nutritional status; in women with advanced lung disease, preterm delivery is very common.

McMullen et al. [26] in 2006 characterized health outcomes in CF pregnant women, comparing them with a group of never-pregnant CF population: this large observational study showed a nonsignificant difference in terms of FEV1 decline between the two groups (6.8% in pregnant group and 4.7% in never-pregnant, *P*=0.61). Respiratory exacerbations and hospitalizations were increased during pregnancy, as well as the number of outpatient visits and administered therapies.

The risk for congenital anomalies in the fetus is not increased in CF gravidas and breastfeeding is possible without complications.

3.3. Risk factors

The pregravid pulmonary function is clearly the greatest outcome predictor in CF women, but there are multiple clinical prognostic markers to consider. Women with poor nutritional status, pulmonary hypertension, and relevant decrease in pulmonary function during the first 3 months of gestation have to be informed about the high risk of maternal mortality and should consider therapeutic abortion [27].

3.3.1. Lung function

FEV1% predicted, PO2, and PCO2 are important predictors of pregnancy outcomes. In 1995, Edenborough et al. [28] reported that a pregravid FEV1 <60% caused greater pulmonary function decrease, a higher frequency of preterm infants, and also a higher mortality. However, successful pregnancies have been reported also in CF patients with compromised lung function ($FEV_1 < 50\%$ of that predicted), and most patients seem to return to baseline pulmonary status after pregnancy.

The only absolute contraindication to pregnancy in CF is represented by pulmonary hypertension, which is correlated with higher rates of mortality in pregnancy. An echocardiogram performed before pregnancy can be useful to individuate underlying pulmonary hypertension and cor pulmonale, in order to advise the patient about the high mortality risk in case of pregnancy [24].

3.3.2. Pancreatic insufficiency and diabetes mellitus

In old literature, pancreatic insufficiency was considered as a major risk factor in pregnancy outcomes. Actually, with the modern pancreatic enzymes supplementations, it is a nonsignificant issue in CF pregnancies.

CF women planning pregnancy have to be tested for glucose intolerance before conception and the test has to be repeated at 20 weeks of gestational age. Insulin therapy is indicated in case of abnormalities in blood glucose monitoring.

3.3.3. Nutritional status

Clinician should advise to reach a pregravid weight before conception up to 90% of the ideal body weight. Poor nutritional status is without any doubt one of the most relevant risk factor for pregnancy outcomes in CF, and a severe malnutrition (BMI <18 kg/m^2) is a relative contraindication to pregnancy. A weight gain of 11–12 kg during pregnancy is recommended [29]; poor outcome is particularly associated with a maternal gain less than 4.5 Kg. A high caloric intake should be maintained and a poor weight gain is an indication for aggressive nutritional intervention (dietary supplementation, nasogastric, or gastrostomy feeding).

3.3.4. Microbiological issues

Burkholderia cepacia complex has been considered for several years a relative contraindication for pregnancy in CF, because this infection seemed to be related with a higher maternal mortality [30]. *B. cepacia* (particularly *B. cenocepacia* and *B. multivorans*) is also considered related to preterm delivery, weight loss, and rapid pulmonary function decline [31], but further studies are needed to better define its role in CF pregnancies.

3.3.5. Pulmonary transplantation

Limited cases of pregnancy after lung transplantation have been reported; most experience comes from renal transplantation. Compared to other solid organ transplants, lung recipients experience more frequent rejections during pregnancy and also a higher rate of graft loss postpartum [32]. Graft dysfunction is unpredictable and may occur anytime during pregnancy, leading to progressive decline and also eventual death after delivery. However, further studies are necessary to determine long-term maternal survival.

Prematurity and neonatal complications in these pregnancies are very high (56% and 33%, respectively), but no long-term consequences on children are reported [33].

3.4. Management of pregnancy in CF women

The management of pregnancy in CF requests necessarily a multidisciplinary approach. Most of the literature on pregnancy in CF is constituted by case reports and a few national centre based reviews. Unfortunately, at the moment, we have no available trials about any aspect of pregnancy management in CF. In 2008, Edenborough et al. [34] published the guidelines for the management of pregnancy in women with CF, based on the review of the literature and experience of pediatricians, adult and transplant physicians, nurses, physiotherapists, dietitians, pharmacists and psychologists experienced in CF, and also anesthetists and obstetricians with experience of CF pregnancy.

3.4.1. Counselling

Counselling consists in helping the CF patient planning pregnancy and her partner to explain the risks of their decision, such as medical implications, treatment options, and also the impact of a toddler on the everyday life of a CF woman.

Genetic features, such as the risk of recurrence of the disease, have also to be discussed with the couple. CF genotype, if not already known, have to be defined and the partner should also be tested before conception. Genetic counsellors should be involved in order to discuss these delicate issues with the couple.

Genetic tests have a sensitivity <100% with detection rates from 70% to 95% of CFTR mutations. If the partner has not been tested, given a CF carrier frequency of 1:25, the risk of an affected infant is 1:50; while if the partner is a CF carrier, the risk is 1:2.

When the partner is a known carrier or if he has not been tested, clinicians should suggest to perform prenatal genetic diagnosis to the couple, with the analysis of chorionic villus sample (CVS) within the first trimester of gestation. This procedure includes technical risks that should be discussed with the couple.

Psychological counselling is also an important part of the counselling activities: CF team should provide information about sexual health and reproduction to all of their patients, particularly teenage girls. Psychologists and clinicians play an important role also in psychological counselling for CF women who want to become pregnant, even if women with advanced disease with a very strong wish to have a child may proceed whatever the advices.

3.4.2. Medications during pregnancy

Most drugs have not been tested on pregnant women. Relevant issues about their use in pregnancy are timing of exposure (periconception, first, second, third trimester, or perinatally), systemic availability of the drug, and its ability to cross the placenta. Side effects can consist in teratogenesis, growth retardation, death, renal insufficiency, neurological disorders, stillbirth, etc.

Many pregnancies are unplanned and drugs could have been taken at the time of conception and continued in the first weeks of pregnancy, and many women with serious illnesses required treatment to be continued. Even if nowadays there is experience to guide prescribing in pregnancy, the principle remains to avoid drug use where possible, except when the risk of the drug is outweighed by the risk of the condition being treated.

The Swedish FASS information catalog provides information on the risks of drugs to the fetus during pregnancy and to the infant during lactation. Each drug is classified to one category of safety:

1. Drugs that have been used widely during pregnancy and are assumed safe for the fetus
2. Drugs not known to cause harm to the human fetus but with insufficient experience to consider them safe. This category can be subdivided into
3. drugs that have been demonstrated to cause no harm in animal studies
4. drugs with insufficient animal data
5. drugs that have been demonstrated to harm the fetus only in animal studies
6. Drugs that could theoretically cause harm to the fetus by their pharmacological actions
7. Drugs known or believed to cause harm to the fetus

Patient's therapy should be reviewed during the discussion of a potential pregnancy, even if most of the routine CF medications are safe and could be continued. Contraindicated drugs have to be discontinued. β-lactams are safe in pregnancy and aminoglycosides at conventional doses have not showed toxic results. Once-daily tobramicin has been tested in second and third trimesters, showing safe results. Ciprofloxacin has been widely used during pregnancy with no certain side effects, but its use is indicated only if vital for the mother.

3.4.3. *Lung function and infections*

CF women can become pregnant in all pulmonary disease stage, but the outcome for the mother and the newborn is closely related to lung function (FEV1 predicted) and clinical stability. Lung function should be optimized and chronic infections may be suppressed before pregnancy: oral flucloxacillin could be administered in case of *Staphylococcus aureus* colonization; for *Pseudomonas aeruginosa* nebulized colistin or aminoglycoside treatment should be employed.

When a pregnancy is unplanned, pregnancy is frequently connected to a worsening in lung function: if necessary, one or more courses of IV antibiotic treatment could be administered in the usual format also during pregnancy (β-lactam + aminoglycoside).

During the first trimester, most patients will feel breathless and the frequency of hospitalizations could rise up: at each visit, physical examination, sputum cultures, weight and oxygen saturation measurement, and pulmonary function test should be performed.

3.4.4. *Physiotherapy*

If the pregnancy is planned, preconceptional period could represent a good opportunity to optimize the daily physiotherapy program. Inhalation therapies and techniques should also be reviewed and optimized; the timing of these treatments in relation to airway clearance therapy (ACT) is a relevant feature during pregnancy, especially in CF patients who produce big volumes of sputum. ACT adherence and technique have to be adapted in pregnant women. Advice on physical exercise and pelvic floor strength should be given as soon as possible.

The breathing pattern is affected by physiological and mechanical changes during pregnancy, and in the last trimester these features can lead to increase in closing volume and determine atelectasis. Physiotherapists should meet the pregnant patients weekly to optimize the physiotherapy regimen, monitor lung function and sputum production in terms of colour and quantity. Also maintaining exercise capacity should be useful during pregnancy and in last trimester.

3.4.5. *Nutrition*

Dietetic counselling is crucial in preconceptional period, because maternal nutritional state is one of the most important factors influencing outcomes for mother and infant. A low pre-pregnancy BMI is strictly associated with reduced birth weight. Preconceptional assessment is similar to non-CF population and should be performed by a CF specialist dietitian, who can advise not only on increasing energy density of the diet but also oral supplements and invasive nutritional support (enteral tube feeding) can be purposed to the patient if nutritional status is unsatisfactory. Vitamin supplementation with folic acid, vitamin A, and vitamin D are recommended.

An overall weight gain of 12.5 Kg is considered normal and in CF it is recommended a weight gain of at least 11 Kg. Also gastro-oesophageal reflux, heartburn, nausea, recurrent vomiting, and constipation may occur more frequently in women with CF and required clinicians monitoring.

3.4.6. Diabetes care

A pre-pregnancy diagnosis of CF-related diabetes and gestational diabetes are associated with a poorer prognosis; in literature, it is reported that an unsatisfactory glycemic control in the first trimester is associated with an increased risk of teratogenesis. During preconceptional counselling an OGTT is recommended, if not already performed, and blood sugars have to be monitored during lung exacerbations. Usually, OGTT is repeated at 20 weeks gestation and glycaemia should be measured at every visit: if random values are high, another OGTT could be repeated at 28 weeks.

Insulin is the recommended treatment for diabetes in CF also during pregnancy. A high calorie intake should also be assessed in diabetic patients.

3.4.7. Termination of pregnancy

Guidelines about when to terminate pregnancy in a woman with advanced CF remain fluid. The indications may be psychosocial (in order to prevent serious injury to the mental health of the pregnant woman) or medical.

The only absolute contraindication to pregnancy is a pre-existing pulmonary hypertension with cor pulmonale; also chronic hypoxia could be considered a contraindication to pregnancy. There are no clear indications about the FEV1 cut-off to recommend pregnancy termination.

There are also some relative contraindications to pregnancy in CF women:

1. Poor nutritional status (BMI <18 kg/m^2; <85% ideal body weight)
2. Uncontrolled CF-related diabetes
3. *Burkholderia cepacia* infection
4. Significant liver disease

3.4.8. Delivery

Most pregnancies in CF end in spontaneous vaginal delivery. Caesarean section is indicated only in case of maternal or fetal sufferance, preferably with spinal anesthesia. In CF, a high proportion (26–46%) of pregnancies end up with a spontaneous or therapeutic preterm delivery, and the usual indication is represented by maternal conditions. Usually, failing lung function and hypoxia occur in patients with a significant low pre-pregnant lung function;

persisting hypoxia and onset of headache are in these cases severe signs and could request oxygen support or non-invasive ventilation.

In peripartum, pain and anxiety can lead to hyperventilation and decrease in alveolar gas exchanges; hypoxia, hypercarbia, and respiratory acidosis occur rapidly in patients with compromised lung function. An adequate analgesia should be performed, because it reduces pain, fear, and fatigue; oxygen support can be useful in case of desaturations.

4. Our experience

In our CF Center, we have 230 patients in regular follow-up and 153 of these are >18 years old. In the last few years, fertility issues increased significantly in our population, surely because of the significant improvement in prognosis and the easier access to the assisted reproduction treatments.

During the last 20 years, 12 of our male patients recurred to in vitro fertilization with sperm obtained by epididymal aspiration and in 6 cases had successful reproduction (with twin pregnancy in 2 cases and in 1 case triplet pregnancy). All the newborns enjoyed good health and no recurrence of CF has been detected (all the partners were tested for CFTR mutations before the conception). In the other six cases in vitro fertilization was not successful and one of these three patients decided to use heterologous fertilization by sperm donor, with a subsequent successful pregnancy.

In the same period four of our female patients recurred to in vitro fertilization with two successful pregnancies (in one case twin pregnancy). Also in these cases the newborns enjoyed good health and no recurrence of CF has been detected (all the partners were tested for CFTR mutations before the conception).

In our population 12 of our patients (10 women and 2 men) had spontaneous conceptions with 18 successful pregnancies. Also in these cases no recurrence of the disease has been detected, even if in some cases the diagnosis of CF in these patients had been performed after the delivery and in most cases the partners had not been tested for CFTR mutations before the conception. Three of our female patients, after several attempts to become pregnant spontaneously, decided and obtained to adopt a child.

Actually, no literature is available about scrotal imaging in males affected by CF. We decided to realize an original study, performing scrotal ultrasound examination with high-definition technique, to better evaluate abnormalities in shape, volume, and structure of the testes, epididymis, and spermatic cord in a group of adult patients (>18 years) affected by CF. Preliminary results seem to show an increased incidence of testicular and epididymal abnormalities in comparison to the general population, but in most cases these seem to be secondary to the obstruction of vas deferens [FigureS 7,8,9].

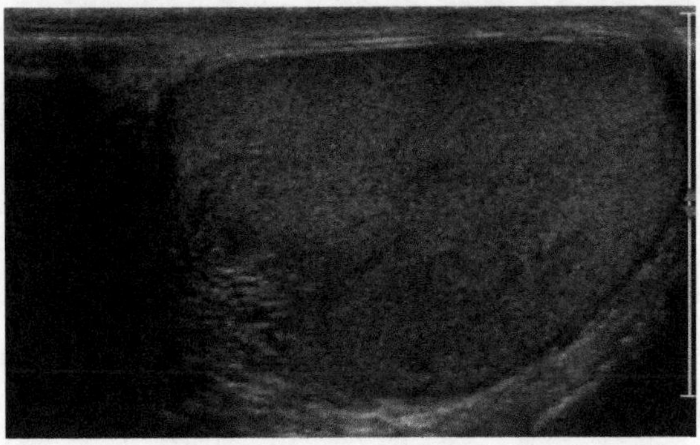

Figure 7. US Figure of rete testis ectasia with structure inhomogeneities in a CF patient

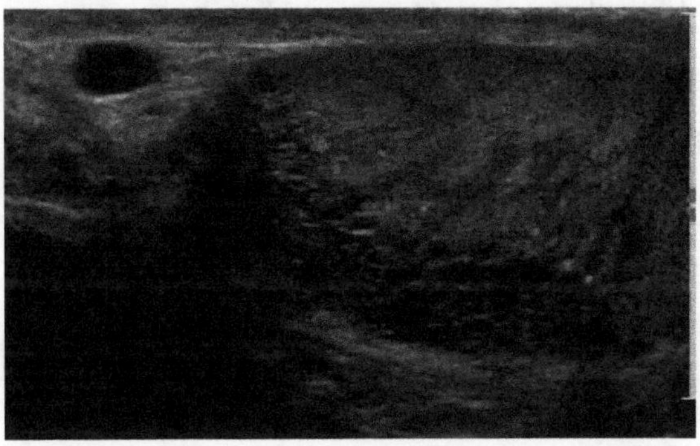

Figure 8. US Figure of rete testis ectasia with structure inhomogeneities with a little epididymal cyst in a CF patient

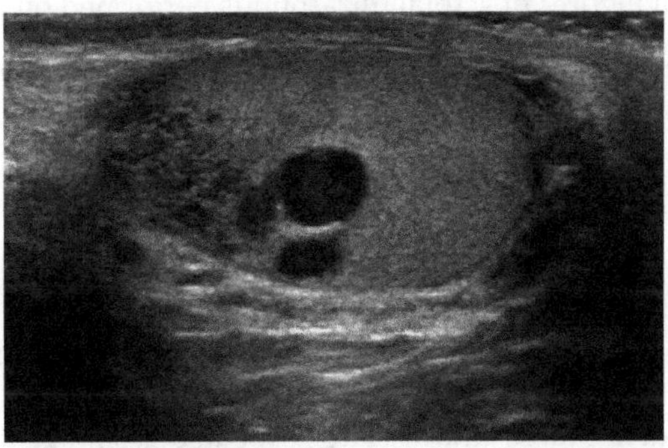

Figure 9. US Figure of intradidymal cysts (one with corpuscular content) in a CF patient

Nomenclature

CF = Cystic fibrosis

CFTR = Cystic fibrosis transmembrane conductance regulator

CBAVD = Congenital bilateral absence of the vas deferens

LH = Luteinizing hormone

FSH = Follicle stimulating hormone

US = ultrasounds

IVF = in vitro fertilization

ICSI = Intracytoplasmic sperm injection

PESA = Percutaneous epididymal sperm aspiration

MESA = Microsurgical epididymal sperm aspiration

TESA = Percutaneous testicular aspiration

TESE = Testicular sperm extraction

FVC = forced vital capacity

FEV1 = Forced expiratory volume in 1 second

PO2 = Partial pressure of oxygen

PCO2 = Partial pressure of carbon dioxide

BMI = Body mass index

Acknowledgements

We want to thank Professor Lorenzo Derchi (IRCCS A.O.U San Martino – IST, Radiology Unit, Genova) for the original Figures of scrotal ultrasounds performed on our CF patients.

We want to thank Dr. Mauro Costa (Ospedale Evangelico Internazionale, Reproduction Medicine Unit, Genova) for the collaboration.

Author details

Rosaria Casciaro*, Federico Cresta, Federica Favilli and Laura Minicucci

*Address all correspondence to: rosariacasciaro@ospedale-gaslini.ge.it

Pneumology Unit – Cystic Fibrosis Center, IRCCS Giannina Gaslini, Genova, Italy

References

[1] Quinton PM. Physiological basis of cystic fibrosis: a historical perspective. Physiol Rev 1999;79(Suppl):S3–22; PMID:9922374.

[2] Taussig LM, Lobeck CC, di Sant'Agnese PA, Ackerman DR, Kattwinkel J. Fertility in males with cystic fibrosis. N Engl J Med 1972;287:586–9; PMID:5055208.

[3] Holsclaw DS, Perlmutter AD, Jockin H, Shwachman H, Genital abnormalities in male patients with cystic fibrosis. J Urol 1971;106:568–74; PMID:4399160.

[4] Meschede D, Dworniczak B, Behre HM, Kliesch S, Claustres M, Nieschlag E, Horst J. CFTR gene mutations in men with bilateral ejaculatory-duct obstruction and anomalies of the seminal vesicles. Am J Hum Genet 1997;61:1200–2.

[5] van der Ven K, Messer L, van der Ven H, Jeyendran RS, Ober C. Cystic fibrosis mutation screening in healthy men with reduced sperm quality. Hum Reprod 1996;11:513–7; PMID:8671256.

[6] Trezise AE, Linder CC, Grieger D, Thompson EW, Meunier H, Griswold MD, Buchwald M. CFTR expression is regulated during both the cycle of the seminiferous epithelium and the oestrous cycle of rodents. Nat Genet 1993;3:157–64; PMID 7684647.

[7] Wang XF, Zhou CX, Shi QX, Yuan YY, Yu MK, Ajonuma LC, Ho LS, Lo PS, Tsang LL, Liu Y, et al. Involvement of CFTR in uterine bicarbonate secretion and the fertilizing capacity of sperm. Nat Cell Biol 2003; 5:902–6; PMID 14515130.

[8] Xu WM, Shi QX, Chen WY, Zhou CX, Ni Y, Rowlands DK, Yi Liu G, Zhu H, Ma ZG, Wang XF, et al. Cystic fibrosis transmembrane conductance regulator is vital to sperm fertilizing capacity and male fertility. Proc Natl Acad Sci USA 2007;104:9816–21; PMID:17519339.

[9] Durieu I, Bey-Omar F, Rollet J, et al. Diagnostic criteria for cystic fibrosis in men with congenital absence of vas deferens. Med (Baltimore) 1995;74:42–7.

[10] Blau H, Freud E, Mussaffi H, Werner M, Konen O, Rathaus V. Urogenital abnormalities in male children with cystic fibrosis. Arch Dis Child 2002 Aug;87(2):135–8.

[11] Wilschanski M, Corey M, Durie P, et al. Diversity of reproductive tract abnormalities in men with cystic fibrosis. JAMA 1996;276:607–8.

[12] Smith HC. Fertility in men with cystic fibrosis assessment, investigations and management. Ped Resp Rev 2010;11:80–3.

[13] Temple-Smith PD, Southwick GJ, Yates CA, Trounson AO, de Kretser DM. Human pregnancy by in vitro fertilization (IVF) using sperm aspirated from the epididymis. J in Vitro Fert Embryo Transf 1985;2:119–22.

[14] Silber SJ, Balmaceda J, Borrero C, Ord T, Asch R. Pregnancy with sperm aspiration from the proximal head of epididymis: a new treatment for congenital absence of the vas deferens. Fertil Steril 1988;50:525–8.

[15] Sherins RJ, Thorsell LP, Dorfmann A, Dennison-Lagos L, Calvo LP, Krysa L, Coulam CB, Schulman JD. Intracytoplasmic sperm injection facilitates pregnancies even in the most severe forms of male infertility. Fertil Steril 1995;Aug 64(2):369–75.

[16] Siegel B, Siegel S. Pregnancy and delivery in a patient with cystic fibrosis of the pancreas. Obstet Gynecol 1960;16:438–40.

[17] Grand RJ, Talamo RC, di San'Agnese PA, et al. Pregnancy in cystic fibrosis of the pancreas. JAMA 1966;195:993.

[18] Edenborough FP, Stableforth DE, Mackenzie WE. The outcome of 72 pregnancies in 55 women with cystic fibrosis in United Kingdom 1977–1986. BJOG 2000;254–61.

[19] Gilljam M, Antoniou M, Shin J, et al. Pregnancy in cystic fibrosis: fetal and maternal outcomes. Chest 2000;118:86–91.

[20] Cystic fibrosis foundation. Patient registry: annual data report 2007. Bethesda, Maryland.

[21] Johannesson M, Csemiczky G, Landgren BM, Hjelte L, Gotllieb C. Female patients with cystic fibrosis suffer from reproductive endocrinological disorders despite good clinical status. Hum Reprod 1998;13:2092–7.

[22] Edenborough FP. Women with cystic fibrosis and their potential for reproduction. Thorax 2001;Aug 56(8):649–55.

[23] Hodges CA, Palmert MR, Drumm ML. Infertility in females with cystic fibrosis is multifactorial: evidence from mouse models. Endocrin. 2008;Jun 149(6):2790–7. DOI: 10.1210/en.2007-1581. Epub 2008 Mar 6.

[24] Whitty JE, Cystic fibrosis in pregnancy. Clin Obstet Gynecol 2010;53(2):369–76.

[25] Goss CH, Rubenfeld GD, Otto K, et al. The effect of pregnancy on survival in women with cystic fibrosis. Chest 2003;124:1460–8.

[26] McMullen AH, Pasta DJ, Frederick PD, et al. Impact of pregnancy on women with cystic fibrosis. Chest 2006;129:3.

[27] Lau EMT, Moriarty C, Ogle R, Bye PT. Pregnancy and cystic fibrosis. Ped Resp Rev 11(2010):90–4.

[28] Edenborough FP, Stableforth DE, Webb AK. Outcome of pregnancy in women with cystic fibrosis. Thorax 1995;50:170–4.

[29] Hilman BC, Aitken ML, Constantinescu M. Pregnancy in patients with cystic fibrosis. Clin Obstet Gynecol 1996;39:70–86.

[30] Tanser SJ, Hodson ME, Geddes DM. Case report of death during pregnancy in patients with cystic fibrosis: three out of four patients were colonized by Burkholderia cepacia. Respir Med 2000;94:1004.

[31] Bose D, Yentis SM, Fauvel NJ. Caeserean section in a parturient with respiratory failure caused by cystic fibrosis. Anaesthesia 1997;52:578–82.

[32] Gyi KM, Hodson ME, Yacoub MY. Pregnancy in cystic fibrosis lung transplant recipients: case series and review. J Cyst Fibros 2006;5:171–6.

[33] Chetty SP, Shaffer BL, Norton ME. Management of pregnancy in women with genetic disorders: Part 2: Inborn errors of metabolism, cystic fibrosis, neurofibromatosis type 1, and Turner syndrome in pregnancy. Obstet Gynecol Surv. 2011;Dec 66(12): 765–76.

[34] Edenborough FP, Borgo G, Knoop C, Lannefors L, et al. Guidelines for the management of pregnancy in women with cystic fibrosis. J Cyst Fibros 2008; 7:S2–32.

5

Medications to Enhance CFTR Activity

Terry W. Chin

Abstract

Since the basic defect in cystic fibrosis (CF) involves a defective cell surface protein controlling chloride channel transport across cell membranes, medications which are developed to enhance the cystic fibrosis transmembrane conductance regulator (CFTR) protein should result in improvement in patients with CF. The presence of over 2000 genetic mutations have made these efforts difficult. However, a classification scheme of these mutations has allowed three basic approaches: to bypass missense mutations by having the cellular translation machinery read through the premature stop codon, to enhance the "gating" function of the CFTR protein on the cell surface, and to correct a defective CFTR protein "trafficking" though the cytoplasm to be inserted properly in the cell membrane. This chapter will review clinical trials using drugs which are designed to enhance CFTR protein activity.

Keywords: Cystic fibrosis, CFTR, CFTR modulators, CFTR potentiators, CFTR correctors, VC-770, ivacaftor, VX-809, lumacaftor, VX-661, PTC124, ataluren

1. Introduction

The identification of the genetic defect in CF allowed the classification of CFTR mutations into six types of mutations. The over 2000 mutations which has been described can be placed in one of these classes: Class I mutations, which may be the result of the genetic mutation resulting in a stop codon or a shift in the reading frame in the messenger RNA which eventually results in a downstream stop codon, do not produce a complete CFTR protein. Class ii mutations result in an altered CFTR protein which is degraded in the endoplasmic reticulum and/or Golgi systems within the cell. Some proteins may be able to make it to the cell surface and have variable levels of function (or Class III, IV, or VI effects). Class III mutations result in amino acid substitutions which affect how the CFTR protein is regulated on the cell surface, usually decreasing the channel opening. Class IV mutations result in amino acid substitutions which affect how the CFTR protein functions in its conduction of chloride ions. Class V mutations result in decreased production of normal functioning CFTR protein. Therefore, there is a reduced amount of normal CFTR protein on the cell surface. Finally, class VI mutations are those which affect the stability of CFTR.

Awareness of the types of genetic mutations affecting the normal functioning of the CFTR protein has resulted in searches for treatments directed at various CFTR dysfunctions. This chapter will review recent attempts to develop treatments specific for the various classes of mutations.

2. Premature termination codons

In approximately 10% of patients with CF, the responsible mutation results in a nonsense mutation that terminates the CFTR protein production due to a premature stop codon in the CFTR messenger ribonucleic acid (mRNA). The resultant truncated protein cannot properly transport chloride ion across the membrane. PTC Therapeutics, Inc. had discovered a small molecule drug ataluren (PTC124®) which enables the mRNA containing the premature stop codon to be read through the ribosome. The molecule is a 1,2,4-oxadiazole with a molecular weight of 284 Daltons. Using cell culture as well as a mouse model of CF, investigators determined that oral administration of ataluren was effective as long plasma concentrations in the range of 2 to 10 mcg/mL will result in functional CFTR activity. [1, 2] There was no evidence of nonspecific read through of normal stop codons. It did not appear to be teratogenic in rats and rabbits. However, there did appear to be inhibition of cytochrome P450 (CYP2C9) at therapeutic concentrations of ataluren. Therefore, monitoring blood levels of medications which are primarily metabolized by this enzyme (such as warfarin or phenytoin) may be needed clinically.

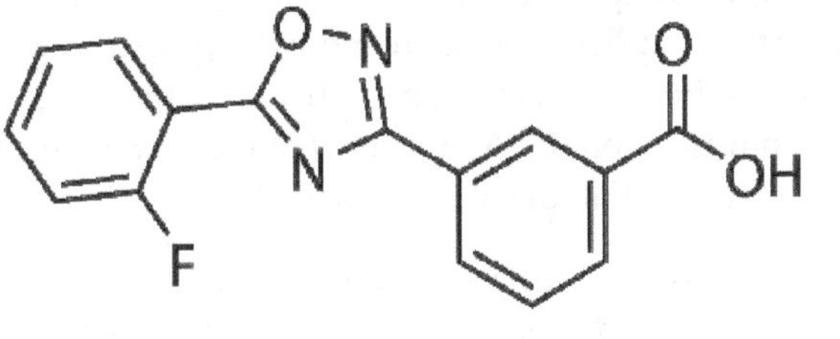

Figure 1. Structural formula of atalaren

Phase 1 studies indicate that serum ataluren levels of 2 to 10 mcg/mL can be achieved with a three times per day (TID) dosing schedule. Since administration with meals can result in prolonged levels in the blood, dosing after a meal appears to be desired.

Phase 2a studies have been conducted in 30 children and 47 adult patients in the United States, Israel, and Europe. [3, 4, 5] Using transepithelial potential difference (TEPD), which assesses transepithelial chloride conductance, as the primary outcome measure, these studies found statistically significant improvements. Pulmonary function testing also showed positive trends with decreased sputum volume and thickness, easier elimination of sputum, decreased coughing, and increased quality of life. There were no serious adverse drug effects. Phase 2a extension study looked at a 3-month administration of ataluren and confirmed its effectiveness and safety. [6] Optimal responses appear to be with doses of 10-, 10-, 20-mg/kg on the TID schedule and were seen with numerous different missense mutations.

The encouraging results of these preliminary studies prompted PTC Therapeutics to conduct a Phase 3, randomized, double-blind, placebo-controlled study to look at the effects of 48 weeks of therapy on pulmonary function and clinical symptoms in CF patients with the appropriate mutation. Over 400 patients were enrolled and showed positive trends favoring ataluren over placebo with an increase in percent of predicted for forced expiratory volume in 1 second (FEV1) and decreased pulmonary exacerbation rate. [7] A subgroup of patients who were not receiving inhaled antibiotics (primarily tobramycin) showed an even greater improvement on ataluren. The study continued to show the drug was well tolerated and had a good safety profile. There were some cases of creatinine elevation which were associated with the combination of potential nephrotoxic antibiotics with ataluren. These results resulted in conducting another international, multicenter study in which patients will not be allowed to receive treatment with chronic inhaled aminoglycosides (such as tobramycin or TOBI) in early 2015. The aim is to randomize approximately 208 patients who will receive either ataluren or placebo for 48 weeks.

3. Potentiators

The presence of some CFTR on the cell surface in mutation classes III, IV, and VI suggests another approach may be to increase the "gating" function of these protein molecules. The most common gating mutation is G551D, a missense mutation that results in the replacement of a glycine for an aspartic acid at position 551 of the CFTR protein. The resulting CFTR protein is present at the cell surface but does not open and close properly, which is called defective channel gating. The effort to find an effective "potentiator" of the channel opening has resulted in the Federal Drug Administration (FDA) approval of the first medication which modulates the function of CFTR, ivacaftor (Kalydeco), in January 2012.

Ivacaftor (or VX-770) was developed by Vertex Pharmaceuticals, Inc., to potentiate the action of the mutated CFTR on the cell surface. It has a molecular weight of 392 and a molecular formula of $C_{24}H_{28}N_2O_3$. Studies with recombinant cell lines with G551D-CFTR indicated that VX-770 did result in increased total chloride transport by greater than 10%. [8] There was evidence to indicate that it acted directly on the mutated CFTR protein to keep the channel open. It apparently has similar activity on other mutant CFTR forms resulting from other CFTR gating mutations. However, since the G551D mutation affects about 5% of all CF patients and

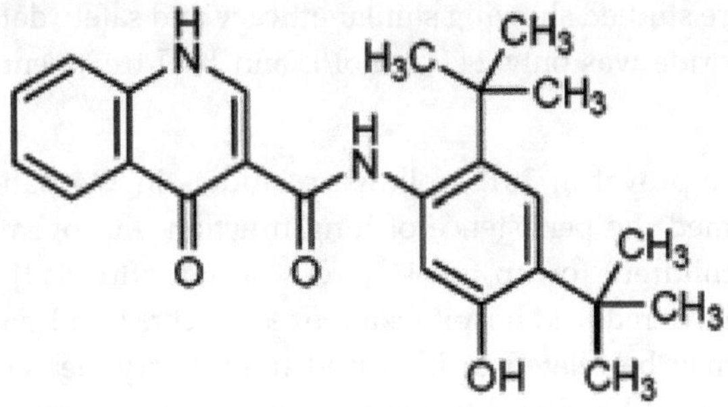

Figure 2. Structural formula of ivacaftor

is the most common gating mutation, initial studies focused on patients with this particular mutation.

Phase 1 studies indicated that ivacaftor is primarily metabolized in the liver and moderate hepatic impairment may reduce its elimination. Since *in vitro* studies indicated that ivacaftor is a substrate of CYP3A4/5 and therefore, strong (e.g., ketoconazole) and moderate (e.g., fluconazole) CYP3A inhibitors as well as strong CYP3A inducers (e.g., rifampin) will affect ivacaftor's metabolism. A detailed list of the numerous drug interactions is found in the package insert of ivacaftor (Kalydeco®) (see http://www.accessdata.fda.gov/drugsatfda_docs/label/2012/203188lbl.pdf).

An initial phase 2 study by Accurso found that the safety profile of ivacaftor in adult patients with at least one G551D mutation was excellent for a wide variety of daily doses (from 50 mg to 500 mg for 2 to 4 weeks). An improvement in FEV1 and drop in sweat chloride were also noted (although these were not primary end points of the study). [9] This prompted two randomized, placebo-controlled, double blind studies eventually resulting in FDA approval. Ivacaftor 150 mg twice daily for 48 weeks was studied in 167 patients 12 years or older with at least one G551D mutation. There was a 10.6% improvement in predicted FEV1 from baseline versus placebo. Additionally, a 55% reduction in pulmonary exacerbation was also observed. Sweat chloride levels dropped to a mean of 47.8 mmol/L compared with 100.0 mmol/L in the placebo group. There was improvement in quality of life measurements as well as a more significant increase in weight gain (4.1 kg increase) in those receiving ivacaftor. [10] An additional pediatric study of 52 patients 6 to 12 years of age showed a 12.5% improvement in FEV1 and a 2.8 kg increase in weight. A decrease in sweat chloride of 54 mmol/L was also seen. [11] In both studies, the incidence of adverse events was similar in both treated and placebo groups.

Similar results were observed in studies examining non-G551D gating mutations. [12] These 36 patients also showed significant improvements in FEV1, sweat chloride measurements, changes in BMI, and quality of life indices. Therefore, the FDA also approved ivacaftor for G178R, S549N, S549R, G551S, G970R, G1244E, S1251N, G1349D, and S1255P mutations in February 2014. Finally, in December 2014, one additional mutation, R117H, was added by the FDA to the list of approved CF mutations for ivacaftor administration after 69 patients greater than 6 years of age were studied showing similar efficacy and safety data. [13] However, their decrease in sweat chloride was only 24.0 mmol/L and BMI treatment differences were not significant.

Since its initial FDA approval in 2012, follow-up studies in 144 patients with the G551D mutation have confirmed the persistence of lung function improvement (9.4% increase in adults and 10.3% in children) for up to 144 weeks on ivacaftor. [14] Additionally, treated patients continued to have reduced hospitalizations and decreased Pseudomonas aeruginosa culture rates, which may be related to increased mucociliary clearance. [15] There was a reduced rate of decline in FEV1. The absolute increase in weight was 5.1 kg in adults and 14.8 kg in children after almost 3 years, indicating that there was an increased rate of weight gain and improved BMI. [16] Not all the nutritional improvement may be attributed to improved lung function since treated patients also showed a normalizing in small bowel pH which may have improved pancreatic enzyme function.[14]

Although the FDA approval was for patients greater than 6 years of age, Davies et al. found ivacaftor to be well-tolerated in 34 children between 6 months and 5 years of age at doses 50 to 75 mg twice a day. [17] They also showed a significant decrease in sweat chloride with a mean drop of 44 mmol/L, and many patients showed improvement in pancreatic function with increases in stool elastase. However, 14.7% showed a higher rate of elevated liver function test results indicating the need to especially monitor these younger patients.

4. Correctors

Most patients with CF have the F508del mutation in which the defective CFTR protein has defective folding and processing in the endoplasmic reticulum, resulting in minimal amounts of CFTR at the cell surface. After screening a large number of molecules, Vertex Pharmaceuticals found two in which the CFTR molecule appears to be "corrected" in its "trafficking" through the cytoplasmic to the cell membrane. Importantly, the F508del-CFTR corrected by VX-809 (subsequently named lumacaftor) appears to have biochemical and functional characteristics similar to normal CFTR such as biochemical susceptibility to proteolysis, time in the plasma membrane, and single-channel openness. [18]

Although there was a statistically significant reduction in sweat chloride values, no effect was seen in CFTR function in the nasal epithelium as measured by nasal potential difference (NPD) or in lung function as measured by FEV1. Therefore, although it appeared to be safe and was well tolerated at all doses, there did not appear to be any significant effect on CFTR function in upper and lower respiratory tracts. Indeed, a phase 2 study with 140 patients did not show any difference in lung function although there was a slight reduction in sweat chloride of 2.9 mmol/L which was barely significant ($p=0.04$).

VX-661 is another corrector with very similar structure to lumacaftor (see Figures 3 and 4). In a Phase 2 study of 128 adult patients with homozygous F508del mutation in whom four doses of VX-661 (10, 30, 100, and 150 mg) dosed once daily were given either alone or with ivacaf-

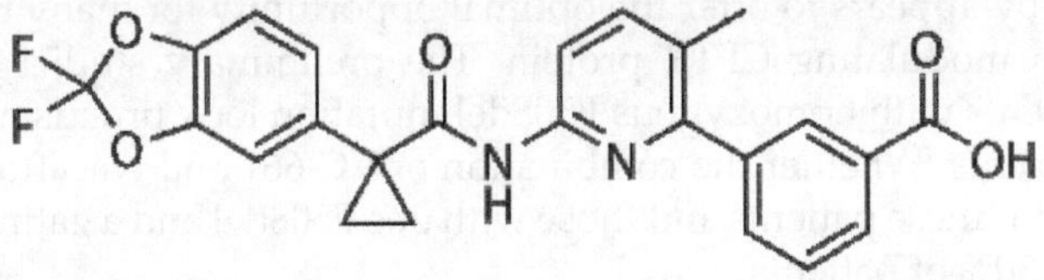

Figure 3. Structural formula of lumacaftor (VX-809)

tor150 mg twice a day for 28 days. Interim results found decreases in sweat chloride with both treatments. However, significant increases in FEV1 were found in both doses 100 mg and 150 mg of VX-661 with ivacaftor at 9% and 7.5% over baseline, respectively. [19]

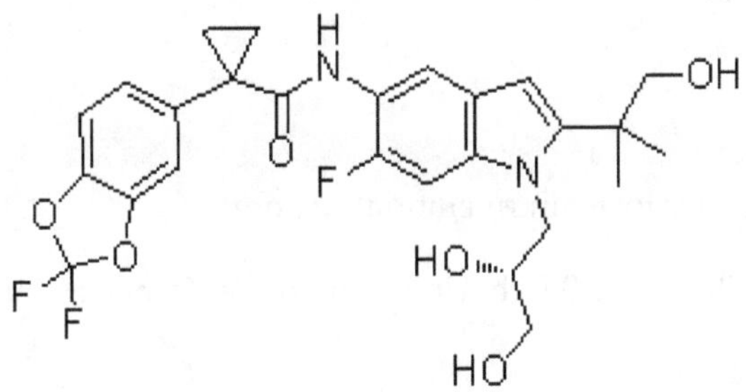

Figure 4. Please Add Caption

[20] There were significant improvements in the mean absolute change in percent predicted of FEV1 and BMI after 24 weeks. Because there appeared to be no difference in two doses studied, the submission to the FDA selected lumacaftor 400 mg BID plus ivacaftor 250 mg BID. An open label roll-over study is still in progress and expected to continue for another 24 weeks.

Patients receiving just VX-661 monotherapy in the Phase 2 study also did not show any improvement, further supporting the strategy of combining a corrector and potentiator in treating patients with F508del mutation. In 2015, Vertex is starting a series of large-scale Phase 3 studies examining the efficacy of the combined therapy with VC-661 and ivacaftor in patients with one or two copies of the F508del mutation.

5. Conclusions

The capability of molecules to enhance CFTR protein activity offers potential new treatment options for patients with CF. Long-term follow-up studies on ivacaftor, the first CFTR modulator to obtain FDA approval, look very promising. However, the drawback with these targeted therapies is the wide range of CFTR dysfunction seen in CF. Expanding the use of ivacaftor to nine other gating mutations only benefit about 10% of the total CF patient population.

Combination therapy appears to offer the optimal opportunity for many more patients with CF to benefit from modulating CFTR protein. The preliminary studies on ivacaftor with lumacaftor for patients with homozygous F508del mutation look promising and may benefit another 50% of patients. Whether the combination of VC-661 and ivacaftor is more effective remains to be seen for these patients and those with one F508del and a gating mutation, which represents another 30% of patients.

Although Vertex has been the first to develop chemicals which correct trafficking of F508del-CFTR and restoring its activity, other companies such as Norvartis are also actively testing other molecules, such as picolinamide-based compounds. [21] It is hoped that with increased competition from other companies, the high cost of these medications can be lessened.

Author details

Terry W. Chin

Address all correspondence to: tchin@memorialcare.org

Miller Children's Hospital, Long Beach, University of California, Irvine, USA

References

[1] Du M, Liu X, Welch EM, et al. PTC124 is an orally bioavailable compound that promotes suppression of the human CFTR-G542X nonsense allele in a CF mouse model. Proc Natl Acad Sci USA. 2008 Feb 12;105(6):2064-9.

[2] Targets genetic disorders caused by nonsense mutations. Nature. 2007 May 3;447(7140):87-91.

[3] Kerem E, Hirawat S, Armoni S, et al. Effectiveness of PTC124 treatment of cystic fibrosis caused by nonsense mutations: aprospective phase II trial. Lancet. 2008 Aug 30;372(9640):719-27. Epub 2008 Aug 20.

[4] Clancy JP, Konstan MW, Rowe SM, et al. A Phase 2 study of PTC124 in cystic fibrosis patients harboring premature stop mutations. Pediatr Pulmonol 2006;40 (Suppl29): 301 (abst #269).

[5] Sermet-Gaudelus I, De Boeck K, Casimir G, et al. Children with nonsense-mutation mediated cystic fibrosis respond to investigational treatment with PTC124. Pediatr Pulmonol. 2008 Oct;43(Suppl S31):313 (abst #316).

[6] Kerem E, YaakovY, Armoni S, et al. PTC124 induces time-dependent improvements in chloride conductance and clinical parameters in patients with nonsense-mutation-mediated cystic fibrosis. Pediatr Pulmonol. 2008 Oct;43(Suppl S31):294 (abst #266).

[7] Rowe SM, Sermet-Gaudelus I, Konstan M, et al. Results of the Phase 3 Study of Ataluren in Nonsense Mutation Cystic Fibrosis (nmCF). Pediatr Pulmonol. 2012 Sep; 47(S35): 290 (abst #193).

[8] Van Goor F, Hadida S, Groothuis PD, et al. Rescue of CF airway epithelial cell function in vitro by a CFTR potentiator, VX-770. Proc Natl Acad Sci U S A. 2009;106(44): 18825-30.

[9] Please Add Reference

[10] Please Add Reference

[11] Davies JC1, Wainwright CE, Canny GJ, et al. Efficacy and safety of ivacaftor in patients aged 6 to 11 years with cystic fibrosis with a G551D mutation. Am J RespirCrit Care Med. 2013 Jun 1;187(11):1219-25. doi: 10.1164/rccm.201301-0153OC.

[12] De Boeck K, Munck A, Walker S, et al. Efficacy and safety of ivacaftor in patients with cystic fibrosis and a non-G551D gating mutation. J Cyst Fibros. 2014 Dec;13(6): 674-80. doi: 10.1016/j.jcf.2014.09.005. Epub 2014 Sep 26.

[13] Moss RB, Flume PA, Elborn JS, et al. Ivacaftor treatment in patientswith cystic fibrosis who have an R117H-CFTR mutation, the KONDUCT study. J Cyst Fibros 2014;13(S2):S44 (abst WS23.6).

[14] McKone EF, Borowitz D2, Drevinek P3, et al. Long-term safety and efficacy of ivacaftor in patients with cystic fibrosis who have the Gly551Asp-CFTR mutation: a phase 3, open-label extension study (PERSIST). Lancet Respir Med. 2014 Nov;2(11):902-10. doi: 10.1016/S2213-2600(14)70218-8. Epub 2014 Oct 9.

[15] Rowe SM, Heltshe SL, Gonska T, et al. Clinical Mechanism of the Cystic Fibrosis Transmembrane Conductance Regulator Potentiator Ivacaftor in G551D-mediated Cystic Fibrosis. Am J RespirCrit Care Med 2014;190(2):175-184. doi: 10.1164/rccm. 201404-0703OC.

[16] Sawicki GS, McKone EF, Pasta DJ, et al.The effect of ivacaftor on weight over three years in patients with CF and a G551K-CFTR mutation. Pediatr Pulmonol 2014; 49(S38):289 (abst #207).

[17] Davies JC, Robertson S, Green Y, et al. An open-label study of the safety, pharmacokinetics, and pharmodynamics of ivacaftor in patients aged 2 to 5 years with CF and a CFTR-gating mutation: the kiwi study. Pediatr Pulmonol 2014; 49(S38):286 (abst #200).

[18] Van Goor F, Hadida S, Grootenhuis PD, et al. Correction of the F508del-CFTR protein processing defect in vitro by the investigational drug VX-809. Proc Natl Acad Sci U S A. 2011 Nov 15;108(46):18843-8. doi: 10.1073/pnas.1105787108. Epub 2011 Oct 5.

[19] Donaldson S, Pilewski J, M. Griese M, et al. VX-661, an investigational CFTR corrector, in combination with ivacaftor, a CFTR potentiator, in patients with CF and ho-

mozygous for the F508Del-CFTR mutation: Interim analysis. J Cystic Fibrosis 2013 June;12(Suppl 1):S14 (abst WS7.3).

[20] Ramsey B, Boyle MP, Elborn J, et al. Effect of lumacaftor in combination with ivacaftor in patients with cystic fibrosis who are homozygous for F508del-CFTR: Transport study. Pediatr Pulmonol 2014;49(S38):305 (abs # 250).

[21] Norman P. Novel picolinamide-based cystic fibrosis transmembrane regulator modulators: evaluation of WO2013038373, WO2013038376, WO2013038381, WO2013038386 and WO2013038390. Expert OpinTher Pat. 2014 Jul;24(7):829-37. doi: 10.1517/13543776.2014.876412. Epub 2014 Jan 7.

6

Outcome Measures for Respiratory Physiotherapy in Cystic Fibrosis – Challenges and Advances

Alda Marques, Joana Cruz, Cristina Jácome and Ana Oliveira

Abstract

Respiratory physiotherapy is part of the routine management of patients with cystic fibrosis. It normally consists of airway clearance techniques and exercise training. The evidence of such interventions has been questioned. Nevertheless, the lack of evidence should not be interpreted as lack of benefit. Instead, attention to methodological issues, such as the selection of the outcome measures, is needed, as they may hamper the establishment of the effectiveness of respiratory physiotherapy techniques. Hence, this chapter presents and discusses the strengths and weaknesses of conventional and emerging outcome measures possibly to be used (i) in clinical practice before, during and after each session of respiratory physiotherapy to monitor its effectiveness; (ii) before and after the respiratory physiotherapy treatment (i.e., normally characterised by weeks of intervention) and (iii) in applied research in respiratory physiotherapy used in the management for cystic fibrosis. A comprehensive overview of the available outcome measures is provided, with particular emphasis on their strengths and limitations that should be recognised when interpreting the results.

Keywords: Respiratory physiotherapy, outcome measures, cystic fibrosis

1. Introduction

Respiratory physiotherapy is a non-pharmacological treatment commonly provided to patients with cystic fibrosis (CF) [1]. According to international guidelines, respiratory physiotherapy is a key element of care for patients with CF, as it aims at both rehabilitation and prevention [2]. Specifically, respiratory physiotherapy is used to deal with the progressive loss of pulmonary function accompanied by symptoms of cough, excessive sputum production, dyspnoea, exercise intolerance, reduced functionality and impaired quality of life. To respond to these multiple problems and needs, respiratory physiotherapy involves a range of strategies and techniques, such as airway clearance, exercise training and breathlessness management, which have an overall aim of reducing the progression of the disease [3, 4].

However, there is a lack of evidence to suggest the superiority of one technique over the other [5] and to determine which strategies promote the adherence of this population to regular physical activity [6]. Nevertheless, the lack of evidence does not mean lack of benefit. Instead, methodological issues, such as the selection of the outcome measures, may hamper the establishment of the effectiveness of the respiratory physiotherapy techniques.

Respiratory physiotherapists use several outcome measures to monitor and evaluate their interventions. Most of the clinically available outcome measures are not specific for the physiotherapy intervention employed and may be affected by other factors. This means that there are no gold standard outcome measures specifically related to respiratory physiotherapy interventions. Thus, in all areas of respiratory physiotherapy, one of the barriers to generate evidence has been the lack of accurate, reliable, sensitive and valid outcome measures. To overcome this problematic issue, new measures have been emerging.

This chapter starts by providing an overview of the problem. It then presents and discusses the strengths and weaknesses of the commonly used clinical outcome measures and other measures that have been gaining interest in the assessment and monitoring of respiratory physiotherapy interventions in CF. The chapter ends with a brief conclusion. A comprehensive overview of the available outcome measures is sought to be provided, with particular emphasis on their strengths and limitations that should be recognised when interpreting the results.

2. Outcome measures for respiratory physiotherapy

Respiratory physiotherapy in CF involves a wide range of interventions and among them airway clearance techniques and exercise training are recognised as the most important. The primary aim of airway clearance techniques is to relieve the airway obstruction by promoting the normal mucociliary clearance mechanism of the lungs and facilitating expectoration, thus reducing the risk of infection and inflammation. A variety of airway clearance techniques have been developed. Some involve airway oscillation, some are independently performed and others require electricity or physical assistance [5]. Exercise training is advocated as an important package of care delivered to patients with CF [5], since exercise intolerance has been associated with reduced survival [45]. Observed benefits of exercise training include slow pulmonary function decline [46], reduced dyspnoea and improved exercise capacity, muscle strength and health-related quality of life (HRQoL) [47].

Although adhering to airway clearance techniques [7] and exercise training is generally regarded as beneficial for patients with CF, there is no consensus about the superiority of one technique over the other [5]. Methodological issues, such as the underpowered samples or the selection of the outcome measures, may explain this lack of evidence and thus hamper the establishment of the effectiveness of these interventions. A clear example of this issue has been the use of forced expiratory volume in the first second (FEV_1) as a gold standard to assess the impact of the mentioned interventions for many years, which is currently considered as not a sensitive measure to be used in respiratory physiotherapy [5].

Most of the clinically available outcome measures are not specifically related to the physiotherapy intervention employed and may be affected by other factors. This means that there is no gold standard outcome measure that is specifically related to respiratory physiotherapy interventions. Moreover, there are many doubts about the accuracy, reliability, sensitivity and validity of the current measures. Given this problematic situation, several researchers have been investigating the potential of other objective, simple and non-invasive measures to be used as outcome measures in respiratory physiotherapy.

The outcome measures most commonly used by respiratory physiotherapists to monitor their interventions and evaluate their practice are: FEV_1, respiratory sounds, sputum weight, measures of oxygenation, chest radiography, dyspnoea, exercise capacity and HRQoL. Computerised respiratory sounds, lung ultrasound, fat-free mass, inspiratory muscle strength and endurance, physical activity and burden of treatment are some examples of these emerging outcome measures to assess and monitor respiratory physiotherapy interventions in CF. Each one of these outcome measures, their strengths and weaknesses are presented in detail below according to their novelty in the field (i.e., conventional and emerging).

2.1. Conventional outcome measures

2.1.1. Forced expiratory volume in the first second

The most common pulmonary function test performed to assess respiratory physiotherapy interventions is the forced spirometry, i.e., the volume and/or flow of air that can be inhaled and exhaled as a function of time. The procedure consists in three distinct phases: (1) maximal inspiration followed by an expiration at functional residual capacity; (2) a "blast" of exhalation; and (3) continued complete exhalation until the end of test [8]. First, the patient should exhale until he or she reaches the functional residual capacity and then be instructed to inhale rapidly and completely. In this phase, the mouthpiece should be placed in the patient's mouth and indications should be given for the patient to blow as much and as fast as possible and to keep blowing until totally emptying the lungs. Spirometry has been described as a cost-effective, simple, reliable, valid and easy-to-interpret bedside measure [8]. The most used pulmonary function parameter is the forced expiratory volume in the first second (FEV_1), followed by the forced vital capacity (FVC) and the ratio between FEV_1/FVC. Measurements are taken considering patient's gender, age, height, weight and race and are then compared with predicted values.

Spirometry, namely FEV_1, has been used to assess the effectiveness of respiratory physiotherapy interventions. However, contradictory findings have emerged. Pfleger et al. (1992) found significant improvements in FEV_1 after autogenic drainage and high-pressure PEP-mask (n=14,

Cohen's d_z 0.09 and 0.22) [9]. Jarad, Powell and Smith (2010) reported a statistically significant reduction in FEV1 following hydro-acoustic therapy (n=19, Cohen's dz=0.12) or flutter (n=19, Cohen's dz=0.06) [10]. Nevertheless, these changes returned to baseline on the second study day [10].

In two recent reviews where conventional physiotherapy [11] and the active cycle of breathing techniques (ACBT) [12] were compared with other airway clearance techniques, no significant differences were observed between the techniques in terms of pulmonary function measured with spirometry [11]. Nevertheless, when oscillating devices for airway clearance were used, significant results were observed in pulmonary function, the FEV_1 being the primary outcome measure more frequently reported [13].

Findings in the literature about the effectiveness of respiratory physiotherapy interventions in CF remain controversial when FEV_1 is considered as the outcome measure. This is in part due to the fact that accuracy and sensitivity of spirometry depends on many factors that are difficult to control and not related to the intervention itself. Some examples of these factors are the transducer characteristics, presence or absence of an in-line filter, presence or absence of a display, patient's mood and motivation to cooperate, relationship between the patient and the technician, among others. Therefore, spirometry might be unsuitable or its reliability may be affected in a number of situations, for example if the equipment or settings change, if patients are unwilling or unable to collaborate (e.g. children, people with dementia), or if pain or discomfort is present. Hence, this measure should be routinely used to characterise the pulmonary function of patients with CF, but not to assess the effectiveness of respiratory physiotherapy interventions.

2.1.2. *Respiratory sounds*

Lung auscultation, performed with conventional stethoscopes, is one of the oldest and most used techniques to diagnose and monitor respiratory diseases [14, 15]. It consists in acquiring acoustic signals from the lung structures during spontaneous or controlled volume or flow breathing, and classifying the respiratory sounds as normal or abnormal (e.g., adventitious respiratory sounds, such as crackles and wheezes) [15]. Auscultation is recognised as an efficient and safe method for the early detection of respiratory diseases as it is non-invasive, practical, low cost and easy to apply in all clinical settings and patients, irrespective of patients' age and severity of the disease [14-16].

The efficiency of this method depends on the hearing ability of the health professionals [17], their capacity to memorise different sound patterns [18] and on the quality of the acoustic properties of the stethoscope being used [17]. Considering these limitations and subjectivity, reliability studies have been performed. In CF there are no reliability studies using conventional stethoscopes. However, in other respiratory diseases, poor to fair correlations between different raters have been reported, either in taped recorded sounds (kappa=0.26 and coefficient of reliability of less than 60%) [19, 20] and real-time auscultation ($-0.02<\text{kappa}<0.77$) [21]. Using digital stethoscopes, one study conducted in adult patients with CF assessed the inter-rater agreement between real-time manual annotation of respiratory sounds and automatic detection of respiratory sounds through a computerised system [22]. Poor to moderate correlations were found (–0.20<kappa<0.60) [22]. Similar results were found in children with respiratory diseases (–0.08<kappa<0.86) [23–25]. Direct comparisons between conventional and digital stethoscopes showed that, although digital stethoscopes have a better sound quality [26], the performance of health professionals to detect respiratory sounds is not enhanced by its use [27].

It is also important to note that, in all the studies, the recognition of crackles was always less accurate than the recognition of wheezes. As respiratory sounds in CF are mainly characterised by the presence of crackles [28] and conventional auscultation has provided poor reliability results, particularly for detection of crackles, it can be concluded that respiratory sounds are not a reliable outcome measure for CF diagnosis and monitoring. Also due to its poor reliability, conventional auscultation has not been used as an outcome measure for respiratory physiotherapy interventions in recent research [7]. Nevertheless, due to its simplicity and wide availability in all clinical settings, it is still recurrently used in clinical practice by physiotherapists to monitor patients with CF and to define therapeutic approaches [3]. Despite these limitations, the advantages of using lung auscultation should not be overlooked, and currently significant research efforts are being conducted to create equipment capable of overcoming the subjectivity associated with conventional auscultation while preserving its main advantages (i.e., portability, patients' minimal cooperation and cost-effectiveness) [16].

2.1.3. Sputum weight

Mucus is transported from the bronchial airways towards the exterior by mucociliary clearance, spontaneous cough and through a range of airway clearance techniques, such as directed huffs and coughs. Subsequently, secretions are either expectorated or swallowed. During respiratory physiotherapy sessions, patients are encouraged to expectorate to a cup. Sputum volume or weight can then be used as an outcome measure for respiratory physiotherapy.

While sputum volume has shown to be difficult to determine with precision, sputum weight (either dry or wet) has shown to be more accurate [29]. In a recent Cochrane review on the effectiveness of respiratory physiotherapy interventions in respiratory diseases, five of the eight studies used sputum weight as an outcome measure, out of which four were conducted in patients with CF [7]. Mortensen et al. (1991) found that patients expectorated 8–8.6g of sputum weight after airway clearance techniques and 0 g during a control day (range 0–2.1 g) [30]. In Pfeger et al. (1992), the mean weight of expectorated mucus with spontaneous cough was approximately 17g whereas with airway clearance techniques ranged from 34 to 45g (n=14) [9]. Although no mean and standard deviation was provided, Rossman et al. (1982) also found a higher volume of expectorated secretions during the different forms of chest physiotherapy compared to a control session (n=6) [31]. However, Jarad et al. (2010) found no significant differences in wet or dry sputum weight between a positive expiratory pressure (PEP) device (flutter) or a placebo [10].

Another study conducted by Osman et al. (2010) compared high-frequency chest wall oscillation with conventional airway clearance techniques in 29 patients with CF using wet sputum weight. Expectorated sputum in a single session was significantly different between the techniques ($p<0.001$; Cohen's $d_z=0.72$) [32].

The problem with sputum weight remains that the lack of expectoration during respiratory physiotherapy techniques does not mean that airway clearance techniques are not effective. It is very common to expectorate after respiratory physiotherapy sessions or to swallow secretions even during the session, which means that sputum weight expectorated during a session may underestimate the effect of airway clearance techniques. On the other hand, expectoration may be contaminated with saliva [30]. Sputum weight can, therefore, be both over- and under-estimated and it is not surprising that contradictory findings have been found in the literature.

Although simple to collect and measure, sputum collected during and following the treatments is not considered a reliable measure of alveolar recruitment, airway clearance or even sensitive to small changes. In fact, this outcome measure has been frequently questioned [29, 30, 33–35] and is no longer considered as a valid outcome measure for studies in airway clearance techniques [36].

2.1.4. *Measures of oxygenation*

Blood gas measurements are used to evaluate a person's lung function and acid–base balance, i.e., it measures the amount of oxygen and carbon dioxide that is in the blood and determines its levels of acidity (pH). The test results provide information about the partial pressure of oxygen (PaO_2), partial pressure of carbon dioxide ($PaCO_2$) and hydrogen ion activity (pH) in arterial blood, as well as indices of bicarbonate concentration, base excess and oxygen saturation. The analysis is performed on the blood collected from a person's artery and is therefore, an invasive and relatively complex procedure. Although it is possible to measure oxygenation more accurately, given the nature of the procedure, it is not practical to be performed on a routine basis to monitor respiratory physiotherapy treatments. Hence, transcutaneous pulse oximetry (reported as the percentage of saturation of arterial haemoglobin by oxygen [SaO_2]) has become the most common method in clinical practice and research for measuring oxygenation [37].

Peripheral oxygen saturation is commonly used as it is simple to perform via pulse oximeters and finger probes. Pulse oximeters monitor the saturation of haemoglobin with oxygen (i.e., oxyhaemoglobin). This is possible because blood changes its colour as haemoglobin absorbs various amounts of light depending on its saturation with oxygen. Oxyhaemoglobin absorbs greater amounts of infrared light and does not absorb much red light, but as the haemoglobin oxygen saturation drops, more and more red light is absorbed and the blood becomes darker. Hence, pulse oximeters emit two wavelengths of light, red at 660 nm and near-infrared at 940 nm from the finger probe [38]. The pulse oximeter directly senses the absorption of light and translates it through complex signal processing to a function of the arterial oxygen saturation. A microprocessor integrates the data and, through an elaborate calibration algorithm based on human volunteer data, the oxygen saturation can be estimated. This measure allows constant monitoring of heart rate as well, being ideal to monitor patient's safety during interventions.

Nonetheless, this measure can provide unreliable readings due to several factors such as haemoglobin level, arterial blood flow to the vascular bed, oximetry sensor location and temperature, fluorescent or direct sunlight, jaundice, discoloration of the nail bed, nail polish, bruising under the nail, motion artefacts, intravascular dyes and skin pigmentation. All these are discussed in detail elsewhere [38].

In two Cochrane reviews about respiratory physiotherapy techniques, insufficient evidence was found regarding peripheral oxygen saturation as an outcome measure [7,12]. Osman et al. (2010) compared high-frequency chest wall oscillation with conventional airway clearance techniques in 29 patients with CF. It was found that, compared to the baseline, non-significant changes in peripheral oxygen saturation were observed during or after any of the treatments applied (Cohen's d_z from 0 to 0.28) [32]. However, in a recent study, the addition of non-invasive ventilation to chest physiotherapy resulted in a significant reduction in the proportion of treatment time with peripheral oxygen saturation below 90% ($p<0.001$) [39].

Controversial evidence exists on the potential of peripheral oxygen saturation as an adequate measure to assess the effectiveness of respiratory physiotherapy. Hence, this measure seems ideal to monitor patients' safety but it may not present the required specificity and/or sensitivity to assess changes caused by respiratory physiotherapy interventions.

2.1.5. Dyspnoea

Dyspnoea is defined as "a subjective experience of breathing discomfort that consists of qualitatively distinct sensations that vary in intensity" [40]. In a study conducted with 123 patients with CF, dyspnoea was reported to be present in 74% of the patients [41] and therefore, it is an important problem to consider in this population. As a subjective experience, adequate assessment depends on patient self-report. Depending on the circumstances in which breathing discomfort occurs and the history of similar sensations, dyspnoea may be perceived as a threat associated with anxiety, fear or depression, and it may be viewed as a sign of disease. This symptom has multidimensional aspects involving physiological, psychological, social and environmental factors that result in a behavioural response. The assessment of multidimensional aspects of dyspnoea has assumed significance in recent years [40].

Dyspnoea has been assessed using scales and questionnaires, however, important differences exists between these instruments, particularly in what they measure (e.g., one instrument may ask what breathing feels like, whereas another may ask how distressing it is or how it impacts on patient's performance or quality of life), in the rating task (i.e., what patients are instructed to rate), and in whether measurements are performed on real time or involve the recall of a specific episode. These differences make comparisons across studies difficult.

In one study exploring the effectiveness of non-invasive ventilation during chest physiotherapy [39], it was found that dyspnoea scores, assessed with the Borg scale, increased in slightly lesser extent following chest physiotherapy assisted with non-invasive ventilation than chest physiotherapy alone (2.26±1.96 vs. 2.69±1.82, $p=0.02$, Cohen's $d_z=0.23$). Marques (2008), however, found that dyspnoea assessed with the modified Borg scale was not significantly different after one session of airway clearance techniques (Cohen's $d_z=0.06$) [42]. Enright et al. (2004) investigated the effect of an 8-week inspiratory muscle training (n=19) and also did not find significant differences is dyspnoea, using the dyspnoea domain of the Chronic Respiratory Disease Questionnaire (Cohen's d_z 0.07 to 0.37) [43].

A combination of unidimensional and multidimensional tools will probably be the best approach for clinical assessment. Measurement of dyspnoea has to be seen in context, taking into consideration the patient's history, physical examination and diagnostic tests [44]. As dyspnoea is a symptom perceived by patients, it has the potential to contribute for early management of the disease, for adjusting the respiratory physiotherapy interventions and, thus, for improving outcomes in patients.

2.1.6. Chest radiography

Several imaging techniques are available to diagnose and monitor a respiratory condition. Within the respiratory field, chest radiography is the most commonly used. Although relatively simple to perform, and in itself being relevant and reliable, the measure presents several important limitations to be used as an outcome measure for respiratory physiotherapy. The interpretation of chest radiography imaging is somewhat complex and presents high levels of inter-observer subjectivity [45], the reports detailing either the presence or the absence of any abnormalities are not commonly available immediately after the exam, its portability is limited to places where health and safety radiation protection standards can be ensured, as considerable doses of radiation are involved and is difficult to perform in non-collaborative populations such as children or people with dementia. These factors prevent the use of this measure to monitor respiratory physiotherapy patients with the required frequency.

In two long-term studies (n=36 and n=32), conducted for approximately one year comparing different respiratory physiotherapy airways clearance techniques in patients with CF, chest radiography was used as an outcome measure. However, no significant differences were shown between interventions [46, 47]. In the most recent Cochrane reviews [11, 12] about physiotherapy in CF, chest radiography is no longer reported as an outcome measure in the included studies.

It therefore, seems that chest radiography is ideal for contributing to diagnosis and providing a measure of improvement or deterioration over time but might not be the most appropriate to be used as an outcome measure for respiratory physiotherapy.

2.1.7. Exercise capacity

The assessment of exercise capacity, expressed as the maximal workload achievable or the peak oxygen consumption on a progressive maximal test, has been used to measure patients' functional capacity and limitation, facilitates a safe exercise prescription and identifies changes in patients' performance as a result of an intervention [48, 49]. There are two types of clinically applicable tests to assess exercise capacity in patients with CF: laboratory-based tests and field tests [50, 51].

Laboratory-based tests, such as the cardiopulmonary exercise testing (CPET) [48, 49], are the gold standard for evaluating the causes of exercise intolerance in patients with respiratory diseases, as they provide a comprehensive assessment of the physiological responses to exercise involving the respiratory, cardiovascular and musculoskeletal systems [52]. CPET consists of a progressive exercise performed at increasing levels of intensity either on a treadmill or cycle ergometer, with simultaneous monitoring of breath-by-breath measures of airflow (e.g., VO_2, VCO_2) along with heart rate, peripheral oxygen saturation and exercise-related symptom responses (e.g. dyspnoea, leg discomfort) [49]. There are a number of protocols that can be used to perform a CPET in patients with CF, but the most commonly reported is the Godfrey protocol [53]. The CPET has been shown to be reproducible in young and adult patients with CF [54, 55]. In patients with CF (n=23) enrolled in a strength and endurance training for 6 months, significant differences were observed in VO_2 peak between 3 and 6 months (Cohen's d_z=2.01) and between 18 and 24 months (Cohen's d_z=2.22) [56]. Despite its sensitivity to change, the application of CPET is still limited in clinical settings [57]. This may be attributable to the need for expensive equipment and technical expertise. For this reason, field tests are more commonly used by physiotherapists to assess changes in exercise capacity [58].

Field tests are simple clinical exercise tests that do not require expensive equipment [59] and, thus, are suitable to be used at different settings of respiratory physiotherapy practice, such as hospitals, private practices, at home or in community environments. In patients with CF, the field tests most frequently used are the 6-minute walk test (6MWT), the 3-min step test (3MST) and the modified shuttle test (MST) [51, 58]. The 6MWT measures the maximal distance that a patient can walk in 6 minutes over a marked course (usually a corridor) following a standardised protocol [60]. The 6MWT has been recommended for patients with CF [60] and is valid and reliable for assessing exercise capacity in children [61, 62] and adults [63] with CF. The product of the distance walked during a 6MWT and body mass have been reported to correlate with aerobic capacity (VO_2max) in children with CF [64], thus supporting the use of this test in clinical settings. Furthermore, the 6MWT was found to be valuable for identifying patients who might experience oxygen desaturation and physical impairment in daily activities [65]. For this reason, the 6MWT has been considered more reflective of activities of daily living than other walk tests [59]. Numerous reference equations of the 6MWT are available for children [66–69] and adults [70].

The 3MST is a simple test that requires the patient to step at a rate of 30 steps per min on and off a step with 15 cm (6 inch) of height, during 3 minutes. This test was developed for children with CF by Balfour-Lynn et al. (1998) [71] based on the original Master two-step exercise test (1929) [72]. One major advantage of the 3MST is that it does not depend on patient's motivation, since the cadence of steps is fixed and determined by a metronome. One limitation concerns to the fact that, as step height and rate are kept constant, the workload varies between patients depending on their height and lower limb length [51, 58]. The 3MST has been found to be repeatable [71] and sensitive to changes in pulmonary function and peripheral oxygen saturation in children with CF following a course of intravenous antibiotics for acute respiratory exacerbations [73]. This is an important finding since even physiotherapists without access to a formal exercise laboratory may evaluate the response to an intervention using a simple field test. When compared to the 6MWT, the 3MST elicited a significantly greater change in heart rate and breathlessness in children with CF, along with a comparable [71] or higher [74] fall in oxygen saturation, suggesting that this test is a more vigorous exercise challenge. Nevertheless, Narang et al. (2003) showed that, in children with mild disease, important information such as the exercise-related desaturation that occurs at higher exercise levels may be missed with this test [75].

While the 6MWT and 3MST may be submaximal tests for patients with mild-to-moderate CF, the MST allows maximal exercise capacity to be reached [58]. The MST [76] consists of a validated adaptation of the Incremental Shuttle Walk Test [77], specifically developed for adults with CF. This adaptation allowed individuals to walk and run at increasing speeds over 15 levels with a maximum speed of 10.2 km/h [76]. Bradley et al. (1999, 2000) studied the validity, reliability and sensitivity of the MST in adults with CF [76, 78]. When compared to a laboratory-based treadmill test, they showed that 90% of the variation of directly measured VO_2 peak was explained by the variation in MST performance [76]. Moreover, the MST was effective in evoking a symptom-limited exercise response (i.e., peak heart rate and peak rating of perceived dyspnoea) similar to what is found in treadmill tests [76]. Thus, it may be a valid alternative when laboratory-based exercise testing cannot be performed. The validity of the MST has also been assessed in children with CF (correlation of the MST distance with VO_2peak, $r=0.663$ $p<0.01$) [79]. In adults with CF, the MST was found to be reliable (correlation between trials for distance completed and symptoms reported, $r=0.99$, $p<0.01$) and repeatable (coefficients of repeatability: distance completed, four shuttles; peak heart rate, 6 beats/min; peak oxygen saturation, 4%) [78]. The sensitivity of the test was assessed by measuring the change in MST performance after 2 weeks of antibiotic therapy in patients admitted to hospital with acute respiratory exacerbations. An effect size of 1.18 was achieved, suggesting that this is a highly sensitive measure [78]. This test has also been used to assess changes in exercise capacity after 2 months of exercise training and significant differences were found (median number of shuttles: from 100 (range 21–150) to 105 (44–150)) [80]. Despite the good measurement properties, it was recently argued that the 15-level MST developed by Bradley et al. (1999) [76] still remained sub-maximal for some patients with CF and, thus, levels were extended to 25 in order to create a truly maximal test [81].

There is no "best" exercise test. The selection of the test will depend upon the aspect of exercise capacity of interest, availability of resources (i.e., time to perform the test, staff and equipment) and patient's characteristics (e.g., age, disease stage) [50, 51]. For example, if the aetiology of a patient's reduced exercise capacity is of interest, a laboratory-based test would be more appropriate, while a field test could be used in large population studies. In addition, a young child (< 7 years old) may not be able to cooperate sufficiently for a formal laboratory exercise testing. Physiotherapists have the important role of selecting the best exercise test for a specific individual according to the specific question being asked and the specificities of each test.

2.1.8. Health-related quality of life

Health-related quality of life (HRQoL) has been extensively studied in patients with CF, especially in the last decades due to the improvement in patients' life expectancy [82]. Several instruments have been used to assess HRQoL in CF, either generic [83-85] or disease-specific

[85-87]. One disadvantage of generic questionnaires is that they lack the sensitivity needed to assess areas of functioning that are critically important for patients with CF [88]. Disease-specific questionnaires were developed in an attempt to better understand CF specific issues in clinical practice and research.

The most commonly used disease-specific questionnaires include the Cystic Fibrosis Questionnaire (CFQ) and the Cystic Fibrosis Quality of Life questionnaire. The CFQ was developed for assessing HRQoL of patients with CF and encompasses general domains of HRQoL (physical functioning, role functioning, vitality, health perceptions, emotional functioning and social functioning), as well as domains specific to CF (body image, eating disturbances, treatment burden, and respiratory and digestive symptoms) [89]. Three versions of the instrument have been developed: one for adolescents aged 14 years or older and adults (CFQ-Teen/Adult), and two for assessing children 6–13 years old, one to be completed by the child (CFQ-Child) and the other by parents (CFQ-Parent) [89, 90]. Each version takes around 15 minutes to fill in. The different versions of the CFQ questionnaire have shown good psychometric properties (validity [88-90], reliability [89, 90], internal consistency [88-90] and responsiveness [90]). Hebestreit et al. (2010) found that patients with CF (n=23) enrolling in strength and endurance training for 6 months improved their subjective health perception (CFQ domain) significantly between months 3 and 6 (Cohen's d_z=0.92) [56]. Schmidt et al. (2011) evaluated a 12-week individually tailored unsupervised aerobic exercise programme in 14 patients with CF and also found significant differences in emotional functioning and treatment burden domains of the CFQ (Cohen's d_z of 0.29 and 1.03) [91]. Thus, this questionnaire may be used in clinical practice to assess HRQoL of patients with CF, document the progression of disease and explore the effects of respiratory physiotherapy interventions.

The Cystic Fibrosis Quality of Life questionnaire was specifically developed for adolescents (14 years old or older) and adults, presenting good validity (concurrent and discriminate), internal consistency, test–retest reliability results and responsiveness [92]. One advantage of this instrument is the inclusion of domains concerning wider impacts of the disease on patient's lives (e.g., interpersonal relationships, career issues and future concerns), which are not found in other CF questionnaires. Though, it is not adaptable to children.

In sum, disease-specific instruments present good psychometric properties and seem appropriate for several different applications in patients with CF, such as to identify problems and intervene on an individual basis, compare different CF groups, or detect changes in patients' HRQoL as a result of disease progression or interventions.

2.2. Emerging outcome measures

2.2.1. Computerised respiratory sounds

Computerised auscultation consists of recording patient's respiratory sounds with a digital stethoscope and automatically analysing and classifying them based on specific signal characteristics [93]. Computerised auscultation allows to objectively detect, characterise and identify both normal and adventitious (i.e., crackles and wheezes) respiratory sounds within the breathing cycle [93].

To assess computerised respiratory sounds, the patient is positioned in the sitting or supine position (for long-term assessments) and instructed to breath from his/her mouth. Successive or simultaneous recordings are taken from the trachea plus six chest locations (i.e., right and left: anterior, lateral and posterior positions), using a single or a multichannel equipment (Figures 1 and 2) [94].

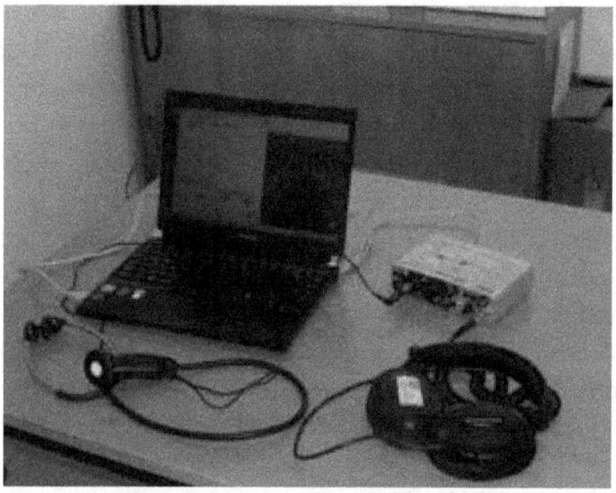

Figure 1. Single-channel equipment for computerised respiratory sound analysis.

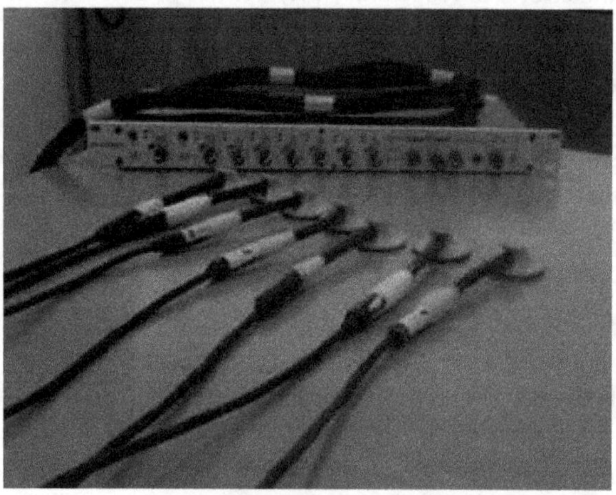

Figure 2. Multi-channel equipment for computerised respiratory sound analysis.

Seven to ten respiratory cycles at tidal breathing or at a flow of 1 to 1.5 L should be recorded to ensure the stability of sound and quality of the analysis [94]. Then, the sound is filtered using a combination of low-pass and high-pass filters in cascade to reduce sound artefacts (e.g., muscle, heart sounds and movement frequencies) and specialised algorithms for respiratory sound detection and analysis are implemented [94].

A wide range of analysis methods exists and new ones are continuously being proposed. However, the ones with more evidence are time-frequency analysis, fast Fourier and wavelet transformations, neural networks, periodogram and auto- regressive models [93, 95-97]. Specifically for patients with CF, a time-frequency wheeze detector has already been validated, demonstrating high levels of sensitivity (77.2%) and specificity (98.4%) [98]. Nevertheless, algorithms for the detection of crackles in patients with CF were not found and, thus, further studies are needed.

The reliability of computerised respiratory sounds has been mainly studied in adults with CF [99] and children with asthma, pneumonia [100] and bronchiolitis [23]. In adults with CF, one study assessed the test–retest reliability of two main parameters of crackles (i.e., the initial defection width and the two cycle duration). The intra-subject reliability of crackle parameters was found to be 'good' to 'excellent' (0.76<intraclass correlation coefficients<0.94) with no systematic bias. The smallest real difference found for the initial defection width was between 0.30 and 0.66 ms, and for the two-cycle duration between 1.57 and 2.42 ms. The reliability of wheezes has only been assessed in children with bronchiolitis, presenting moderate to good agreement (0.77<kappa<0.79) [99]. The reliability of computerised respiratory sounds to assess wheezing in adults and its overall reliability in children with CF is still unexplored.

Due to its simplicity and increasing reliability, computerised respiratory sounds have been used as outcome measures for pharmacological and respiratory physiotherapy interventions in children and adult patients with several respiratory diseases, including CF [93]. Marques et al. (2008) investigated the effect of one single session of respiratory physiotherapy using the ACBT in 17 adult patients with CF [42]. The initial defection width and two cycle duration of crackles were analysed. Considering the mean of all participants, no significant differences were found in the analysed parameters. However, when the individual data of each participant was considered, significant changes were observed in the initial defection width of 9 patients (53%) and in the two-cycle duration of 10 participants (59%).

Considering the detection of wheezes and their analysis, one study assessing the sensitivity of computerised respiratory sounds to defect bronchial hyperactivity in 23 children with CF, following an induced methacholine challenge, found a sensitivity of 50% and a specificity of 100% [101]. Studies in patients with lower respiratory tract infection, a common form of exacerbation in CF [102], have shown that computerised respiratory sounds are effective in detecting changes following pharmacological and respiratory physiotherapy interventions [93]. Small to large effects were found in the number of crackles (Cohen's d_z: 0.14 to 1.65), peak frequency (Cohen's d_z: 0.11 to 0.47), two-cycle duration (Cohen's d_z: 0.83 to 0.85) and initial/largest deflection width (Cohen's d_z: 0.38 to 1.25). Better results have been found in the detection and characterisation of wheezes, with medium to large effect sizes for the number and occupation rate of wheezes (Cohen's d_z: 0.34 to 4.30) [93].

One of the disadvantages of computerised respiratory sounds concerns the complexity and costs associated with the equipment and subsequent sound analysis. Nevertheless, an emerging body of health and engineer researchers have been gathering efforts to produce more simple and efficient hardware/software that can be used in clinical practice [101, 103].

Despite the scarce evidence of computerised respiratory sounds in CF, it seems that this measure might offer potential to assess the short- and long-term effects of respiratory physiotherapy interventions in these patients. However, more research is still required to determine the parameters of computerised respiratory sounds (i.e., number, frequency, duration) that are more sensitive to change after an intervention and to establish the reference values that will allow physiotherapists to interpret with confidence the results obtained from the computerised auscultation.

2.2.2. Lung ultrasound

Lung ultrasound (LU) is a simple, non-invasive and radiation-free methodology [104] mainly used in critical care, emergency medicine, trauma surgery and pulmonary medicine for diagnostic purposes [105]. However, due to its practical and secure character, which enables its use as often as required, LU has become an attractive alternative imaging technique for monitoring patients on whom thoracic computed tomography (CT) cannot be performed on a routine basis or where chest X-ray presents serious limitations in terms of sensitivity and specificity [106]. In fact, the international evidence-based guidelines for LU recommend this technique to monitor aeration changes and the effects of therapy in a number of acute respiratory diseases, including acute pulmonary edema, acute respiratory distress syndrome, acute lung injury, community-acquired pneumonia, ventilator-associated pneumonia and recovery from lavage of alveolar proteinosis (level A) [105].

Usually, LU is performed using a 3–5 MHz convex transducer to visualise deeper lung structures [107, 108]. A high-frequency 5–12 MHz linear probe is most effective in visualising the chest wall, pleura and the lung peripheral parenchyma [108]. A complete examination of the chest requires longitudinal, transversal and oblique-array probes to be placed along the rib spaces, proceeding from top to bottom in the ventral-dorsal direction, along of 12 regions of interest (parasternal, medial clavicular, anterior axillary, medial, and posterior right and left chest walls) [106, 108]. Anterior examination should be performed with the patient in the supine or semi-lateral position [106] while posterior examination should take place with the patient seated [107].

LU has shown to be reliable in the diagnosis of several acute respiratory conditions, such as pneumothorax (sensitivity of 65–100%; specificity of 78–100%) [108-110], including the diagnosis of this condition in patients with CF (specificity of 100%) [109], interstitial syndrome (sensitivity and specificity of 94%), lung consolidation (sensitivity of 90 to 95%; specificity of 95%), pleural effusion (sensitivity of 90 to 100%; specificity of 100%) [110] and atelectasis (sensitivity of 88%; specificity of 89%) [104]. One study assessed the inter-subject reliability of LU in the detection of atelectasis and reported a very good agreement (kappa=0.90; 95%CI 0.75 to 1) [104]. When compared with other imaging equipment (e.g. chest X-ray and MRI), this measure showed similar or even better reliability results [104, 107, 110].

No data has been found regarding the use of LU to monitor respiratory physiotherapy interventions in stable or exacerbated patients with CF. Nevertheless, considering its high accuracy in detecting signals commonly presented in CF exacerbations, such as atelectasis and consolidation [111], and its increasing impact in the management of acute respiratory conditions [105], it is reasonable to conclude that LU may be a promising measure to monitor the effectiveness of respiratory physiotherapy in patients with acute exacerbations of CF. Considering stable CF, one study used LU to characterise diaphragm thickness as a way to infer about its muscle mass. The authors reported an excellent inter- and intra-subject agreement (90% and 91%, respectively) and showed that LU was capable of detecting differences between patients with low and high rates of fat-free mass [112]. From these findings, it can be hypothesised that LU may also play a role in the assessment of the effectiveness of inspiratory muscle training and general exercise training programmes in increasing the diaphragm thickness of patients with stable CF, and thus, its muscle mass. Nevertheless, studies assessing the LU validity, reliability and responsiveness to change are needed before it can be recommended as an outcome measure for respiratory physiotherapy interventions.

At this point, there is no evidence to recommend LU as an outcome measure for respiratory physiotherapy in patients with CF. However, the advantages presented by LU over other imaging measures and its good performance as a diagnostic tool, should motivate further investigation on the validity and reliability of this measure to assess respiratory physiotherapy interventions in this population.

2.2.3. *Fat-free mass*

Fat free mass (FFM) is the component of body mass that represents muscle mass and protein stores [113] and it is a critical determinant of maximal exercise capacity [114]. It is known that, in patients with CF, lower FFM is also associated with lower FEV_1 percentage predicted and more frequent respiratory exacerbations [115, 116]. Maintaining appropriate levels of FFM is therefore crucial for maintaining the overall functional capacity in patients with CF [114].

The gold standard to assess FFM are the 4-C models, which divide body weight into fat, water and remaining fat-free dry tissue, with the last item further divided into proteins and minerals. The 4-C models require measurements of body weight, body water, body volume and bone mineral [117] and thus several specialised equipment, such as dual-energy X-ray, measures of air displacement plethysmography (BOD POD) and D_2O analysis, are needed. The partial measures are then pulled together in a predictive equation [118]. Although all devices involved are valid and reliable (intraclass correlation coefficient>0.99), the improved accuracy of the 4-C models may be offset by the potential propagation of errors due to the inherent measurement error of each device used to assess each variable [118]. Also, it appears not to be suitable for widespread clinical use due to the need for specialised equipment, experienced personnel and large amount of time. Thus, its main value lies in the quality of its evidence in supporting treatment approaches, rather than in routine practical application [117, 119].

For application of respiratory physiotherapy clinical practice, 2-C models, which require only the use of one device, are the most recommended and have shown large correlations with the 4-C models. These are bioelectrical impedance ($r>0.79$, $R^2=0.70$), CT scans ($r>0.83$, $R^2=0.96$), MRI ($r>0.91$), and specially dual-energy X-ray ($r>0.91$) [120, 121]. Indirect strategies involving calculations based on anthropometric measurements, such as skinfold thickness analysis, are controversial. Measuring FFM by measurement of skinfolds implies that no index of this component of weight is directly measured, and thus it is based on the assumption that measuring fatness reflects lean body mass as well. Therefore, its use has not been recommended [117]. Nevertheless, studies that show medium correlations between measurements of skinfold thickness and 4-C models (R^2=0.62) exist [120] and support the usability of this measure to monitor FFM irrespective of the clinical severity of CF [122].

FFM has been used as an outcome measure in respiratory physiotherapy interventions for children and adults with CF, mainly for the assessment of different types of exercise training. In the study of Selvadurai et al. (2002), 66 children with exacerbated CF significantly increased their FFM after five sessions of exercise training (aerobic or resistance training) or chest physiotherapy, independently of the protocol applied (Cohen's d_z: 1.65 to 5.22) [123]. Sosa et al. (2012) did not find improvements in the percentage of FFM of children with stable CF following an 8-week exercise training protocol (78.1 to 79.4%; Cohen's d_z 0.47) [119], however, significant differences were reached when a component of inspiratory muscle training was added (81.6 to 82.6%; Cohen's d_z 0.85) [124]. Gruber et al. (2014) compared the effect of a 6-week interval exercise training vs. standard exercise training in 43 adults with CF [125]. Significant improvements in FFM were only observed in the standard exercise training group (41.7 to 43.3 kg; Cohen's d_z 0.29). These four studies, with its medium and large effect sizes, demonstrated that FFM is an adequate outcome measure to assess the effectiveness of respiratory physiotherapy or just exercise training protocols in patients with CF.

Despite the limited evidence available, FFM assessed with 2-C or 4-C models appears to be a valid, reliable and usable measure to assess respiratory physiotherapy interventions in CF.

2.2.4. *Inspiratory muscle strength*

One of the functions of the muscles is to develop strength. In the specific case of the inspiratory muscles, strength is usually estimated as pressure [126]. Several techniques have been described to measure inspiratory muscle strength, however, the maximum static inspiratory pressure at the mouth (Pimax) is one of the most widely used [126].

The assessment of Pimax requires patients to make a maximum inspiratory (Mueller manoeuvre) effort at or near the residual volume, maintained for at least 1–1.5 seconds. These tests are volitional and require patient's full cooperation. For these reasons, this technique is usually performed by an experienced health professional to assure adequate instruction and encouragement. The manoeuver is repeated until the variation between measures is less than 20%. Pimax is usually expressed in absolute values (cmH_2O) or as a percentage of the predicted values.

Pimax is a simple, low-cost and well tolerated technique. In addition, through the hand-held and portable electronic pressure transducers, the technique is easily used by physiotherapists in a wide range of clinical settings (e.g., primary care, hospital wards, intensive care units). Another advantage of using this technique is the availability of reference values for healthy children, adults and the elderly, enabling the interpretation of results [127, 128].

The reliability of this measure is well established in people with non-CF bronchiectasis [129] and healthy people [130]. In patients with CF, only one study was found assessing the test–retest reliability of Pimax [131]. Pimax had an excellent coefficient of reliability (89%) and intraclass correlation coefficient (0.88) in patients with CF (n=20), in line with the results obtained in healthy individuals (coefficient of reliability 91%; intraclass correlation coefficient 0.87) [131]. One of the disadvantages of this study is the fact that it was conducted only with adult patients with CF (22.7±3.4 years old). The reliability of Pimax in children with CF is still unexplored.

Due to its simplicity and adequate reliability, Pimax has been used as an outcome measure of inspiratory muscle training programmes. In the study by de Jong et al. (2001), seven patients with CF improved their Pimax from 105 to 123cmH_2O after 6 weeks of inspiratory muscle training (Cohen's d_z 0.82) [132]. Enright et al. (2004) investigated the effect of an 8-week inspiratory muscle training with a high (n=9) and low (n=10) training intensity. Large effects were found using the Pimax, with improvements from 114–134cmH_2O to 155–159cmH_2O (Cohen's d_z 1.01 and 1.34) [43]. Amelina et al. (2006), after a 6-week inspiratory muscle training, found that patients with CF (n=10) had a mean improvement from 77% to 91% of the predicted Pimax (p=0.023; Cohen's d_z 0.73) [133]. These three studies, with its medium and large effect sizes, demonstrated that Pimax is an adequate outcome measure to assess the effectiveness of inspiratory muscle training.

Pimax has also been used as an outcome measure to determine the effectiveness of non-invasive ventilation during chest physiotherapy [39]. It was found that Pimax was maintained following ACBT assisted with non-invasive ventilation, resulting in a significant difference compared with ACBT alone (mean difference from standard treatment 9.04cmH_2O, 95%CI 4.25 to 13.83, p=0.006) [39].

Despite the limited evidence available, it seems that physiotherapists can confidently rely on Pimax to assess the effectiveness of respiratory physiotherapy interventions in patients with CF.

2.2.5. *Inspiratory muscle endurance*

Inspiratory muscles, in addition to developing strength, have to be able to sustain muscular tasks over time – also known as endurance [126]. Inspiratory muscle endurance is a highly complex ability, which provides insight about the resistance to fatigue of inspiratory muscles and about the function of the inspiratory pump.

Dyspnoea, one of the primary complaints of patients with CF, has been related to inspiratory muscle fatigue. In adults with CF (n=18), inspiratory muscle endurance was found to be strongly correlated with exercise dyspnoea (r=–0.72) and explained 48% of the variability of this symptom [134]. In patients with advanced CF, the assessment and monitoring of inspiratory muscle endurance may have a greater importance since, in these patients, activities of daily living may be limited by their ability to sustain ventilation. Therefore, the measure of inspiratory muscle endurance seems to be useful to evaluate the determinants of dyspnoea and fatigue in patients with CF.

A number of distinct techniques have been employed to measure endurance of the inspiratory muscles [126]. In CF, two main techniques have been employed: (i) ventilatory endurance tasks [43, 112, 131] and (ii) endurance to external loads [132, 134].

In ventilatory endurance tasks, inspiratory muscle endurance has been measured through the sustained maximum inspiratory pressure (SMIP). This sustained pressure is determined using an electronic manometer, with a fixed leak via a 2 mm diameter during the inspiratory manoeuver, and a specific computer software. The leak sets a maximum flow during the inspiratory effort and allows continuous measurement of pressure over a full range of lung volumes, until no further pressure can be generated. During this technique, patients are asked to take a maximal and sustained inspiratory effort from residual volume to total lung capacity. SMIP is measured as the area under the pressure–time curve and is generally expressed in absolute values (pressure–time units) [43, 112, 131].

The coefficient of reliability for measurements of SMIP in CF was previously established as 90% [131]. Albinni et al. (2004) reported that inspiratory muscle endurance, measured by the SMIP, improved significantly in patients with CF (n=16) after 12 weeks of inspiratory muscle training (p=0.0002) [135]. Enright et al. (2004) investigated the effect of an 8-week inspiratory muscle training with a training intensity of either 80% of maximal inspiratory effort (n=9) or 20% of maximal inspiratory effort (n=10) [43]. The SMIP improved significantly in the two groups (from 654–782 to 808–923 pressure–time units; Cohen's d_z 0.46 and 0.51) [43].

In endurance to external loads, inspiratory muscle endurance has been determined with incremental loading tests using threshold devices. During these tests, patients have to generate sufficient inspiratory pressure to open the valve and allow inspiratory flow. The test starts with an inspiratory load of 20–30% of Pimax for 2 min. The load is then increased every 2 min in increments of 10% of Pimax. The maximal load is defined by the maximal inspiratory pressure sustained for 1 or 2 min (Plim), which can be expressed in absolute values and as a percentage of the Pimax [132, 134].

The reliability of the Plim in CF has not yet been explored. In patients with COPD and in healthy people, however, it has been demonstrated that the reproducibility of the inspiratory pressure of the threshold was excellent, with small coefficients of variation in both groups (<1%) [136]. Future studies should assess the reliability and test–retest reliability of the Plim in the CF population.

Only one small study was found using Plim as an outcome measure in CF population. In this study, patients with CF (n=7) were submitted to a 6-week inspiratory muscle training. Plim, expressed as a percentage of the Pimax, increased significantly from 49% to 66% (Cohen's d_z 1.29) [132]. Using Plim, inspiratory muscle training was also found to have large effect sizes in patients with COPD (n=16; Cohen's d_z 0.83) [137] and with chronic heart failure (n=16; Cohen's d_z 1.09) [138]. Further research is needed to assess the sensitivity and responsiveness of Plim to inspiratory muscle training in patients with CF.

Both SMIP and Plim appear to be adequate outcome measures to assess the effectiveness of inspiratory muscle training in the inspiratory endurance of patients with CF. Nevertheless, this evidence emerges from few studies with small sample sizes. More research is needed to determine the responsiveness of these two outcome measures to inspiratory muscle training, as well as to other respiratory interventions, such as respiratory retraining.

2.2.6. *Physical activity*

Given the clinical implications of regular physical activity in patients' pulmonary function [139], exercise tolerance [140] and airway clearance [141], its assessment and monitoring in patients with CF has also become a topic of great interest in research and clinical practice. An assessment of physical activity (and inactivity) in the free living environment can be performed using subjective and objective methods [142, 143], although no gold standard is still available.

Subjective methods rely on the individuals' self-report through physical activity questionnaires. These instruments are simple, inexpensive and easy to employ for routine assessment of patients' physical activity levels [142]. Examples of questionnaires used in CF include the Habitual Activity Estimation Scale [144] and the Seven Day Physical Activity Recall [145]. Although the Habitual Activity Estimation Scale has presented good test–retest reliability results (intraclass correlation coefficients of 0.72) in patients with CF [146], a previous systematic review concluded that these two instruments were not able to generate valid activity data or provide a valid assessment of aerobic fitness at the individual level [147]. Thus, the use of these questionnaires for individual assessment and counselling may provide imprecise data. For these purposes, objective measures are recommended.

Objective measures to assess daily physical activity include heart rate monitoring devices and motion sensors, such as pedometers, accelerometers and multisensor devices [143, 148]. These measures have been used in studies involving patients with CF [149-151] and show promising results in evaluating the impact of respiratory physiotherapy interventions [56, 123]. Given the small size of the devices, low participant burden and relatively low cost, objective measures are appropriate for use in research and clinical practice [148]. Heart rate monitoring devices enable the assessment of patients' level of exertion since heart rate increases in a linear fashion with oxygen consumption, especially in moderate to strenuous intensity activities [152]. As such, these devices have been mostly used as a feedback tool to ensure patients' compliance with the intensity recommendations when exercising at home [56, 153]. Regarding motion sensors, there are a large number of options available that makes the choice of the best device challenging. Pedometers are designed to measure the number of steps taken by an individual by detecting vertical movement at the hip or waist. They may be desirable in simpler studies due to their lower cost and limited data [143]. Furthermore, since pedometers provide immediate feedback to the user [143], they may be valuable in self-monitoring interventions delivered to patients with CF. Despite their potential applications, no data is still available regarding the validity and reliability of pedometers in CF [154]. Still, pedometers have provided good reliability results in healthy and chronic respiratory diseases except when walking at slower speeds [155].

Although more expensive than pedometers, accelerometers provide a more detailed analysis of daily physical activity by capturing the frequency, duration and intensity of physical activity through the collection of body accelerations during movements [143]. They have also the advantage of storing the data for several weeks [143]. Multisensor devices combine accelerometry data with physiologic information collected from other sensors, such as heart rate and skin temperature, and also have a memory function. The use of accelerometers and multisensor devices in CF has increased dramatically in recent years [140, 146, 156–158] and this will likely continue with the technology advances. The clinimetric properties of these devices in CF are described in a recent systematic review [154]. The authors found that only one accelerometer (ActiGraph model 7164) and one multisensor device (BodyMedia SenseWear armband) were tested. The ActiGraph presented good convergent validity [157, 159], test–retest reliability (intraclass correlation coefficient of 0.63) and feasibility [146, 157] in adolescent and adult patients with CF. Discriminate validity [160] and responsiveness [123] were only evaluated in children with CF. Selvadurai et al (2002), exploring the effects of exercise training in children with CF admitted to hospital (n=66), found a significant improvement in activity levels after five sessions of endurance training (8.64%, $p<0.001$, Cohen's d_z 0.82) or resistance training (3.81%, $p<0.001$, Cohen's d_z 0.85) measured by accelerometry [123]. Therefore, accelerometers may be a useful tool to assess changes in physical activity levels of patients with CF in response of respiratory physiotherapy interventions. Regarding the SenseWear armband device, its validity (discriminate, convergent and concurrent) [140, 161] was only determined for adult patients with CF and no data on reliability and responsiveness exist. Further research is needed to determine which motion sensors provide the best clinimetric properties in CF in order to improve physiotherapy assessment. Moreover, as children have typically higher physical activity levels than adults [162], validation studies should be conducted in children and adults with CF. Finally, it would be useful to develop specific guidelines for the use (e.g., number of monitoring days, duration) of these motion sensors in CF, in order to standardise the collection of activity data and optimise their interpretation.

2.2.7. *Burden of treatment*

The concept of burden of treatment has been receiving increasing attention in patients with CF. Burden of treatment is described as the increased demand experienced from performing self-care activities required to undertake treatment regimens and monitor health outcomes [163]. Recent evidence demonstrated, however, that from a patient's perspective, treatment burden is beyond the workload arising from treatment regimens, being experienced in three disruption domains: biological (physical side effects), biographical (sense of self) and relational (impact on valued relationships) [164].

A large observational cohort study explored treatment complexity in patients with CF (n=7252) over a 3-year period [165]. It may be hypothesised that treatment regimens would be more complex only among patients with more severe disease. Indeed, in this cohort, the highest treatment complexity was presented by patients with more severe disease. Nevertheless, over the 3-year period, the complexity of treatment regimens increased in all age and disease severity groups. This study showed that the recommended management of CF resulted in high burden of treatment for patients.

In the specific case of respiratory physiotherapy, vigorous airway clearance and exercise regimens are recommended for patients with CF [166], which may result in increased burden of treatment. Burden of treatment, in turn, is associated with non-adherence and poor health outcomes [158, 163, 167–169]. This is particularly important for physiotherapists since the level of adherence to exercise and physiotherapy is generally reported to be poor (40–55%) [170, 171], in contrast with moderate to high adherence to nebulised medications, pancreatic enzymes and antibiotics (65–95%) [170, 172].

These levels of adherence suggest that patients with CF make decisions based on the complexity of recommended therapies they can complete, while fulfilling their responsibilities and commitments to family and work. As the number of adjunct therapies increase in CF, there may be a point at which perceived treatment burden outweighs the benefits of new or adjunct therapies, adversely affecting patient's adherence. Physiotherapists therefore, need to be sensitive recognising, understanding and supporting the reduction of burden of treatment, in order to balance the potential benefits and burdens of physiotherapy interventions and maximise adherence [158, 173].

The recognition of this concept led to the development of specific instruments for assessing burden of treatment. Burden of treatment has been incorporated into the CFQ [89]. Specifically, the burden of treatment domain is comprised of three questions: 'to what extent do your treatments make your daily life more difficult?', 'how much time do you currently spend each day on your treatments?' and 'how difficult is it for you to do your treatments each day?'. The score ranges from 0 to 100, with lower scores representing higher burden of treatment.

The burden of treatment domain of the CFQ has been used in recent studies evaluating the effectiveness of novel interventions [91, 174]. In a trial with patients with CF (n=12), assessing the effect of a nebulised hypertonic saline therapy, a significant improvement was found in respiratory symptoms together with an increased in perceived burden of treatment (Cohen's d_z 3.05) [174]. Schmidt et al. (2011) evaluated a 12-week individually tailored unsupervised aerobic exercise programme in patients with CF (n=14) [91]. Patients were instructed to exercise at least 30 minutes, three times a week with a heart rate target above 70% of their maximum. This study showed that an exercise programme could significantly increase VO_2max and, at same time, significantly decrease the perceived burden of treatment (Cohen's d_z 1.03) [91]. These two studies, despite being distinct, show that the burden of treatment domain of the CFQ is sensitive to change over time and demonstrate large effect sizes. Physiotherapists can, therefore, confidently rely on the burden of treatment domain of the CFQ to assess their interventions.

One of the disadvantages of the burden of treatment domain is the fact that it mainly addresses the complexity and time consuming routine of self-care. However, recent research has demonstrated that burden of treatment goes beyond these aspects and is experienced as biological, biographical and relational disruptions [164]. Therefore, when designing future instruments and methods for assessing burden of treatment, these three disruption domains should also be taken into account. This highlights the relevance of assessing burden of treatment as an outcome measure of respiratory physiotherapy in CF. The evaluation of burden of treatment will also inform the development of new and minimally disruptive interventions.

3. Conclusions

This chapter presented and discussed the strength and weaknesses of the outcome measures currently applied or emerging in CF respiratory physiotherapy interventions. It provided a comprehensive overview of the most commonly used, and also addressed the less used and some even emerging, outcome measures, which show potential to overcome some of the barriers to build an evidence base for respiratory physiotherapy practice in patients with CF.

The chapter presented outcome measures possibly to be applied (i) in clinical practice before, during and after each session of respiratory physiotherapy to monitor its effectiveness; (ii) before and after the respiratory physiotherapy treatment (i.e., normally characterised by weeks of intervention) and (iii) clinically, but which main interest is fundamental and/or applied research in CF respiratory physiotherapy.

In a time where the relationship between "best care" versus "burden of treatment" is discussed, two factors seem crucial for respiratory physiotherapy: (1) to take into consideration family and patient's preferences when providing treatments and (2) build a sound evidence base. For the latter, a shift of the commonly used outcome measures, namely FEV_1, is essential, and a strong consideration to start applying new outcome measures is recommended.

Author details

Alda Marques[1,2*], Joana Cruz[1,2], Cristina Jácome[1,2] and Ana Oliveira[1,2]

*Address all correspondence to: amarques@ua.pt

1 Lab 3R - Respiratory Rehabilitation Research Laboratory, School of Health Sciences, University of Aveiro (ESSUA), Aveiro, Portugal

2 Center for Health Technology and Services Research (CINTESIS), School of Health Sciences, University of Aveiro, Aveiro, Portugal

References

[1] McIlwaine MP, Lee Son NM, Richmond ML. Physiotherapy and cystic fibrosis: what is the evidence base? Curr Opin Pulm Med. 2014;20(6):613–7.

[2] Holland AE, Button BM. Physiotherapy for cystic fibrosis in Australia: knowledge and acceptance of the Consensus Statement recommendations. Respirology. 2013;18(4):652–6.

[3] Bradley JM, Moran FM, Stuart Elborn J. Evidence for physical therapies (airway clearance and physical training) in cystic fibrosis: an overview of five Cochrane systematic reviews. Respir Med. 2006;100(2):191–201.

[4] Bott J, Blumenthal S, Buxton M, Ellum S, Falconer C, Garrod R, et al. Guidelines for the physiotherapy management of the adult, medical, spontaneously breathing patient. Thorax. 2009;64(Suppl 1):i1–i52.

[5] Main E. Airway clearance research in CF: the 'perfect storm' of strong preference and effortful participation in long-term, non-blinded studies. Thorax. 2013;68(8):701–2.

[6] Cox NS, Alison JA, Holland AE. Interventions for promoting physical activity in people with cystic fibrosis. Cochrane Database Syst Rev. 2013;12:CD009448.

[7] Warnock L, Gates A, van der Schans CP. Chest physiotherapy compared to no chest physiotherapy for cystic fibrosis. Cochrane Database Syst Rev. 2013;9:CD001401.

[8] Miller MR, Hankinson J, Brusasco V, Burgos F, Casaburi R, Coates A, et al. Standardisation of spirometry. Eur Respir J. 2005;26(2):319–38.

[9] Pfleger A, Theissl B, Oberwaldner B, Zach MS. Self-administered chest physiotherapy in cystic fibrosis: a comparative study of high-pressure PEP and autogenic drainage. Lung. 1992;170(6):323–30.

[10] Jarad NA, Powell T, Smith E. Evaluation of a novel sputum clearance technique – hydro-acoustic therapy (HAT) in adult patients with cystic fibrosis: a feasibility study. Chron Respir Dis. 2010;7(4):217–27.

[11] Main E, Prasad A, Schans C. Conventional chest physiotherapy compared to other airway clearance techniques for cystic fibrosis. Cochrane Database Syst Rev. 2005(1):Cd002011.

[12] McKoy NA, Saldanha IJ, Odelola OA, Robinson KA. Active cycle of breathing technique for cystic fibrosis. Cochrane Database Syst Rev. 2012;12:Cd007862.

[13] Morrison L, Agnew J. Oscillating devices for airway clearance in people with cystic fibrosis. Cochrane Database Syst Rev. 2009(1):Cd006842.

[14] Xavier GN, Duarte ACM, Melo-Silva CA, dos Santos CEVG, Amado VM. Accuracy of pulmonary auscultation to detect abnormal respiratory mechanics: A cross-sectional diagnostic study. Med Hypotheses. 2014;83(6):733–4.

[15] Abbas A, Fahim A. An automated computerized auscultation and diagnostic system for pulmonary diseases. J Med Syst. 2010;34(6):1149–55.

[16] Bohadana A, Izbicki G, Kraman SS. Fundamentals of lung auscultation. N Engl J Med. 2014;370(8):744–51.

[17] Sovijärvi ARA, Vanderschoot J, Earis JE. Standardization of computerized respiratory sound analysis. Eur Respir Rev. 2000;10(77):974–87.

[18] Marques A, Bruton A, Barney A. Clinically useful outcome measures for physiotherapy airway clearance techniques: a review. Physi Ther Rev. 2006;11(4):299–307.

[19] Brooks D, Wilson L, Kelsey C. Accuracy and reliability of 'specialized' physical therapists in auscultating tape-recorded lung sounds. Physiother Can. 1993;45(1):21–4.

[20] Allingame S, Williams T, Jenkins S, Tucker B. Accuracy and reliability of physiotherapists in the interpretation of tape-recorded lung sounds. Aust J Physiother. 1995;41(3):179–84.

[21] Brooks D, Thomas J. Interrater reliability of auscultation of breath sounds among physical therapists. Phys Ther. 1995;75(12):1082–8.

[22] Marques A, Oliveira A, Jácome C, Dinis J, Pinho C. 236 Agreement between real-time auscultation and computerised respiratory analyses. J Cyst Fibros.12:S108.

[23] Elphick HE, Lancaster GA, Solis A, Majumdar A, Gupta R, Smyth RL. Validity and reliability of acoustic analysis of respiratory sounds in infants. Arch Dis Child. 2004;89(11):1059–63.

[24] Morrow B, Angus L, Greenhough D, Hansen A, McGregor G, Olivier O, et al. The reliability of identifying bronchial breathing by auscultation. International Journal of Therapy and Rehabilitation. 2010;17(2):69–75.

[25] Puder LC, Fischer HS, Wilitzki S, Usemann J, Godfrey S, Schmalisch G. Validation of computerized wheeze detection in young infants during the first months of life. BMC Pediatr. 2014;14:257.

[26] Tourtier JP, Libert N, Clapson P, Tazarourte K, Borne M, Grasser L, et al. Auscultation in flight: comparison of conventional and electronic stethoscopes. Air Med J. 2011;30(3):158–60.

[27] Hoffmann C, Falzone E, Verret C, Pasquier P, Leclerc T, Donat N, et al. Brief report: pulmonary auscultation in the operating room: a prospective randomized blinded trial comparing electronic and conventional stethoscopes. Anesth Analg. 2013;117(3): 646–8.

[28] Zemanick ET, Harris JK, Conway S, Konstan MW, Marshall B, Quittner AL, et al. Measuring and improving respiratory outcomes in cystic fibrosis lung disease: opportunities and challenges to therapy. J Cyst Fibros. 2010;9(1):1–16.

[29] Falk M, Kelstrup M, Andersen JB, Kinoshita T, Falk P, Stovring S, et al. Improving the ketchup bottle method with positive expiratory pressure, PEP, in cystic fibrosis. Eur J Respir Dis. 1984;65(6):423–32.

[30] Mortensen J, Falk M, Groth S, Jensen C. The effects of postural drainage and positive expiratory pressure physiotherapy on tracheobronchial clearance in cystic fibrosis. Chest. 1991;100(5):1350–7.

[31] Rossman CM, Waldes R, Sampson D, Newhouse MT. Effect of chest physiotherapy on the removal of mucus in patients with cystic fibrosis. Am Rev Respir Dis. 1982;126(1):131–5.

[32] Osman LP, Roughton M, Hodson ME, Pryor JA. Short-term comparative study of high frequency chest wall oscillation and European airway clearance techniques in patients with cystic fibrosis. Thorax. 2010;65(3):196–200.

[33] Braggion C, Cappelletti LM, Cornacchia M, Zanolla L, Mastella G. Short-term effects of three chest physiotherapy regimens in patients hospitalized for pulmonary exacerbations of cystic fibrosis: a cross-over randomized study. Pediatr Pulmonol. 1995;19(1):16–22.

[34] Kluft J, Beker L, Castagnino M, Gaiser J, Chaney H, Fink RJ. A comparison of bronchial drainage treatments in cystic fibrosis. Pediatr Pulmonol. 1996;22(4):271–4.

[35] Oermann CM, Sockrider MM, Giles D, Sontag MK, Accurso FJ, Castile RG. Comparison of high-frequency chest wall oscillation and oscillating positive expiratory pressure in the home management of cystic fibrosis: a pilot study. Pediatr Pulmonol. 2001;32(5):372–7.

[36] Pryor JA, Tannenbaum E, Scott SF, Burgess J, Cramer D, Gyi K, et al. Beyond postural drainage and percussion: Airway clearance in people with cystic fibrosis. J Cyst Fibros. 2010;9(3):187–92.

[37] Elphick HE, Mallory G. Oxygen therapy for cystic fibrosis. Cochrane Database Syst Rev. 2013;7:CD003884.

[38] Chan ED, Chan MM, Chan MM. Pulse oximetry: understanding its basic principles facilitates appreciation of its limitations. Respir Med. 2013;107(6):789–99.

[39] Holland AE, Denehy L, Ntoumenopoulos G, Naughton MT, Wilson JW. Non-invasive ventilation assists chest physiotherapy in adults with acute exacerbations of cystic fibrosis. Thorax. 2003;58(10):880–4.

[40] Parshall MB, Schwartzstein RM, Adams L, Banzett RB, Manning HL, Bourbeau J, et al. An official American Thoracic Society statement: update on the mechanisms, assessment, and management of dyspnea. Am J Respir Crit Care Med. 2012;185(4):435–52.

[41] Stenekes SJ, Hughes A, Gregoire MC, Frager G, Robinson WM, McGrath PJ. Frequency and self-management of pain, dyspnea, and cough in cystic fibrosis. J Pain Symptom Manage. 2009;38(6):837–48.

[42] Marques A. The use of computer aided lung sound analysis to characterise adventitious lung sounds: a potential outcome measure for respiratory therapy. Southampton: University of Southampton; 2008.

[43] Enright S, Chatham K, Ionescu AA, Unnithan VB, Shale DJ. Inspiratory muscle training improves lung function and exercise capacity in adults with cystic fibrosis. Chest. 2004;126(2):405–11.

[44] Bausewein C, Booth S, Higginson IJ. Measurement of dyspnoea in the clinical rather than the research setting. Curr Opin Support Palliat Care. 2008;2(2):95–9.

[45] Neuman MI, Lee EY, Bixby S, Diperna S, Hellinger J, Markowitz R, et al. Variability in the interpretation of chest radiographs for the diagnosis of pneumonia in children. J Hosp Med. 2012;7(4):294–8.

[46] McIlwaine PM, Wong LT, Peacock D, Davidson AG. Long-term comparative trial of conventional postural drainage and percussion versus positive expiratory pressure physiotherapy in the treatment of cystic fibrosis. J Pediatr. 1997;131(4):570–4.

[47] McIlwaine PM, Wong LT, Peacock D, Davidson AG. Long-term comparative trial of positive expiratory pressure versus oscillating positive expiratory pressure (flutter) physiotherapy in the treatment of cystic fibrosis. J Pediatr. 2001;138(6):845–50.

[48] Clinical exercise testing with reference to lung diseases: indications, standardization and interpretation strategies. ERS Task Force on Standardization of Clinical Exercise Testing. European Respiratory Society. Eur Respir J. 1997;10(11):2662–89.

[49] ATS/ACCP Statement on cardiopulmonary exercise testing. Am J Respir Crit Care Med. 2003;167(2):211–77.

[50] Orenstein DM. Exercise testing in cystic fibrosis. Pediatr Pulmonol. 1998;25(4):223–5.

[51] Rogers D, Prasad SA, Doull I. Exercise testing in children with cystic fibrosis. J R Soc Med. 2003;96(Suppl 43):23–9.

[52] Palange P, Ward SA, Carlsen K-H, Casaburi R, Gallagher CG, Gosselink R, et al. Recommendations on the use of exercise testing in clinical practice. Eur Respir J. 2007;29(1):185–209.

[53] Godfrey S, Mearns M. Pulmonary function and response to exercise in cystic fibrosis. Arch Dis Child. 1971;46(246):144–51.

[54] McKone EF, Barry SC, FitzGerald MX, Gallagher CG. Reproducibility of maximal exercise ergometer testing in patients with cystic fibrosis. Chest. 1999;116(2):363–8.

[55] Saynor ZL, Barker AR, Oades PJ, Williams CA. Reproducibility of maximal cardiopulmonary exercise testing for young cystic fibrosis patients. J Cyst Fibros. 2013;12(6):644–50.

[56] Hebestreit H, Kieser S, Junge S, Ballmann M, Hebestreit A, Schindler C, et al. Long-term effects of a partially supervised conditioning programme in cystic fibrosis. Eur Respir J. 2010;35(3):578–83.

[57] Stevens D, Oades PJ, Armstrong N, Williams CA. A survey of exercise testing and training in UK cystic fibrosis clinics. J Cyst Fibros. 2010;9(5):302–6.

[58] Urquhart D. Exercise testing in cystic fibrosis: why (and how)? J R Soc Med. 2011;104(suppl 1):S6–S14.

[59] Solway S, Brooks D, Lacasse Y, Thomas S. A qualitative systematic overview of the measurement properties of functional walk tests used in the cardiorespiratory domain. Chest. 2001;119(1):256–70.

[60] ATS statement: guidelines for the six-minute walk test. Am J Respir Crit Care Med. 2002;166(1):111–7.

[61] Gulmans VAM, van Veldhoven NHMJ, de Meer K, Helders PJM. The six-minute walking test in children with cystic fibrosis: reliability and validity. Pediatr Pulmonol. 1996;22(2):85–9.

[62] Cunha MT, Rozov T, de Oliveira RC, Jardim JR. Six-minute walk test in children and adolescents with cystic fibrosis. Pediatr Pulmonol. 2006;41(7):618–22.

[63] Gruet M, Brisswalter J, Mely L, Vallier J-M. Use of the peak heart rate reached during six-minute walk test to predict individualized training intensity in patients with cystic fibrosis: validity and reliability. Arch Phys Med Rehabil. 2010;91(4):602–7.

[64] Lesser DJ, Fleming MM, Maher CA, Kim SB, Woo MS, Keens TG. Does the 6-min walk test correlate with the exercise stress test in children? Pediatr Pulmonol. 2010;45(2):135–40.

[65] Ziegler B, Rovedder PM, Lukrafka JL, Oliveira CL, Menna-Barreto SS, Dalcin Pde T. Submaximal exercise capacity in adolescent and adult patients with cystic fibrosis. J Bras Pneumol. 2007;33(3):263–9.

[66] Priesnitz CV, Rodrigues GH, da Silva Stumpf C, Viapiana G, Cabral CP, Stein RT, et al. Reference values for the 6-min walk test in healthy children aged 6–12 years. Pediatr Pulmonol. 2009;44(12):1174–9.

[67] Klepper SE, Muir N. Reference values on the 6-minute walk test for children living in the United States. Pediatr Phys Ther. 2011;23(1):32–40.

[68] Kanburoglu MK, Ozdemir FM, Ozkan S, Tunaoglu FS. Reference values of the 6-minute walk test in healthy turkish children and adolescents between 11 and 18 years of age. Respir Care. 2014;59(9):1369–75.

[69] Ulrich S, Hildenbrand F, Treder U, Fischler M, Keusch S, Speich R, et al. Reference values for the 6-minute walk test in healthy children and adolescents in Switzerland. BMC Pulm Med. 2013;13(1):49.

[70] Dourado VZ. Equações de referência para o teste de caminhada de seis minutos em indivíduos saudáveis. Arq Bras Cardiol. 2011;96:e128–e38.

[71] Balfour-Lynn IM, Prasad SA, Laverty A, Whitehead BF, Dinwiddie R. A step in the right direction: assessing exercise tolerance in cystic fibrosis. Pediatr Pulmonol. 1998;25(4):278–84.

[72] Master AM, Oppenheimer ET. A simple exercise tolerance test for circulatory efficiency with standard tables for normal individuals. Am J Med Sci. 1929;177(2):223–43.

[73] Pike SE, Prasad SA, Balfour-Lynn IM. Effect of intravenous antibiotics on exercise tolerance (3-min step test) in cystic fibrosis*. Pediatr Pulmonol. 2001;32(1):38–43.

[74] Aurora P, Prasad SA, Balfour-Lynn IM, Slade G, Whitehead B, Dinwiddie R. Exercise tolerance in children with cystic fibrosis undergoing lung transplantation assessment. Eur Respir J. 2001;18(2):293–7.

[75] Narang I, Pike S, Rosenthal M, Balfour-Lynn IM, Bush A. Three-minute step test to assess exercise capacity in children with cystic fibrosis with mild lung disease. Pediatr Pulmonol. 2003;35(2):108–13.

[76] Bradley J, Howard J, Wallace E, Elborn S. Validity of a modified shuttle test in adult cystic fibrosis. Thorax. 1999;54(5):437–9.

[77] Singh SJ, Morgan MD, Scott S, Walters D, Hardman AE. Development of a shuttle walking test of disability in patients with chronic airways obstruction. Thorax. 1992;47(12):1019–24.

[78] Bradley J, Howard J, Wallace E, Elborn S. Reliability, repeatability, and sensitivity of the modified shuttle test in adult cystic fibrosis. Chest. 2000;117(6):1666–71.

[79] Rogers D, Smith P, John N, Oliver W, IJM D. Validity of a modified shuttle walk test as a measure of exercise tolerance in paediatric CF patients. J Cys Fibros. 2002;1(Suppl 11):139.

[80] Paranjape SM, Barnes LA, Carson KA, von Berg K, Loosen H, Mogayzel Jr PJ. Exercise improves lung function and habitual activity in children with cystic fibrosis. J Cyst Fibros. 2012;11(1):18–23.

[81] Elkins MR, Dentice RL, Bye PT. Validation of the MST-25: an extension of the modified shuttle test (MST). J Cyst Fibros. 2009;8, Supplement 2(0):S70.

[82] Royce FH, Carl JC. Health-related quality of life in cystic fibrosis. Curr Opin Pediatr. 2011;23(5):535–40.

[83] Britto MT, Kotagal UR, Hornung RW, Atherton HD, Tsevat J, Wilmott RW. Impact of recent pulmonary exacerbations on quality of life in patients with cystic fibrosis. Chest. 2002;121(1):64–72.

[84] Congleton J, Hodson ME, Duncan-Skingle F. Quality of life in adults with cystic fibrosis. Thorax. 1996;51(9):936–40.

[85] Thomas C, Mitchell P, O'Rourke P, Wainwright C. Quality-of-life in children and adolescents with cystic fibrosis managed in both regional outreach and cystic fibrosis center settings in Queensland. J Pediatr. 2006;148(4):508–16.

[86] Gee L, Abbott J, Conway SP, Etherington C, Webb AK. Quality of life in cystic fibrosis: the impact of gender, general health perceptions and disease severity. J Cyst Fibros. 2003;2(4):206–13.

[87] Abbott J, Hart A, Morton A, Gee L, Conway S. Health-related quality of life in adults with cystic fibrosis: the role of coping. J Psychosom Res. 2008;64(2):149–57.

[88] Modi AC, Quittner AL. Validation of a disease-specific measure of health-related quality of life for children with cystic fibrosis. J Pediatr Psychol. 2003;28(8):535–46.

[89] Quittner AL, Buu A, Messer MA, Modi AC, Watrous M. Development and validation of the cystic fibrosis questionnaire in the United States: A health-related quality-of-life measure for cystic fibrosis. Chest. 2005;128(4):2347–54.

[90] Henry B, Aussage P, Grosskopf C, Goehrs JM. Development of the Cystic Fibrosis Questionnaire (CFQ) for assessing quality of life in pediatric and adult patients. Qual Life Res. 2003;12(1):63–76.

[91] Schmidt AM, Jacobsen U, Bregnballe V, Olesen HV, Ingemann-Hansen T, Thastum M, et al. Exercise and quality of life in patients with cystic fibrosis: a 12-week intervention study. Physiother Theory Pract. 2011;27(8):548–56.

[92] Gee L, Abbott J, Conway SP, Etherington C, Webb AK. Development of a disease specific health related quality of life measure for adults and adolescents with cystic fibrosis. Thorax. 2000;55(11):946–54.

[93] Marques AS, Oliveira AL, Jacome CI. Computerized adventitious respiratory sounds as outcome measures for respiratory therapy: a systematic review. Respir Care. 2014;59(5):765–76.

[94] Rossi M, Sovijarvi ARA, Piirila P, Vannuccini L, Dalmasso FVJ. Environmental and subject conditions and breathing manoeuvres for respiratory sound recordings. Eur Respir Rev. 2000;10(77):611–5.

[95] Oliveira A, Marques A. Respiratory sounds in healthy people: a systematic review. Respir Med. 2014;108(4):550–70.

[96] Gurung A, Scrafford CG, Tielsch JM, Levine OS, Check W. Computerized lung sound analysis as diagnostic aid for the detection of abnormal lung sounds: a systematic review and meta-analysis. Respir Med. 2011;105(9):1396–403.

[97] Reichert S, Gass R, Brandt C, Andres E. Analysis of respiratory sounds: state of the art. Clinical medicine Circulatory, respiratory and pulmonary medicine. 2008;2:45–58.

[98] Oliveira D, Pinho C, Marques A, Dinis J. Validation of a time-frequency wheeze detector in cystic fibrosis: a pilot study. Eur Respir J. 2011;38(55):237s.

[99] Marques A, Bruton A, Barney A. The reliability of lung crackle characteristics in cystic fibrosis and bronchiectasis patients in a clinical setting. Physiol Meas. 2009;30(9): 903–12.

[100] Prodhan P, Dela Rosa RS, Shubina M, Haver KE, Matthews BD, Buck S, et al. Wheeze detection in the pediatric intensive care unit: comparison among physician, nurses, respiratory therapists, and a computerized respiratory sound monitor. Respir Care. 2008;53(10):1304–9.

[101] Sanchez I, Powell RE, Pasterkamp H. Wheezing and airflow obstruction during methacholine challenge in children with cystic fibrosis and in normal children. Am Rev Respir Dis. 1993;147(3):705–9.

[102] van Ewijk BE, van der Zalm MM, Wolfs TFW, van der Ent CK. Viral respiratory infections in cystic fibrosis. J Cyst Fibros. 2005;4, Supplement 2(0):31–6.

[103] Pinho C, Oliveira A, Oliveira D, Dinis J, Marques A. Lungsounds@UA Interface and Multimedia Database. Int J E-Health Med Commun. 2014;5(1):81–95.

[104] Acosta CM, Maidana GA, Jacovitti D, Belaunzaran A, Cereceda S, Rae E, et al. Accuracy of transthoracic lung ultrasound for diagnosing anesthesia-induced atelectasis in children. Anesthesiology. 2014;120(6):1370–9.

[105] Volpicelli G, Elbarbary M, Blaivas M, Lichtenstein DA, Mathis G, Kirkpatrick AW, et al. International evidence-based recommendations for point-of-care lung ultrasound. Intensive Care Med. 2012;38(4):577–91.

[106] Xirouchaki N, Kondili E, Prinianakis G, Malliotakis P, Georgopoulos D. Impact of lung ultrasound on clinical decision making in critically ill patients. Intensive Care Med. 2014;40(1):57–65.

[107] Reissig A, Copetti R, Mathis G, Mempel C, Schuler A, Zechner P, et al. Lung ultrasound in the diagnosis and follow-up of community-acquired pneumonia: a prospective, multicenter, diagnostic accuracy study. Chest. 2012;142(4):965–72.

[108] Gardelli G, Feletti F, Nanni A, Mughetti M, Piraccini A, Zompatori M. Chest ultrasonography in the ICU. Respir Care. 2012;57(5):773–81.

[109] Slater A, Goodwin M, Anderson KE, Gleeson FV. COPD can mimic the appearance of pneumothorax on thoracic ultrasound. Chest. 2006;129(3):545–50.

[110] Xirouchaki N, Magkanas E, Vaporidi K, Kondili E, Plataki M, Patrianakos A, et al. Lung ultrasound in critically ill patients: comparison with bedside chest radiography. Intensive Care Med. 2011;37(9):1488–93.

[111] Ng MY, Flight W, Smith E. Pulmonary complications of cystic fibrosis. Clin Radiol. 2014;69(3):e153–e62.

[112] Enright S, Chatham K, Ionescu AA, Unnithan VB, Shale DJ. The influence of body composition on respiratory muscle, lung function and diaphragm thickness in adults with cystic fibrosis. J Cyst Fibros. 2007;6(6):384–90.

[113] Matel JL, Milla CE. Nutrition in cystic fibrosis. Semin Respir Crit Care Med. 2009;30(5):579–86.

[114] Klijn PH, van der Net J, Kimpen JL, Helders PJ, van der Ent CK. Longitudinal determinants of peak aerobic performance in children with cystic fibrosis. Chest. 2003;124(6):2215–9.

[115] Engelen MP, Schroder R, Van der Hoorn K, Deutz NE, Com G. Use of body mass index percentile to identify fat-free mass depletion in children with cystic fibrosis. Clin Nutr. 2012;31(6):927–33.

[116] Bolton CE, Ionescu AA, Evans WD, Pettit RJ, Shale DJ. Altered tissue distribution in adults with cystic fibrosis. Thorax. 2003;58(10):885–9.

[117] Wells JC, Fewtrell MS. Measuring body composition. Arch Dis Child. 2006;91(7):612–7.

[118] Moon JR, Stout JR, Smith-Ryan AE, Kendall KL, Fukuda DH, Cramer JT, et al. Tracking fat-free mass changes in elderly men and women using single-frequency bioimpedance and dual-energy X-ray absorptiometry: a four-compartment model comparison. Eur J Clin Nutr. 2013;67 Suppl 1:S40–6.

[119] Santana Sosa E, Groeneveld IF, Gonzalez-Saiz L, Lopez-Mojares LM, Villa-Asensi JR, Barrio Gonzalez MI, et al. Intrahospital weight and aerobic training in children with cystic fibrosis: a randomized controlled trial. Med Sci Sports Exerc. 2012;44(1):2–11.

[120] Mijnarends DM, Meijers JM, Halfens RJ, ter Borg S, Luiking YC, Verlaan S, et al. Validity and reliability of tools to measure muscle mass, strength, and physical performance in community-dwelling older people: a systematic review. Journal of the American Medical Directors Association. 2013;14(3):170–8.

[121] Atherton RR, Williams JE, Wells JC, Fewtrell MS. Use of fat mass and fat free mass standard deviation scores obtained using simple measurement methods in healthy children and patients: comparison with the reference 4-component model. PLoS ONE. 2013;8(5):e62139.

[122] de Meer K, Gulmans VA, Westerterp KR, Houwen RH, Berger R. Skinfold measurements in children with cystic fibrosis: monitoring fat-free mass and exercise effects. Eur J Pediatr. 1999;158(10):800–6.

[123] Selvadurai HC, Blimkie CJ, Meyers N, Mellis CM, Cooper PJ, Van Asperen PP. Randomized controlled study of in-hospital exercise training programs in children with cystic fibrosis. Pediatr Pulmonol. 2002;33(3):194–200.

[124] Santana-Sosa E, Gonzalez-Saiz L, Groeneveld IF, Villa-Asensi JR, Barrio Gómez de Aguero MI, Fleck SJ, et al. Benefits of combining inspiratory muscle with 'whole

muscle' training in children with cystic fibrosis: a randomised controlled trial. Br J Sports Med. 2013. Epub: 2013/05/16.

[125] Gruber W, Orenstein DM, Braumann KM, Beneke R. Interval exercise training in cystic fibrosis – effects on exercise capacity in severely affected adults. J Cyst Fibros. 2014;13(1):86–91.

[126] ATS/ERS Statement on Respiratory Muscle Testing. Am J Respir Crit Care Med. 2002;166(4):518–624.

[127] Enright PL, Kronmal RA, Manolio TA, Schenker MB, Hyatt RE. Respiratory muscle strength in the elderly. correlates and reference values. Cardiovascular Health Study Research Group. Am J Respir Crit Care Med. 1994;149(2 Pt 1):430–8.

[128] Wilson SH, Cooke NT, Edwards RH, Spiro SG. Predicted normal values for maximal respiratory pressures in caucasian adults and children. Thorax. 1984;39(7):535–8.

[129] Moran F, Piper A, Elborn JS, Bradley JM. Respiratory muscle pressures in non-CF bronchiectasis: repeatability and reliability. Chron Respir Dis. 2010;7(3):165–71.

[130] McConnell AK, Copestake AJ. Maximum static respiratory pressures in healthy elderly men and women: issues of reproducibility and interpretation. Respiration. 1999;66(3):251–8.

[131] Enright S, Unnithan VB, Davies D. Reproducibility of measurements of inspiratory work capacity in cystic fibrosis patients. Respir Physiol Neurobiol. 2006;150(1):35–43.

[132] de Jong W, van Aalderen WM, Kraan J, Koeter GH, van der Schans CP. Inspiratory muscle training in patients with cystic fibrosis. Respir Med. 2001;95(1):31–6.

[133] Amelina E, Cherniak A, Chikina S, Krasovsky S, Appaeva A. Inspiratory muscle training (IMT) in cystic fibrosis adults. Eur Respir J. 2006:716s.

[134] Leroy S, Perez T, Neviere R, Aguilaniu B, Wallaert B. Determinants of dyspnea and alveolar hypoventilation during exercise in cystic fibrosis: impact of inspiratory muscle endurance. J Cyst Fibros. 2011;10(3):159–65.

[135] Albinni S, Rath R, Renner S, Eichler I. Additional inspiratory muscle training intensifies the beneficial effects of cycle ergonometer training in patients with cystic fibrosis. J Cyst Fibros. 2004;Suppl1:S63.

[136] Gosselink R, Wagenaar RC, Decramer M. Reliability of a commercially available threshold loading device in healthy subjects and in patients with chronic obstructive pulmonary disease. Thorax. 1996;51(6):601–5.

[137] Hill K, Jenkins SC, Philippe DL, Cecins N, Shepherd KL, Green DJ, et al. High-intensity inspiratory muscle training in COPD. Eur Respir J. 2006;27(6):1119–28.

[138] Dall'Ago P, Chiappa GR, Guths H, Stein R, Ribeiro JP. Inspiratory muscle training in patients with heart failure and inspiratory muscle weakness: a randomized trial. J Am Coll Cardiol. 2006;47(4):757–63.

[139] Schneiderman JE, Wilkes DL, Atenafu EG, Nguyen T, Wells GD, Alarie N, et al. Longitudinal relationship between physical activity and lung health in patients with cystic fibrosis. Eur Respir J. 2014;43(3):817–23.

[140] Troosters T, Langer D, Vrijsen B, Segers J, Wouters K, Janssens W, et al. Skeletal muscle weakness, exercise tolerance and physical activity in adults with cystic fibrosis. Eur Respir J. 2009;33(1):99–106.

[141] Baldwin DR, Hill AL, Peckham DG, Knox AJ. Effect of addition of exercise to chest physiotherapy on sputum expectoration and lung function in adults with cystic fibrosis. Respir Med. 1994;88(1):49–53.

[142] Andre D, Wolf DL. Recent advances in free-living physical activity monitoring: a review. J Diabetes Sci Tech (Online). 2007;1(5):760–7.

[143] Strath SJ, Kaminsky LA, Ainsworth BE, Ekelund U, Freedson PS, Gary RA, et al. Guide to the Assessment of Physical Activity: Clinical and Research Applications: A Scientific Statement from the American Heart Association. Circulation. 2013. Epub 2013/10/14.

[144] Hay J, Cairney J. Development of the habitual activity estimation scale for clinical research: A systematic approach. Pediatric Exercise Science. 2006;18(2):193–202.

[145] Sallis JF, Haskell WL, Wood PD, Fortmann SP, Rogers T, Blair SN, et al. Physical activity assessment methodology in the Five-City Project. Am J Epidemiol. 1985;121(1): 91–106.

[146] Wells GD, Wilkes DL, Schneiderman-Walker J, Elmi M, Tullis E, Lands LC, et al. Reliability and validity of the habitual activity estimation scale (HAES) in patients with cystic fibrosis. Pediatr Pulmonol. 2008;43(4):345–53.

[147] Hulzebos E, Dadema T, Takken T. Measurement of physical activity in patients with cystic fibrosis: a systematic review. Expert Rev Respir Med. 2013;7(6):647–53.

[148] Trost SG, O'Neil M. Clinical use of objective measures of physical activity. Br J Sports Med. 2013. Epub 2013/12/05

[149] Aznar S, Gallardo C, Fiuza-Luces C, Santana-Sosa E, López-Mojares LM, Santalla A, et al. Levels of moderate–vigorous physical activity are low in Spanish children with cystic fibrosis: A comparison with healthy controls. J Cyst Fibros. 2014;13(3):335–40.

[150] Quon BS, Patrick DL, Edwards TC, Aitken ML, Gibson RL, Genatossio A, et al. Feasibility of using pedometers to measure daily step counts in cystic fibrosis and an assessment of its responsiveness to changes in health state. J Cyst Fibros. 2012;11(3): 216–22.

[151] Ward N, White D, Rowe H, Stiller K, Sullivan T. Physical activity levels of patients with cystic fibrosis hospitalised with an acute respiratory exacerbation. Respir Med. 2013;107(7):1014–20.

[152] American College of Sports Medicine. ACSM's resource manual for guidelines for exercise testing and prescription. 9th ed. Philadelphia: Lippincott Williams & Wilkins; 2014.

[153] Johnson MR, Ferkol TW, Shepherd RW. Energy cost of activity and exercise in children and adolescents with cystic fibrosis. J Cyst Fibros. 2006;5(1):53–8.

[154] Bradley JM, Kent L, Elborn JS, O'Neill B. Motion sensors for monitoring physical activity in cystic fibrosis: what is the next step? Physical Therapy Reviews. 2010;15(3): 197–203.

[155] Turner LJ, Houchen L, Williams J, Singh SJ. Reliability of pedometers to measure step counts in patients with chronic respiratory disease. J Cardiopulm Rehabil Prev. 2012;32(5):284–91.

[156] Dias A, Gorzelniak L, Jörres RA, Fischer R, Hartvigsen G, Horsch A. Assessing physical activity in the daily life of cystic fibrosis patients. Perv Mobile Comput. 2012;8(6): 837–44.

[157] Hebestreit H, Kieser S, Rüdiger S, Schenk T, Junge S, Hebestreit A, et al. Physical activity is independently related to aerobic capacity in cystic fibrosis. Eur Respir J. 2006;28(4):734–9.

[158] Savi D, Quattrucci S, Internullo M, De Biase RV, Calverley PMA, Palange P. Measuring habitual physical activity in adults with cystic fibrosis. Respir Med. 2013;107(12): 1888–94.

[159] Janz KF, Cassady SL, Barr RN, Kelly JM. Monitoring exercise in children and adolescents with cystic fibrosis: validation of the CSA accelerometer. Cardiopulm Phys Ther J. 1995;6(2):3–8.

[160] Selvadurai HC, Blimkie CJ, Cooper PJ, Mellis CM, Van Asperen PP. Gender differences in habitual activity in children with cystic fibrosis. Arch Dis Child. 2004;89(10): 928–33.

[161] Dwyer TJ, Alison JA, McKeough ZJ, Elkins MR, Bye PTP. Evaluation of the SenseWear activity monitor during exercise in cystic fibrosis and in health. Respir Med. 2009;103(10):1511–7.

[162] Troiano RP, Berrigan D, Dodd K, Mâsse L, Tilert T, McDowell M. Physical Activity in the United States Measured by Accelerometer. Med Sci Sports Exerc. 2008;40(1):181–8.

[163] May C, Eton D, Boehmer K, Gallacher K, Hunt K, MacDonald S, et al. Rethinking the patient: using burden of treatment theory to understand the changing dynamics of illness. BMC Health Serv Res. 2014;14(1):281.

[164] Demain S, Goncalves AC, Areia C, Marques A, Marcos AJ, Oliveira R, et al. Living with and managing treatment burden in long-term conditions: A systematic review of qualitative research. PLoS Med. 2015;in press.

[165] Sawicki GS, Ren CL, Konstan MW, Millar SJ, Pasta DJ, Quittner AL. Treatment complexity in cystic fibrosis: trends over time and associations with site-specific outcomes. J Cyst Fibros. 2013;12(5):461–7.

[166] Flume PA, Robinson KA, O'Sullivan BP, Finder JD, Vender RL, Willey-Courand DB, et al. Cystic fibrosis pulmonary guidelines: airway clearance therapies. Respir Care. 2009;54(4):522–37.

[167] Gallacher K, May CR, Montori VM, Mair FS. Understanding patients' experiences of treatment burden in chronic heart failure using normalization process theory. Ann Fam Med. 2011;9(3):235–43.

[168] Karamanidou C, Weinman J, Horne R. A qualitative study of treatment burden among haemodialysis recipients. J Health Psychol. 2014;19(4):556–69.

[169] Eton DT, Ramalho de Oliveira D, Egginton JS, Ridgeway JL, Odell L, May CR, et al. Building a measurement framework of burden of treatment in complex patients with chronic conditions: a qualitative study. Patient Rel Outcome Meas. 2012;3:39–49.

[170] Conway SP, Pond MN, Hamnett T, Watson A. Compliance with treatment in adult patients with cystic fibrosis. Thorax. 1996;51(1):29–33.

[171] Abbott J, Dodd M, Bilton D, Webb AK. Treatment compliance in adults with cystic fibrosis. Thorax. 1994;49(2):115–20.

[172] Kettler L, Sawyer S, Winefield H, Greville H. Determinants of adherence in adults with cystic fibrosis. Thorax. 2002;57(5):459–64.

[173] Jordan S, Philpin S, Warring J, Cheung WY, Williams J. Percutaneous endoscopic gastrostomies: the burden of treatment from a patient perspective. J Adv Nurs. 2006;56(3):270—81.

[174] Donaldson SH, Bennett WD, Zeman KL, Knowles MR, Tarran R, Boucher RC. Mucus Clearance and Lung Function in Cystic Fibrosis with Hypertonic Saline. N Engl J Med. 2006;354(3):241–50.

7

Factors Affecting Prognosis and Prediction of Outcome in Cystic Fibrosis Lung Disease

Cormac McCarthy, Orla O'Carroll,
Alessandro N. Franciosi and Noel G. McElvaney

Abstract

Cystic fibrosis (CF) is a multisystem disorder with a significantly shortened life expectancy with the major cause of mortality related to lung disease. Inflammation is seen in the CF airways from a very early age and contributes significantly to symptoms and disease progression. As the condition worsens over time, lung function declines, usually measured by Forced Expiratory Volume in 1 second (FEV1)% predicted, and extra-pulmonary complications often manifest. While the life expectancy in CF is still short, the median age of death and predicted survival age are continually increasing. Therapeutic interventions for CF have improved significantly in the last 20 years and now there are targeted therapies towards specific elements in CF that may impact upon exacerbation frequency, symptoms, and eventually mortality due to lung disease.

As life expectancy in CF increases, the need for predicting prognosis becomes more and more important. Numerous factors affect prognosis in CF and can be used to ultimately predict outcomes. These factors can be constant or dynamic variables ranging from genetic mutation and gender to clinical measurements including pulmonary function and weight. Further variables that affect prognosis in CF include Diabetes Mellitus, sex, and pancreatic insufficiency. Furthermore, genotype is becoming more and more important as novel targeted therapies are developed that may affect survival and improve prognosis.

While prognosis in CF has traditionally been associated with FEV1% predicted, decrements in lung function that are associated with recurrent pulmonary exacerbations are increasingly important, and these are increasingly common as CF lung disease progresses. What drives these pulmonary exacerbations is bacterial colonisation, particularly *Pseudomonas aeruginosa*, with early eradication shown to improve prognosis. Nutrition and weight are also very important in CF and low body mass index has been shown to predict poor outcomes. There are several clinical prediction tools in CF, both radiological and clinical and many are too complex to be used routinely in patient care. However, newer tools aimed at predicting outcomes based on readily available objective measure are now available, including the CF-ABLE score.

In this chapter we outline, firstly, how prognosis in CF has changed over the last decade as a result of changes in treatment, better diagnostics, and improved care. Secondly, we describe the effects that genotype, pancreatic status, gender, and diabetic status have upon outcome. Thirdly, this chapter highlights the usefulness and importance of clinical measurements, including lung function, radiology, bacteriology, and blood and sputum biomarkers of disease and inflammation in predicting outcomes and how changes in these parameters influence prognosis. Finally, we summarise the prediction tools that have been utilised in CF to predict survival and how these may be utilised in clinical practice.

In conclusion, the most sensitive way of predicating prognosis currently remains a multifaceted approach, including several markers of disease and the use of all factors and a composite clinical prediction tool is suggested to stratify patient risk.

Keywords: Prognosis, prediction, survival, outcome, cystic fibrosis

---

1. Introduction

Cystic fibrosis (CF) is a multisystem inflammatory condition that is associated with a significantly shortened life span, primarily as a result of the pulmonary manifestations of the disease [1]. For many years pulmonary function measurements have been utilised as the primary surrogate of disease severity, with forced expiratory volume in 1 second (FEV1) used to assess clinical status of both patients and to predict mortality [2, 3]. However, in the last two decades there has been a significant improvement in survival in CF and this subsequently has consequences on how to treat patients and predict prognosis in this complex condition. With longer life expectancy it is essential to better predict outcome and prognosticate in CF, thus the use of survival or death as an outcome measure has become almost negligible in clinical trials or indeed in studies to predict prognosis. Hence, the development of surrogate markers or disease severity is increasingly important in CF; these range from physiological measurements of lung function, biomarkers, radiological measures, and composite scoring systems and are becoming essential in CF care and development of new drugs. With groundbreaking therapeutic breakthroughs in CF over the last decade, particularly in the modulation of CFTR function [4], the use of surrogate outcomes has become more apparent. This has led to development of new imaging modalities such as flurodeoxyglucose positron emission tomography (FDG-PET) imaging [5-7] and hyperpolarised helium magnetic resonance imaging (He3-MRI) [8], as well as increased use of multiple breath washout (MBW) and lung clearance index (LCI) to assess disease severity [9]. Moreover, there has been huge progress in the research into and development of biomarkers of inflammation in CF [10–12], both systemic and pulmonary inflammation that correlates with clinical condition and can predict outcome, further highlighting the deeper understating of the pathophysiological changes in CF and the translational research ongoing in this area. Furthermore, the use of new composite scoring systems, taking into account many aspects of this multisystem condition have been developed to aid with the classification of disease severity and predict outcome over a defined period [13].

In this chapter we will outline, firstly, how prognosis in CF has changed over the last decade as a result of changes in treatment, better diagnostics, and improved care. Secondly, the chapter will describe the effects genotype, such as pancreatic status, gender, and diabetic status, have upon outcome. Thirdly, this chapter will highlight the usefulness and importance of clinical measurements, including lung function, radiology, bacteriology, and blood and sputum biomarkers of disease and inflammation in predicting outcomes and how changes in these parameters influence prognosis. Finally, the chapter will summarise the prediction tools that have been created in CF, both clinical and research tools, which utilise measurements of disease and radiological evidence of bronchiectasis to predict survival and how these may be utilised in clinical practice.

2. Prognosis in cystic fibrosis

Life expectancy in patients with cystic fibrosis is in a constant state of change. Whilst there are undoubtedly significant further gains to be made, the improvement in predicted survival in cystic fibrosis sufferers has been a relative success story since its original description as a clinical entity in 1938. Median life expectancy, the time period in which half of a given population will die, has increased from a few months in the 1940s to as high as 41 years old in the current era [14] at present in many countries. The predicted median survival of people born with CF today continues to rise.

Numerous factors have contributed to the changing statistics in CF prognosis. Earlier and more sensitive detection methods, centralised specialist multidisciplinary care and evidence-based research have provided patients, their families, and clinicians with an environment that facilitates the long-term management of this complex multisystem disorder. Identification of increasing numbers of CF genotypes (many of which are characterised by phenotypically milder variants) has also contributed to increasing the CF population and this consequently affects the overall statistics on outcome and prognosis.

What is relevant to a patient diagnosed in infancy with a severe form of CF may not be relevant to a patient diagnosed in middle adulthood. Equally, statistics on survival from one country may not relate accurately to another, not because of difference in treatment alone, but because of differences in the predominating demographics in the two cohorts and methodologies used in assessing outcomes. As such, a "one size fits all" approach to prognosticating is not appropriate. In this chapter, we review the evidence regarding prognosis based on key clinical and demographic parameters, and the biomarkers and prediction tools that may be used to predict outcome.

3. Influence of genotype on prognosis in cystic fibrosis

CF is the most common lethal genetic disease of Caucasian populations and is caused by genetic mutations of the cystic fibrosis transmembrane regulator (CFTR) gene. The CFTR gene encodes an ATP- and CAMP-dependent chloride channel expressed on the apical membrane of epithelial and certain non-epithelial cells throughout the body. To date, greater than 1,000 CFTR mutations have been discovered. In the lung, it also regulates the activity of the ENaC channel (an apical sodium transport channel) defects in which mediate the majority of pathogenic processes in the main target organ in CF sufferers.

Commonly, the multitude of various CFTR mutations are classified into 6 distinct groups based on their ultimate effects on a range of cellular mechanisms such as transcription, processing within the cell, localization of the channel, and quantity of correctly functioning protein. Class I includes mutations with complete lack of production of protein while Class VI involves unstable functional protein being produced that is then degraded at the cell surface (Table 1).

Class	Effect	Mutation Type	Example
I	No functional protein produced	Premature stop codons: nonsense; splicing; deletions	W128X; R553X; G542X
II	Defective processing and maturation	Missense; small deletions or insertions	F508del; N1303K
III	Defects in regulation of channel opening	Missense; small deletions or insertions	G551D; G551S; G1349D
IV	Defective Chloride transport	Missense; small deletions or insertions	R117H; R334W, R347P
V	Reduction of wild-type mRNA	Partial splicing	A455E
VI	Increased turnover of unstable protein at cell surface	Missense; nonsense	120del23; N287Y; 4279insA

Table 1. List of CFTR Mutations.

The most common CFTR mutation worldwide is delF508 that accounts for upwards of 70% of cases of CF and has long been associated with more severe disease and less favourable clinical outcomes [15-17]. Conversely, several mutations have been found to be associated with more favourable outcomes and milder clinical phenotypes. In a study based on the US CF Registry in 2003, it was found that significantly different mortality rates were observed when CFTR genotype was classified according to the effects on quantitative protein production. The authors proposed that groups with severely reduced levels of CFTR (I-III) had a more severe clinical phenotype and higher mortality than groups with some residual CFTR function (IV-VI) [18]. A follow up study found that 'high risk' patients (I-III) had a two-fold greater risk of death when compared to 'low risk' (IV-VI) patients [19] and this risk was not fully explained by lung function, pancreatic insufficiency, *Pseudomonas aeruginosa* (PA) colonisation, or nutritional factors. Hence, CFTR genotype may be useful as an initial measure of prognosis in early CF diagnosis when it is often the only available information about the disease. Knowledge of the genetic processes involved in CF is leading the way for new targeted therapies that ideally will improve mortality. One such therapy is ivacaftor, a potentiator drug that enhances gating at the cell surface in patients with the class III G551D mutation. This novel medication has been associated with sustained increases in FEV1 of up to 10%, reduced frequency of pulmonary exacerbation, weight gain, and subjective improvements in quality of life (CFQ-R) scores [4, 20, 21]. However, there is wide phenotypic variance observed frequently among patients with identical genotypes. This is observed in the clinical realms of lung function, pancreatic and diabetic status, nutritional status, and response to medications and this leads to reluctance to link genotype too closely with phenotype in terms of predicting clinical outcomes and prognosis.

4. Impact of gender on prognosis

It has long been recognized that there is a significant gender difference in terms of both morbidity and mortality in cystic fibrosis. Many studies, throughout early and current cystic fibrosis research, have focused on the poorer outcomes observed in female patients when compared with their male counterparts. This dichotomy endures across the areas of microbial colonization, lung function, frequency of exacerbations, and overall survival. However, an explanation for this vast difference remains to be found.

A notable early study conducted in Canada investigated the effects of numerous variables on mortality and found that on average, males had overall increased survival rates of greater than 5 years when compared with female cohorts from the same time period (1970-1989) [22]. These results were echoed across international cohorts for similar time frames and were postulated to relate to the lower bone mineral density observed in female populations. Over time, as survival in cystic fibrosis increased, this gender difference has persisted with Rosenfeld et al. in 1997 confirming a gender difference in CF survival (25.3 vs. 28.4 females vs. males) in a cohort of over 20,000 patients [23], and Harness-Brumley et al. in more recent 2014 study observed this difference in greater than 32,000 North American patients (36.0 years vs. 38.7 years, females vs. males) [24]. Despite accounting for variables known to influence CF-related mortality, it was demonstrated that female gender is an independent significant risk factor for death. Furthermore, women were found to be colonized at an earlier age with various pathogens and that their clinical course was much worse when colonized with common CF pathogens [24].

Though the relationship between gender and adverse outcomes has been described in a multitude of studies over a vast period of time, a full explanation of this dichotomy remains elusive. Much current research now centres on the role of estrogen in female CF patients. The primary female sex hormone is 17β-estradiol (E_2) and circulates in the body bound to sex hormone binding globulin, interacting with target tissues through a range of estrogen receptors (ERs) expressed on the cell surface. E_2 levels naturally vary over the course of the normal menstrual cycle and E_2 further dehydrates the already compromised airway surface liquid seen in CF and peak levels of E_2 lead to an increased risk of infection and subsequent exacerbation [25]. Furthermore, high levels of E_2 have been shown to promote TLR hyporesponsiveness to a range of bacteria driven by an inhibition of interleukin-8 (IL-8) release [26]. In a study targeted to investigate the effects of E_2 on *Pseudomonas Aeruginosa* (PA). it was found that high levels of E_2 promotes mucoid conversion, alginate synthesis, and genetic mutations in mucins lending increased infectivity and virulence to PA in those exposed to E_2 [15]. An interesting addendum to this study was the observation that the individuals studied had lower rates of exacerbation and required a lower number of antibiotic courses if they were using the combined oral contraceptive pill [15]. As exacerbation rate is commonly quoted as a predictor for mortality, there is scope here to assess the role of targeted estrogen therapies on mortality and the gender dichotomy in CF.

5. Relationship between exocrine disease and prognosis in cystic fibrosis

Pancreatic insufficiency is an extremely common complication of CF and affects over 85% of patients at some point during the course of their disease [27]. Loss of pancreatic exocrine function leads to malabsorption of fat, protein, and micronutrients, which in turn causes failure to thrive, steatorrhoea symptoms, and fat-soluble vitamin deficiencies. This arises as a consequence of obstruction of proximal intralobular ducts in the pancreas due to inspissated mucus plugs and tends to arise early in the disease. Chronic pancreatitis is another less common manifestation generally associated with milder (IV-VI) CF genotypes [28, 29], as residual pancreatic acinar tissue is a prerequisite for pancreatitis to develop. Pancreatitis affects over 10% of CF patients and tends to occur in a chronic relapsing and remitting fashion. It is thought to be due to a combination of obstructive tubulopathy and acidification of the acinar lumen due to reduced ductal bicarbonate secretion. Those with symptomatic pancreatitis can often become pancreatic insufficient as their disease progresses. A recent review of the European Cystic Fibrosis registry demonstrated that pancreatic insufficiency was associated with a statistically significant decreases in FEV1%, with pancreatic insufficient patients twice as likely as sufficient patients to experience severe lung disease, defined as FEV < 40% predicted [30]. This indicates that lack of pancreatic exocrine function is associated with worsening prognosis.

6. Cystic fibrosis-related diabetes is associated with poor prognosis

Cystic fibrosis-related diabetes (CFRD) is a common comorbidity with an estimated prevalence of 20% in adolescents and 40%–50% in adults [31]. As with other disease-related comorbidities, incidence of CFRD continues to increase as life expectancy improves. It encompasses a spectrum of disease from impaired glucose tolerance to CFRD with fasting hyperglycaemia. Impaired chloride channel function leads to thick pancreatic secretions that cause obstructive damage to the exocrine pancreas and subsequent architectural disturbance in islet cells with loss of endocrine function. Insulin deficiency is compounded by insulin resistance that occurs during pulmonary exacerbations as a consequence of increased levels of growth hormone, cortisol, catecholamines, and inflammatory cytokines [32]. Not all patients with CF go on to develop CFRD, and it has been demonstrated that multiple extrinsic factors contribute to disease pathogenesis such as malabsorption, immunosuppressant therapy following lung transplantation, use of glucocorticosteroids, and the presence of liver disease.

CFRD has a significant impact upon clinical parameters of disease and thus impacts upon prognosis. Insulin deficiency and hyperglycaemia negatively affects pulmonary function with the rate of decline in FEV1% over a 4 year period found to be related to the severity of insulin deficiency [33]. Moreover, insulin replacement therapy can improve both nutritional status and pulmonary function in patients with CFRD [34]. Hyperglycaemia also impacts clinically, with moderately elevated blood glucose levels leading to increased airway glucose concentrations, which in turn promotes the growth of various respiratory pathogens and can increase exacerbation rate [35]. CFRD also impacts, predictably, on nutritional status with both insulin deficiency and hyperglycaemia exerting effects. The classical complications of diabetes mellitus also contribute to morbidity in patients with CFRD. Macrovascular complications have not been documented, despite the increasing life expectancy of these patients. However, microvascular complications are common and include mild neuropathy as the most common manifestation with prevalence rates similar to those for non-CF diabetics [36]. Furthermore in one study, retinopathy occurred in 16% of CFRD patients and microalbuminaemia in 14% in a cohort of patients who had diabetes for more than 10 years [36].

In terms of direct mortality, CFRD has been shown to have a negative prognostic effect, with increased mortality seen in association with poorer nutritional status and greater severity of lung disease [37, 38]. In addition, CFRD mortality has been shown to be increased in female cohorts when compared to males [39]. However, over time there have been sustained improvements in CFRD-associated mortality with both female and male mortality decreasing in the period between 1992 and 2003 [31], this effect is presumably a reflection of increased awareness of the importance of CFRD and improvements in diagnosis and treatment strategies. CFRD is a common and complex co-morbidity in CF which negatively impacts on clinical outcomes and mortality. There is evidence to show that early treatment of CFRD can promote improved nutritional status, pulmonary function, and ultimately improve outcome.

7. Cystic fibrosis-related liver disease and prognosis

As the life expectancy of patients with CF continues to improve, cystic fibrosis-related liver disease (CFLD) is becoming increasingly more prevalent with an incidence estimated of up to 30%, according to multiple studies. Liver disease firstly manifests in its most simple form as biochemical derangements in liver enzymes. Structural disease develops next and manifests as fatty infiltration on ultrasound scan or increased bile content in liver parenchyma. Decompensated liver disease occurs last, which can involve portal hypertension, ascites, variceal disease, and impaired coagulation. These disease processes occur as a consequence of altered viscous bile due to abnormal CFTR-regulated ion transport across cholangiocytes. Consequently, biliary flow is reduced and there is obstruction of intrahepatic bile ducts. This causes damage to hepatocytes and cholangiocytes through inflammatory processes, bile duct proliferation, and portal tract fibrosis. The pathogenesis of fatty liver disease in CF is less well understood and has been loosely attributed to fatty acid deficiency, malnutrition, and insulin resistance [40].

Attempts have been made to link the development of CFLD with the presence of certain underlying CFTR mutations, the assumption being that CFLD would be seen with increasing frequency in patients with the classically severe or high-risk phenotypes as described above. However, this relationship has not been demonstrated to date. Non-CFTR modifier genes have been proposed to increase susceptibility to development of CFLD and it is thought that identifying these genetic modifiers may allow early identification of patients at risk. To date only polymorphisms in the SERPINA1 allele, which codes for an alpha-1 antitrypsin, has been demonstrated to be significantly related to CFLD and portal hypertension [41].

Liver disease is widely cited as the third most common cause of death in CF patients after respiratory failure and transplant complications, with a mortality rate estimated at 2.5% [30] and a higher mortality risk is observed in those with liver disease than in those without [40]. However, there continues to be massive variability in the severity of CFLD without adequate explanation as to why it affects only certain patients, thus it is a complex prognostic index.

8. Clinical measurements of disease severity and how they predict prognosis

Whilst recognising the importance of tailoring care of patients with CF to the individual genotypes and associated co-morbidities is essential, many of these factors are established and in many ways less dynamically modifiable than others in clinical practice.

The prognostic value of more dynamic markers of clinical condition offer more practical long-term targets around which to focus treatment and goals in the individual patient. On a day to day basis, these parameters guide practice and stratify patients in terms of expected outcomes.

9. Pulmonary function and how it predicts prognosis

Spirometric measurement of lung function, specifically FEV1, has been the pre-eminent surrogate marker of disease staging in CF for a long time. As it is reproducible, readily available, and cheap, it provides longitudinal measurement of airflow obstruction over years.

Seminal work by Kerem et al. in 1992 suggested that as an independent factor, FEV1 reliably predicts the relative risk of mortality, with a baseline FEV1 of less than 30% predicted giving a 50% two-year mortality [3, 42]. Following on from this work, further studies suggested that rate of decline of FEV1 could more accurately identify the most at risk patients [2, 43, 44]. Interestingly there is evidence that high baseline FEV1 is a risk factor for greater FEV1 decline and that this phenomenon may be explained by less aggressive prescribing patterns in patients with preserved lung function [45].

Few would argue that FEV1 is invaluable in clinical practice; however, it does fall short in identifying early lung disease where spirometry is often normal. This is especially the case in paediatric CF centres, where lung disease is often in its early stages or where technical limitations in performing reliable expiratory manoeuvres are more common. Recent interest has arisen in lung disease assessment using the Lung Clearance Index (LCI), a measurement derived from the multiple-breath inert gas washout. Whilst this technique is time consuming and less readily available, there is growing evidence that it may be more sensitive than FEV1 in diagnosing early lung disease [46, 47] and that abnormal LCI in the setting of normal FEV1 may predict future FEV1 decline [9]. Moreover, LCI correlates with high resolution computerised tomography (HRCT) findings [48] and predicts exacerbations and time to first exacerbation [49]. As such LCI may prove to be an appealing tool for more sensitively detecting improvements in lung health when assessing novel therapeutic options [50] and become a useful prognostic index.

10. Microbial colonisation in cystic fibrosis and its effect upon prognosis

Bacterial colonisation of the airways is the catalyst for cyclical infectious exacerbations of CF, leading to acute, subacute, and chronic inflammation. The identification of organism and subsequent in-vitro sensitivity testing helps in guiding treatment, antibiotic choices, and even infection control measures. The individual impact of specific organisms on prognosis and survival has been a focus of interest in clinical research for some time.

11. *Pseudomonas aeruginosa*

The most prominent pathogen with a specific affinity for the CF lung is *Pseudomonas Aeruginosa* (PA). Though its prevalence in CF populations varies with age [51], it is the most common airway pathogen in adult CF patients. PA colonisation predicts lower FEV1 at the time of culture [52, 53] and greater rate of decline in pulmonary function over time [54-56] when compared with Methicillin Sensitive *Staphylococcus Aureus* colonised (MSSA) and non-colonised patients. Moreover, evidence suggests that patients in whom PA colonisation is eradicated in a systematic manner have a significant reduction in treatment burden and days spent in hospital. This, in turn, can result in reduced expense on treatment of exacerbations [57].

12. *Staphylococcus aureus*

Amongst the earliest pathogens to become clinically prominent in the life of patients with CF is *Staphylococcus Aureus* (SA) [58]. Its prevalence globally is 44%–56% (2008) in its methicillin sensitive form (MSSA) and 8%–23% for methicillin resistant strains (MRSA). The difficulty in accurately establishing the relevance of SA as a pathogen in CF may lie in the complexity involved in characterising the specific virulence of the strains involved. MSSA, *Small colony variant MSSA* (SCV-MSSA) and MRSA (both community acquired-MRSA and healthcare associated MRSA) all differ in resistance patterns and apparent virulence. A study by Hoffman et al. in 2006 [59] suggested that co-colonisation with MSSA and PA favoured the formation of SCV-MSSA. Subsequent work by Besier et al. [60] associated colonisation with SCV-MSSA with worse lung function, more PA co-infection and more antibiotic resistance than those with MSSA. This is especially telling when colonisation with PA and SA is not uncommon. During a 1990s US-based clinical trial [61] an analysis of baseline sputum found 43% of participants to culture both PA and SA. Current evidence suggest that patients culturing MRSA have worse lung function and require more antibiotics than those with MSSA [62] and that PA/MRSA co-colonisation is associated with more pronounced decline in lung function than PA/MSSA co-colonisation [63]. Controversy still exists surrounding the long established practice of prescribing prophylactic antimicrobials with activity against MSSA. Although studies have suggested reduced cough and less culture positivity in the setting of prophylaxis, no clear benefits in terms of outcomes have been observed. Furthermore, several studies have pointed to increased and earlier incidence of PA culture in patients undergoing MSSA suppression therapy [64]. Whilst guidelines published by international bodies vary on their recommendation regarding chronic anti-staphylococcal use, a recent Cochrane review found no convincing evidence for treatment [65] and reiterated concerns around the increase in PA colonisation.

13. *Burkholderia cepacia* complex

Long mistaken for a *Pseudomonas*, *Burkholderia* species were identified more accurately in the 1980s and 1990s as diagnostic techniques improved. Now recognised as perhaps the most virulent pathogens in CF, they present a major treatment challenge. The *Burkholderia Cepacia Complex* (BCC) is comprised of at least 17 distinct species of gram-negative bacteria. Termed Genomovars, these species vary in prevalence and apparent virulence. The most common BCC strains identified are *B.Cenocepacia* and *B.Multivorans*. Evidence from 2002 revealed a four-fold mortality risk in patients colonised with epidemic *B.Cenocepacia*, associated with a more rapid rate of lung function decline versus others (FEV1 -1.9% vs. -0.3% per annum) [66]. Further data from 2004 showed *B.Cenocepacia* was associated with a statistically significant higher rate of lung function decline (-140 ml/year vs. -32 ml/year (p=0.01)) and reduction in BMI when compared to PA and *B.Multivorans* [67]. Whilst evidence is mounting that specific BCC genomovars have a hierarchy of virulence with *B.Cenocepacia* associated with the highest morbidity, it is worth noting that progressive disease can be caused by a multitude of strains. "*Cepacia Syndrome*", a constellation of sepsis, fevers, and leucocytosis and fulminant decline most often resulting in death, has been described with genomovars other than *B.Cenocepacia* [68]. The true determinant of virulence may best be assessed by identification of specific epidemic strains within distinct genomovars. Moreover, strains associated with poor outcomes in the native lungs of CF sufferers may not cause the worst outcomes in post-transplant patients. A 2008 study assessing mortality in CF patients on transplant waiting list and post-transplant revealed a higher waiting-list five year mortality in *B.Multivorans* and non-epidemic strain *B.Cenocepacia* carriers than those with epidemic strains of *B.Cenocepacia*. Furthermore, 5-year post-transplant mortality was highest in the non-epidemic *B.Cenocepacia* cohort and carriers of *Burkholderia Gladioli*, an organism not included in the *BCC* group, and generally considered less relevant as a CF pathogen [69]. Clearly a deeper understanding of the relevance and prognostic implications of specific BCC colonisation is needed. Despite the significant risk posed by *Burkholderia* species in the CF population, evidence for eradication protocols and recommended antibiotic regimens is lacking, which is concerning as it possibly has the most significant effect upon prognosis of all bacterial colonisers [70].

14. Non-tuberculous Mycobacteria (NTM)

A 2013 study by Bryant et al. [71] demonstrating patient to patient transmission of *Mycobacterium Abscessus* (*subspecies Massiliense*) in a CF centre re-focused attention on the clinical management and implications of NTM colonisation. Prevalence (6%-14%) of NTM organisms is variable and changing with time [72] and patient phenotype appears to dictate colonisation with younger, more malnourished patients with more severe genotypes culturing more *Mycobacterium Abscessus Complex* (MBASC) organisms than *Mycobacterium Avium Complex* (MAC) [73, 74]. Recurrent NTM culture positive status has been shown to be associated with progression of HRCT changes [75], however, despite these findings, statistical evidence indicating worse outcomes in pulmonary function or mortality is lacking. With the employment of prophylactic macrolide treatment for reduction of exacerbations, significant concerns were raised regarding the possibility of developing macrolide resistance in colonising NTM species; hence, NTM culture positivity is a contraindication to macrolide prophylaxis. Long-term macrolide use may, however, have a protective effect in reducing incidence of NTM culture positivity as highlighted by Coolen et al. in 2015 [76]. This finding could have a significant impact on prognosis and treatment options, as NTM colonisation is still considered a contraindication to transplant in some centres despite growing evidence that outcomes post-transplant in this cohort are acceptable [77].

15. Other microbial organisms in cystic fibrosis

Aspergillus Fumigatus (AspF) is a common airway fungus found in the CF lung. Previous treatment was aimed largely at patients meeting criteria for diagnosis of Allergic Broncho-pulmonary Aspergillosis (ABPA). More recent evidence, however, suggests that AspF carriage correlates with more severe changes on HRCT [78] and can predict greater rate of FEV1 decline in patients who are a) colonised but not sensitised, b) sensitised but do not meet ABPA diagnostic criteria, and c) those with a diagnosis of ABPA [79]. Suitable studies assessing the value of AspF eradication in patients with CF not meeting ABPA criteria are lacking.

Stenotrophomonas Maltophilia (SM) and its relevance has been a point of debate for some time. Previously regarded as a bystander in the CF microbiome there is growing belief that it represents a true pathogen with potentially significant impact of mortality [80]. Antibiotic options for the treatment of SM are limited and dedicated studies assessing treatment effectiveness are lacking [81].

Candida Species are highly prevalent in CF airway culture [82]. Difficulty arises in differentiating oropharyngeal contamination from bronchial colonisation without bronchoscopic sampling. Data from 2010 suggests that colonisation with *Candida Albicans* is associated with increased exacerbation rate and significant decline in FEV1 [83]. There is a paucity of data relating to the benefits of treating *Candida Species* routinely in CF.

16. Impact of respiratory failure on prognosis in cystic fibrosis

Despite being a predictable outcome of progressive lung disease, the management of respiratory failure in CF, both hypoxic (Type 1 Respiratory Failure) and hypercapnic (Type 2 Respiratory Failure), is lacking in terms of an evidence base [84]. Prescribing habits for oxygen (nocturnal, ambulatory, or resting) borrow largely from guidelines for other conditions. Hypoxia as a determinant of prognosis therefore has not been assessed, although there are suggestions that patients at higher mortality risk have an association with worsening six minute walk test results [85]. However, baseline hypercapnia has been shown to be an independent risk factor for death, even in patients with an FEV1 greater than 30% predicted [86]. There is a paucity of reliable data regarding the benefits of maintenance non-invasive bi-level positive airway pressure ventilation (BIPAP) in CF. One randomised placebo controlled trial from 2008 [87] did show significant benefits with nocturnal BIPAP in terms of symptoms (quality of life questionnaires scores, dyspnoea indices, and chest symptoms), improvements in modified shuttle walk test distances, and improved nocturnal (but not diurnal) arterial hypercapnia, but no significant improvements were shown in lung function. Data does suggest, however, that in the setting of acute respiratory failure requiring admission to intensive care units, non-invasive ventilation (NIV) was associated with significantly improved outcomes when compared to intubation and mechanical ventilation in patients with CF [88-90]. Hence, the importance of respiratory failure in predicting prognosis needs further study in CF.

17. Nutritional status and weight in determining outcome in cystic fibrosis

The impact of malnutrition in CF is of great interest; exocrine and endocrine dysfunction, coupled with high basal metabolic requirements in the setting of chronic disease, exposes patients to a high risk of malnourishment. Low BMI in CF is known to increase in incidence with age and be closely implicated in worsening lung function [91, 92] and predicts worse outcome over a 4-year period [93]. Furthermore, patients awaiting lung transplantation who require nutritional intervention have been shown to have a higher risk of death [86] and improving the nutritional status of malnourished patients may ultimately improve lung function, even in cohorts with relatively advanced lung disease [94-96].

18. Bone mineral density in cystic fibrosis

Low bone mineral density (BMD) and subsequently osteopenia and osteoporosis are common in CF. Thus far, no convincing association has been shown between lung function and BMD and predictors of low BMD include BMI, weight, and age [97, 98]. Despite much research focus in this area, recent evidence raises the possibility that, unlike lung function and life expectancy, there has not been a significant improvement inter-generationally in BMD [99]. The lack of clinical data proving concrete improvements in outcomes with bisphosphonate therapy, other than BMD change itself, has left a clinical conundrum regarding the management of low BMD in CF [100]. Further studies are needed to guide clinical decisions which are currently dictated by experience and judgement. However, there is no prognostic value in BMD scores in CF patients.

19. Biomarkers of disease severity and how they predict prognosis

19.1. Sputum and bronchoalveolar lavage fluid biomarkers

The need for useful and clinically relevant biomarkers is vital, and their use as predictors of prognosis as well as surrogates of clinical response to treatment is increasingly important. Numerous different sputum biomarkers have been investigated and used to correlate with clinical condition, including correlating with exacerbation frequency, pulmonary function, microbiological colonisation and overall prognosis. The use of sputum biomarkers is ideal in CF as patients produce significant amounts of sputum, hence samples are easy to obtain and samples are routinely collected to assess bacterial colonisation as part of best practice care.

Several studies have demonstrated how neutrophil elastase (NE) activity is significantly increased in the CF lung and a recent study by Sly et al. revealed how NE activity is an early biomarker for the development of bronchiectasis in CF [101]. The levels of NE in CF bronchoalveolar lavage fluid (BALF) correlate inversely with FEV1 [10] and furthermore the higher the level of NE detectable the more rapid the decline in lung function [12], neutrophil counts also correlate well with these measures. These results support the use of NE levels and activity as a useful biomarker available from BALF or sputum, and many other potential biomarkers are benchmarked against this measure as well as clinical correlation. Several inflammatory cytokines which are known to be elevated in the CF lung have potential to be useful biomarkers also, particularly interleukin-8 (IL-8) and tumour necrosis alpha (TNF-α). IL-8 is a neutrophil chemo-attractant and elevated levels are seen in CF BALF [102] and levels measured in sputum correlate inversely with FEV1 [10]. IL-8 and TNF- α levels are elevated at the time of an acute pulmonary exacerbation, and have been shown to significantly decrease in response to antibiotic treatment in an inverse pattern compared to lung function measurements [103]. Furthermore, the levels of IL-8 found in the lungs of CF patients correlates with microbial colonisation, with higher levels identifiable in patients colonised with *Pseudomonas Aeruginosa* (PA) and *Staphylococcus Aureus* (SA) compared to non-colonised CF patients and healthy controls [104]. Further support for the usefulness of these cytokines as markers is how they correlate with symptoms of deterioration as reported by patients [105], hence IL-8 and TNF-α are markers of degree of lung damage and bacterial colonisation. There are limitations to the use of sputum and BALF biomarkers such as these, as they do not always correlate with all clinical measurements of disease; in one study IL-8 did not correlate [106] with modified Bhalla scores [107], or other reversible changes on high resolution computed tomography (HRCT) that did correlate with lung function measurements.

Glycosaminoglycans (GAGs) are involved in the modulation of IL-8 activity in BALF and increased expression of GAGs is related to the sustained inflammation in the CF lung, hence the levels of GAGs may be a potential biomarker of disease progression in CF as their expression is related to the neutrophil chemotaxis in the lung [108]. Other cytokines including IL-10 and IL-4 are also significantly elevated in CF BALF compared to healthy controls [109]. However, fewer studies have been done on these cytokines.

Several other sputum and BALF biomarkers have been studied and some have more potential future utility than others. Some of the early sputum biomarkers investigated were nitrites, with sputum NO_2/NO_3 shown to be significantly higher in CF patients with acute exacerbations [110] and correlated with neutrophil counts and inversely with FEV1 [111]. However, the levels did not return to normal despite intensive antibiotic treatment, hence negating their potential use as a marker of response to treatment [110]. Biomarkers that correlate to PA colonisation also include club cell secretory protein (CCSP), which is inversely related to the NE concentration in CF sputum and patients with pseudomonas aeruginosa have significantly lower CCSP than non-colonised individuals [112]. Furthermore, levels of leukotriene B4 (LTB4) correlate with PA colonisation in CF compared to other organisms [104].

To date, the most accurate sputum and BALF biomarker in CF remains NE activity and levels, hence several other biomarkers have been compared to this to demonstrate their usefulness. Other proteases such as matrix metalloproteinases 2 (MMP-2) and MMP-9 correlate well with increased levels noted in BALF which possessed increased NE activity [109], while cathepsins do not correlate with PA colonisation or exacerbations [113]. Biomarkers specific to pulmonary exacerbations are ideal as defining the response to treatment is very difficult in CF,; these include mucins MUC5AB and MUC5AC which are degraded at the time of exacerbation and demonstrate increased sialylation compared to controls [114]. Granulocyte-macrophage colony-stimulating factor (GM-CSF) levels at the time of pulmonary exacerbation predicts a larger acute decline in FEV1[115], which is highly predictive of poor prognosis [13], hence this may be a useful marker of future disease progression. Finally, calprotectin, a neutrophil derived protein, may also be a useful biomarker, where levels both in sputum and serum have been demonstrated to decrease significantly following treatment of an acute exacerbation and predicted time to next exacerbation [116], this is extremely useful as both exacerbations and lung function decline are the most sensitive markers of disease progression in CF.

19.2. Serum biomarkers as markers of systemic inflammation

Similar to sputum biomarkers, the use of serum biomarkers is highly appealing to monitor disease progression and also predict outcomes. Several studies have investigated in CF an array of potentially useful peptides and cytokines measurable in serum that correlate with exacerbation severity, length and recurrence as well as lung function and microbiological colonisation. While there are many studies of biomarkers of inflammation in CF and it further strengthens our understanding of the disease, the use of biomarkers has not become routine clinical practice, hence the need for accurate measurements of both pulmonary and systemic inflammation, which makes serum levels a key factor in this process as they may also be useful in measuring the response to treatment and predicting prognosis especially as new therapeutic options emerge.

As discussed previously, markers of neutrophil activity and elastase levels and activity in the lung correlate excellently with clinical condition, hence the use of neutrophil markers from serum would be ideal as biomarkers. One such biomarker is calprotectin, a neutrophil derived protein that is released during neutrophil activation, which has been shown to correlate with the resolution of exacerbations [116], as well as correlating with radiological scores and pulmonary symptoms [117]. CD16b is a receptor expressed by human neutrophils which binds immunoglobulins and is involved in the inflammatory response in CF. Levels of alpha-1 antitrypsin (AAT) complexed to CD16b (AAT:CD16b complex) have been shown to be significantly higher in CF patients than healthy controls, and correlate to other pro-inflammatory cytokines including IL-8 and TNF-α [11]. Plasma concentrations of AAT:CD16b complex at the time of acute pulmonary exacerbation responded to antibiotic treatment and demonstrated a significant correlation to FEV1 improvement. These results suggest this may be a potentially useful biomarker of acute exacerbations and hence a useful prognostic tool.

The use of cytokines, similarly to sputum, is often viewed as an ideal surrogate of disease state, and many have been studied. Immunoglobulin G (IgG) and IL-6 have been shown previously to correlate with mortality, however, when adjusted for confounding factors, in particular FEV1, this correlation did not remain independent [118]. There is significant cross correlation between inflammatory markers such as TNF-α, IL-8 and cathepsins as well as IL-6 and IgG. However, none have shown any significant correlation with mortality. As survival becomes longer in this disease, the need increases for biomarkers that correlate together with other indices of disease such as pulmonary function, bacterial colonisation, exacerbation frequency, and radiological changes.

Leucocyte ribonucleic acid (RNA) measurements may be one such biomarker for potential future use. In identifying the presence of airway infection, whole blood levels of leucocyte RNA is an accurate measure and is more sensitive than FEV1 or c-reactive protein (CRP), and together with FEV1 is highly sensitive [119]. Other novel biomarkers include anti-neutrophil cytoplasmic antibodies specific for bactericidal/permeability-increasing protein (BPI-ANCA).

Bactericidal/permeability-increasing protein (BPI) is one of the most potent endogenously produced antibacterials secreted by neutrophils, and autoantibodies against this protein are present in up to 90% of CF patients [120]. Levels of BPI-ANCA correlate strongly with markers of lung disease and it may indicate a pathogenic role in CF [121] and a recent study has shown that the presence of BPI-ANCA correlated significantly with a poor outcome, being death or requiring a lung transplantation. Furthermore, in patients colonised with PA the outcome was significantly worse if associated with this biomarker [122].

While no single biomarker of disease severity exists from either sputum or serum, there are several potential biomarkers that need further study and more robust results to support their routine use in clinical practice.

One biomarker that has recently re-emerged as a useful index of disease severity is the measurement of CFTR function. This may be measured by nasal potential difference (NPD) and sweat chloride concentration. It is important as a biomarker as it has been shown that CFTR and sweat chloride concentration at diagnosis predicts long term prognosis [123]. NPD is now reproducible in a more robust manor than previously, as it was difficult to accurately to so in the past [124]. The use of this biomarker has been further established in the recent clinical trials of CFTR modulators and correctors such as ivacaftor, with a change in NPD and sweat chloride seen as marker of improvement and correlating with improvements in lung function and BMI, whether this will be a long-term prognostic indictor remains to be seen [4].

20. Radiological methods to predict prognosis

Due to the complexity of CF lung disease, multiple modalities are needed to fully assess the extent of disease severity, including radiological imaging. Several imaging techniques have been employed and studied in CF; with plain radiograph, CT, and MRI all having varying abilities to predict prognosis, as well as correlate with clinical condition, and a number of scoring systems exist to qualify the extent of pulmonary involvement. High-resolution CT imaging of the lungs is currently the most sensitive method of assessing the structural changes in CF. HRCT permits airway thickness measurements and the extent of bronchiectactic changes, and these changes closely correlate with FEV1 and often adult patients with CF show more acute changes in HRCT abnormalities than decline in spirometric results [125]. The progression of bronchiectasis also correlates with CFTR genotype and levels of neutrophilic inflammation [126], while also significantly predicting exercise capacity in CF patients [127].

Newer methods to image the lungs in CF include hyperpolarised helium magnetic resonance imaging (He3-MRI) [8] and flurodeoxyglucose positron emission tomography (FDG-PET) imaging [5-7]. Both modalities correlate closely with abnormalities seen on HRCT and improve with antibiotic treatment, making them both sensitive useful tools in the acute setting. He3-MRI may identify early ventilatory changes in paediatric disease before identifiable changes on HRCT [128] and may better correlate with spirometry in assessing response after exacerbation treatment [8]. These modalities are not currently in widespread use due to both cost and availability, however, He3-MRI may become more routine in the future as life expectancy increases and the risk associated with increased cumulative exposure to ionising radiation associated with CT and FDG-PET [129].

A number of different radiological scoring systems have been developed to assess disease burden in CF. Older scoring systems were based on chest radiograph changes, and these included the Brasfield [130], National Institutes of Health (NIH) chest radiograph [131], and the Royal Children's Hospital (RCH) chest radiograph score [132]. While these were somewhat useful, they correlated poorly with spirometry and with clinical condition [133]. With the continual improvement in CT imaging modalities, HRCT has become the gold standard for assessing structural abnormalities, and several robust validated scoring systems exist for CT abnormalities. These include the Brody II score [134] and the CF-CT score [135], while one of the older original scoring tools, the Bhalla score, for bronchiectasis is still widely used in modified versions [107]. The Bhalla scoring system is an objective measure incorporating all aspects of CF structural abnormalities and has been validated and correlates with spirometry[136], clinical condition [127, 137], and has some correlation with health related quality of life [138], however, there is little correlation between these scores and other biomarkers of inflammation [106].

Radiological scoring systems are useful in assessing the extent of structural changes in CF, and correlate with certain aspects of the disease, however, they alone are not sufficient to predict prognosis and are likely more beneficial when used as part of composite clinical prediction tools.

21. Usefulness of clinical prediction tools in cystic fibrosis

As previously outlined in this chapter, life expectancy continues to improve in patients with CF due to a combination of improvements in treatment, level of care, and diagnostic tools, as well as multidisciplinary input and the development of disease-specific centres. With continually improving clinical outcomes, the need arises to better predict the prognosis of CF at an individual and group level. This need was first identified in 1958 with the development of the Shwachman-Kulczycki (SK) score to assess the severity of CF [139]. This score formed part of a study which monitored 105 patients for 5 years, the first of its kind to assess the long term progress of young CF patients. It was seen that there was increased frequency of CF patients surviving to adolescence and young adulthood and demonstrated a need to assess disease severity in order to predict the likely course of the disease.

There are many criticisms of the SK score as it is largely a subjective measure that depends on the clinical estimation of the examiner. Another drawback is that it does not include evaluations of pulmonary function. It was also devised with reference to a paediatric population in a time when life expectancy was drastically decreased. However, there have been a range of studies since its conception that have validated this score against a host of parameters increasingly used to measure prognosis. For example, Brasfield et al. observed a significant correlation between the SK score and chest radiography in an evaluation of over 640 chest radiogrpahs of 118 CF patients [130]. A more recent evaluation of the usefulness of this score to assess disease severity was undertaken by Stollar et al. in 2011 where [140] significant correlations were demonstrated between FEV1, chest radiograph, HRCT, 6-minute walk test (6MWT), and SK score. It was felt that the SK score adequately reflects radiographic and functional impairments in patients with greater impairment of lung function, however, the score was less useful in patients with preserved lung function (FEV1 >70%). Regardless of its shortcomings, the SK score is regarded as a milestone in the history of CF and continues to serve as a somewhat tool in the determination of disease severity.

This score formed the basis for the development of a multitude of clinical prediction tools, the majority of which involve clinical parameters, radiological parameters, or a combination of both. One such early radiological scoring system is the Brasfield score [130], which is based on the chest radiograph findings of patients with CF and encompasses a maximum score of 25, with points scored according to the severity of air trapping, linear markings, nodular cystic lesions, large lesions, and an impression of the overall general severity of the radiograph. However, it similarly is a subjective scoring system and there can be inter-rater differences. The Brasfield score does correlate with pulmonary function tests and the SK score and is reproducible. A disadvantage of the Brasfield score is that it was developed to include radiographs assessed by a team of radiologists and clinicians, while the Northern score [141] is an advance on the Brasfield score which allows for a single examiner to determine the radiographic severity based on assessing chest radiographs divided into lung quadrants. The maximum score is 20, with higher scores reflecting poorer outcomes due to increased severity of disease. This score was validated against the Brasfield score and an earlier score, Chrispin-Norman [142], and was found to be equal in terms of consistency, reproducibility, and accuracy in reflecting overall clinical status as measured by the SK score.

The development of widespread use of computed tomography in clinical practice has led to the inclusion of HRCT in prognostic tools for CF. Nathanson et al. proposed the first such score which involved dividing the lung CT into 12 distinct zones in order to classify the severity of bronchiectasis on a 5-point scale in each zone [143]. This, once again, was validated against the SK and Brasfield scoring systems along with the results of pulmonary function tests carried out on the subjects. As discussed, Bhalla et al. [107] further developed the idea of CT scoring systems in order to aid selection for lung transplantation and put forward a score based on the severity of 9 different radiological parameters including peribronchial thickening, extent of bronchiectasis, and extent of mucus impaction. This score is very reproducible and correlates strongly with pulmonary function, hence is the gold standard for HRCT evaluation.

Clinically-based prognostic tools play a central role in the management of CF patients and serve to direct treatments, investigations, and multidisciplinary input. The National Institute of Health scale, developed in 1973, proposed a comprehensive scoring system which included multiple parameters including baseline demographics, various measures of lung function, and presence of common complications encountered in the disease [131]. A 100-point scale derived from these measurements correlated with severity of disease, the higher scores being associated with poorer outcomes. It is a complex and cumbersome scale that reduces the likelihood for its application across the broader clinical setting. However, it is a reliable and reproducible score which encompasses many aspects of the disease and this has led to its continued use in CF-related research.

With the advancement of CF survival and life expectancy a need to develop simple and reliable prognostic tools for use in the clinical setting became apparent. In 1997, Hayllar et al. developed a predictive index based on research from over 400 patients and studied and correlated the index result with a mortality curve [144]. In this way, a simple calculation could be made to estimate 6-month and 1-year survival rates for a given score. The score was based on height, presence of hepatomegaly, white blood cell count, FEV1, and forced vital capacity (FVC). This, and scores like it, revolutionised the approach to prognosis in previously unchartered territory and survival estimates became central to prognostic tools. Liou et al. advanced on the NIH and Hayllar scores to present a 5-year prognostic tool, the longest range survival model in the field at its time of development [145]. It is based on a composite score of 8 clinical factors, as well as measurement of FEV1 and is a comprehensive, reproducible, reliable prognostic tool. However, it remains a complicated score to perform clinically and so focus has shifted in recent times to the development of simplified prediction tools that can be used within the time constraints of the current clinical setting. The CF-ABLE score was devised with this in mind and it involves the measurement of 4 of the major clinical parameters encountered in day to day practice [93]. Age, BMI, FEV1, and frequency of pulmonary exacerbations have been evaluated on a 7-point scale for correlation with prognosis and it has been found that patients with higher scores have a 26% chance of a poor outcome (death or transplantation) within 4 years of measurement. This score has been validated on a national registry and highlights the applicability of simple prediction tools that can be employed in the clinical environment.

Clinical and radiological prediction tools have emerged as a vital resource in the treatment of CF. They allow us to stratify patients by disease severity and to a certain extent allow us to predict likely adverse outcomes in patients with poor prognostic indices. A multitude of prognostic tools have been developed since the original SK score as CF research has continued to expand, each reflecting the changing face of CF treatment and diagnostic tools. Clinical practice favours the use of simple reliable scoring systems which take into account easily measurable parameters, such as the Hayllar score and the more up to date CF-ABLE score. Future research will need to involve the development of further prognostic tools to reflect the changes occurring in the management of CF (Table 2).

Name of Score	Year Published	Number of patients in cohort	Parameters Used	Strengths	Limitations
Shwachman-Kulzcizy [139]	1958	105 CF patients followed for 5 years	- General activity - Physical exam - Nutrition - Chest radiograph	- Uncomplicated assessment - Reproducible - High correlation with pulmonary function	- Subjective - No inclusion of measurement of pulmonary function

Name of Score	Year Published	Number of patients in cohort	Parameters Used	Strengths	Limitations
				-High correlation with Brasfield score	- Developed in paediatric population
NIH Score [131]	1973	73 patients aged 3 to 30 years followed for a period between 3 and 6 years	100 point scale of severity of lung and general parameters as well as common complications: - Chest Radiograph - Pulmonary function - Pulmonary exacerbations - Pneumothorax - Haemoptysis - Pulmonary surgery - Cor Pulmonale - Lung auscultation - Cough and expectoration - Weight - Activity - General attitude - ABG - GI complications - Infertility - Salt depletion - Osteoarthropathy	- Comprehensive - Demonstrated to be useful in prognosis and assessment of disease evolution	- Complex scoring system - Overestimates rare clinical elements - Does not include patients younger than 5 years of age - High variability in pulmonary function evaluation
Brasfield [130]	1979	643 chest radiographs in 118 CF patients	Composite score of presence and severity of each of the following: - Air trapping - Linear markings - Nodular cystic lesions - Large lesions - Overall impression of severity	- Reproducible - Strong correlation with clinical severity - Uncomplicated assessment	- Somewhat subjective in measurement of overall severity - Inflexible - Designed for team of radiologists
Nathanson [143]	1991	28 HRCT of CF patients	Severity of bronchiectasis and mucous impaction on a 5 point scale as measured in 12 distinct lung zones	- Good correlation with existing radiographic scores and clinical outcomes	- No studies in reproducibility

Name of Score	Year Published	Number of patients in cohort	Parameters Used	Strengths	Limitations
Bhalla [107]	1991	HRCT scans of 14 patients studies by 3 radiologists	3-point severity score of the following parameters: - Bronchiectasis severity - Peribronchial thickening - Bronchiectasis extent - Extent of mucoid impaction - Abscesses - General impression - Number of blisters - Emphysema extent - Collapse/consolidation	- Excellent agreement between examiners - Reproducible - High correlation with pulmonary function tests	- Extensive number of parameters - Complex scoring system
Northern Score [141]	1994	45 chest radiographs read by 10 clinical physicians	Severity of radiographic alterations in each lung quadrant: - 0: normal - 1: minimally increased linear signs or nodular cystic lesions - 2: moderately diffuse nodular cystic lesions, more pronounced linear signs - 3: severe; profuse cystic lesions, extensive collapse/ consolidation - 4: very severe; small areas of visible lung with dense infiltrates throughout	- Allows for single-examiner approach - Better agreement seen among examiners - Reproducible - Uncomplicated	- May overly simplify picture and extent of lung disease - No strong correlation with clinical measures
Hayllar [144]	1997	Retrospective data analysed on 403 patients over 18 year period	Predictive index based on measurement of: - Height - Hepatomegaly - FVC (%) - FEV1 (%) - White blood cell count Mortality curve developed to relate predictive index to survival probability	- Directly relates clinical measures to an estimate of survival - Externally validated - Reproducible	- Excludes some known predictors of mortality - Developed based on data in 1970s and 1980s; does not reflect improved diagnostic techniques

Name of Score	Year Published	Number of patients in cohort	Parameters Used	Strengths	Limitations
Liou Predictive 5-year survivorship model of Cystic Fibrosis [145]	2001	Retrospective data collected 5820 patients in US registry between 1986 and 1993	Composite score of the presence or value of following parameters to predict 5-year survival: - Age - Gender (M=0, F=1) - FEV1 (%) - Weight-for-age z score - Pancreatic insufficiency - Diabetes mellitus - Staphylococcus aureus - Burkholderia cepacia - No. of acute exacerbations (0-5)	- Comprehensive - Widely applicable - Validated - User-friendly	- Does not account for radiological findings - Prediction rule is derived from the same cohort as the validation group
CF-ABLE Score [93]	2013	49 CF patients followed over a 7-year period. Validated in 370 patients collected from national registry over 5 years	7-point scale based on evaluation of: - Age <24 = 1 point - BMI <20.1 kg/m² = 1 - FEV1 (%) < 52% = 3.5 - Number of exacerbations in past 3 months > 1 = 3.5 points Score of >5 indicates 26% chance of poor outcome in the next 4 years	- Common clinical measurements used - Easy to caluclate - Validated	- Difficult to define pulmonary exacerbation - Adult only score

Table 2. Summary of Clinical Prediction Tools in Cystic Fibrosis.

22. Conclusion

Over the last two decades, prognosis has improved significantly in CF and this has led to the need to better predict outcomes. Subsequently, many studies have looked at all aspects of the disease and identified modifiable risks, as well as identified biomarkers to follow disease progression. This increased knowledge of the condition has allowed improved treatment and more phenotypically specific therapy to be developed. Many different clinical features and markers predict outcome and this is a complex area, and a multifaceted approach to risk stratifying patients is needed. However, what must be not overlooked as the survival increases in CF are the extrapulmonary manifestations and the significant psychosocial issues associated with chronic illness. It is important to note that up to 22% of CF patients demonstrate symptoms of depression, 10% report anxiety symptoms, and up to 5% report suicidal thoughts [146]. The incidence of depression and anxiety is 2–3 times higher than age matched community control individuals [147]. This is highly important and there is an association between depression and lower FEV1 [146]. Also, patients with well-preserved spirometry who have depression demonstrate more significant decline in lung function than those with no depressive symptoms [148]. Depression is associated with negative medication beliefs leading to lower medication adherence, which ultimately may lead to poorer prognosis, hence it is important to evaluate patients holistically beyond the medical complications of CF when assessing prognosis [149]. Other important factors that are easily overlooked are socio-economic issues that impact upon survival, including lower household income and socio-economic status [150-152], larger family size with more than one person with CF [153], and exposure to cigarette smoke [154] all predicting a poor outcome. These risk factors are sometimes more difficult to quantify and hence are often overlooked. They are also difficult to measure as part of composite prediction tools, but they must be taken into account when assessing the prognostic indices of each individual with CF.

As survival continues to improve, the use of composite scoring systems and multi-disciplinary approach to improving care is essential in CF. Many clinical prediction tools exist for CF and some are more useful in clinical practice than others, however, these are underutilised in general and should be employed in more clinical trials, as well as routine care.

In summary, the prognosis of CF has improved significantly over the last two decades and may improve further as newer medications are developed. The need to accurately predict prognosis is essential as the decision for lung transplantation or to aggressively treat certain aspects of disease may be more tailored and appropriate per individual, this improving survival further. The most sensitive way of predicating prognosis currently remains a multi-faceted approach, including several markers of disease and the use of all factors and a composite clinical prediction tool is suggested to stratify patient risk.

Author details

Cormac McCarthy*, Orla O'Carroll, Alessandro N. Franciosi and Noel G. McElvaney

*Address all correspondence to: cmccarthy@rcsi.ie

Respiratory Research Division, Department of Medicine, Royal College of Surgeons in Ireland, Education and Research Centre, Beaumont Hospital, Dublin, Ireland

References

[1] Ramsey, B.W., *Management of pulmonary disease in patients with cystic fibrosis.* N Engl J Med, 1996. 335(3): p. 179-88.

[2] Rosenbluth, D.B., et al., *Lung function decline in cystic fibrosis patients and timing for lung transplantation referral.* Chest, 2004. 126(2): p. 412-9.

[3] Kerem, E., et al., *Prediction of mortality in patients with cystic fibrosis.* N Engl J Med, 1992. 326(18): p. 1187-91.

[4] Ramsey, B.W., et al., *A CFTR potentiator in patients with cystic fibrosis and the G551D mutation.* N Engl J Med, 2011. 365(18): p. 1663-72.

[5] Klein, M., et al., *18F-fluorodeoxyglucose-PET/CT imaging of lungs in patients with cystic fibrosis.* Chest, 2009. 136(5): p. 1220-8.

[6] Amin, R., et al., *Cystic fibrosis: detecting changes in airway inflammation with FDG PET/CT.* Radiology, 2012. 264(3): p. 868-75.

[7] Chen, D.L., J.J. Atkinson, and T.W. Ferkol, *FDG PET imaging in cystic fibrosis.* Semin Nucl Med, 2013. 43(6): p. 412-9.

[8] McMahon, C.J., et al., *Hyperpolarized 3helium magnetic resonance ventilation imaging of the lung in cystic fibrosis: comparison with high resolution CT and spirometry.* Eur Radiol, 2006. 16(11): p. 2483-90.

[9] Aurora, P., et al., *Lung clearance index at 4 years predicts subsequent lung function in children with cystic fibrosis.* Am J Respir Crit Care Med, 2011. 183(6): p. 752-8.

[10] Mayer-Hamblett, N., et al., *Association between pulmonary function and sputum biomarkers in cystic fibrosis.* Am J Respir Crit Care Med, 2007. 175(8): p. 822-8.

[11] Reeves, E.P., et al., *A novel neutrophil derived inflammatory biomarker of pulmonary exacerbation in cystic fibrosis.* J Cyst Fibros, 2012. 11(2): p. 100-7.

[12] Sagel, S.D., et al., *Sputum biomarkers of inflammation and lung function decline in children with cystic fibrosis.* Am J Respir Crit Care Med, 2012. 186(9): p. 857-65.

[13] McCarthy, C., et al., *The CF-ABLE Score: A Novel Clinical Prediction Rule for Prognosis in Cystic Fibrosis.* Chest, 2012.

[14] *Cystic Fibrosis Foundation Patient Registry Annual Data Report 2013.* 2013; Available from: http://www.cff.org/UploadedFiles/research/ClinicalResearch/PatientRegistryReport/2013_CFF_Patient_Registry_Annual_Data_Report.pdf.

[15] Kerem, E., et al., *The relation between genotype and phenotype in cystic fibrosis--analysis of the most common mutation (delta F508).* N Engl J Med, 1990. 323(22): p. 1517-22.

[16] Johansen, H.K., et al., *Severity of cystic fibrosis in patients homozygous and heterozygous for delta F508 mutation.* Lancet, 1991. 337(8742): p. 631-4.

[17] Santis, G., et al., *Independent genetic determinants of pancreatic and pulmonary status in cystic fibrosis.* Lancet, 1990. 336(8723): p. 1081-4.

[18] McKone, E.F., et al., *Effect of genotype on phenotype and mortality in cystic fibrosis: a retrospective cohort study.* Lancet, 2003. 361(9370): p. 1671-6.

[19] McKone, E.F., C.H. Goss, and M.L. Aitken, *CFTR genotype as a predictor of prognosis in cystic fibrosis.* Chest, 2006. 130(5): p. 1441-7.

[20] Davies, J.C., et al., *Efficacy and safety of ivacaftor in patients aged 6 to 11 years with cystic fibrosis with a G551D mutation.* Am J Respir Crit Care Med, 2013. 187(11): p. 1219-25.

[21] McKone, E.F., et al., *Long-term safety and efficacy of ivacaftor in patients with cystic fibrosis who have the Gly551Asp-CFTR mutation: a phase 3, open-label extension study (PERSIST).* Lancet Respir Med, 2014. 2(11): p. 902-10.

[22] Corey, M. and V. Farewell, *Determinants of mortality from cystic fibrosis in Canada, 1970-1989.* Am J Epidemiol, 1996. 143(10): p. 1007-17.

[23] Rosenfeld, M., et al., *Gender gap in cystic fibrosis mortality.* Am J Epidemiol, 1997. 145(9): p. 794-803.

[24] Harness-Brumley, C.L., et al., *Gender differences in outcomes of patients with cystic fibrosis.* J Womens Health (Larchmt), 2014. 23(12): p. 1012-20.

[25] Coakley, R.D., et al., *17beta-Estradiol inhibits Ca2+-dependent homeostasis of airway surface liquid volume in human cystic fibrosis airway epithelia.* J Clin Invest, 2008. 118(12): p. 4025-35.

[26] Chotirmall, S.H., et al., *17Beta-estradiol inhibits IL-8 in cystic fibrosis by up-regulating secretory leucoprotease inhibitor.* Am J Respir Crit Care Med, 2010. 182(1): p. 62-72.

[27] Nousia-Arvanitakis, S., *Cystic fibrosis and the pancreas: recent scientific advances.* J Clin Gastroenterol, 1999. 29(2): p. 138-42.

[28] Ahmed, N., et al., *Molecular consequences of cystic fibrosis transmembrane regulator (CFTR) gene mutations in the exocrine pancreas.* Gut, 2003. 52(8): p. 1159-64.

[29] Ooi, C.Y., et al., *Type of CFTR mutation determines risk of pancreatitis in patients with cystic fibrosis.* Gastroenterology, 2011. 140(1): p. 153-61.

[30] Kerem, E., et al., *Factors associated with FEV1 decline in cystic fibrosis: analysis of the ECFS patient registry.* Eur Respir J, 2014. 43(1): p. 125-33.

[31] Moran, A., et al., *Cystic fibrosis-related diabetes: current trends in prevalence, incidence, and mortality.* Diabetes Care, 2009. 32(9): p. 1626-31.

[32] Hardin, D.S., et al., *Insulin resistance is associated with decreased clinical status in cystic fibrosis.* J Pediatr, 1997. 130(6): p. 948-56.

[33] Milla, C.E., W.J. Warwick, and A. Moran, *Trends in pulmonary function in patients with cystic fibrosis correlate with the degree of glucose intolerance at baseline.* Am J Respir Crit Care Med, 2000. 162(3 Pt 1): p. 891-5.

[34] Nousia-Arvanitakis, S., A. Galli-Tsinopoulou, and M. Karamouzis, *Insulin improves clinical status of patients with cystic-fibrosis-related diabetes mellitus*. Acta Paediatr, 2001. 90(5): p. 515-9.

[35] Galutira, D., P.W. Allderdice, and W.S. Davidson, *HaeIII RFLP for salivary proline-rich protein gene probe (pPRPII2.2RP)*. Nucleic Acids Res, 1991. 19(23): p. 6667.

[36] Schwarzenberg, S.J., et al., *Microvascular complications in cystic fibrosis-related diabetes*. Diabetes Care, 2007. 30(5): p. 1056-61.

[37] Koch, C., et al., *Presence of cystic fibrosis-related diabetes mellitus is tightly linked to poor lung function in patients with cystic fibrosis: data from the European Epidemiologic Registry of Cystic Fibrosis*. Pediatr Pulmonol, 2001. 32(5): p. 343-50.

[38] Apparailly, F., et al., *Adeno-associated virus pseudotype 5 vector improves gene transfer in arthritic joints*. Hum Gene Ther, 2005. 16(4): p. 426-34.

[39] Milla, C.E., J. Billings, and A. Moran, *Diabetes is associated with dramatically decreased survival in female but not male subjects with cystic fibrosis*. Diabetes Care, 2005. 28(9): p. 2141-4.

[40] Moyer, K. and W. Balistreri, *Hepatobiliary disease in patients with cystic fibrosis*. Curr Opin Gastroenterol, 2009. 25(3): p. 272-8.

[41] Bartlett, J.R., et al., *Genetic modifiers of liver disease in cystic fibrosis*. JAMA, 2009. 302(10): p. 1076-83.

[42] Grasemann, H., H.G. Wiesemann, and F. Ratjen, *[The importance of lung function as a predictor of 2-year mortality in mucoviscidosis]*. Pneumologie, 1995. 49(8): p. 466-9.

[43] Milla, C.E. and W.J. Warwick, *Risk of death in cystic fibrosis patients with severely compromised lung function*. Chest, 1998. 113(5): p. 1230-4.

[44] Konstan, M.W., et al., *Design and powering of cystic fibrosis clinical trials using rate of FEV(1) decline as an efficacy endpoint*. J Cyst Fibros, 2010. 9(5): p. 332-8.

[45] Morgan, W.J., et al., *Probability of treatment following acute decline in lung function in children with cystic fibrosis is related to baseline pulmonary function*. J Pediatr, 2013. 163(4): p. 1152-7 e2.

[46] Lum, S., et al., *Early detection of cystic fibrosis lung disease: multiple-breath washout versus raised volume tests*. Thorax, 2007. 62(4): p. 341-7.

[47] Gustafsson, P.M., P. Aurora, and A. Lindblad, *Evaluation of ventilation maldistribution as an early indicator of lung disease in children with cystic fibrosis*. Eur Respir J, 2003. 22(6): p. 972-9.

[48] Gustafsson, P.M., et al., *Multiple-breath inert gas washout and spirometry versus structural lung disease in cystic fibrosis*. Thorax, 2008. 63(2): p. 129-34.

[49] Vermeulen, F., et al., *Lung clearance index predicts pulmonary exacerbations in young patients with cystic fibrosis.* Thorax, 2014. 69(1): p. 39-45.

[50] Davies, J., et al., *Assessment of clinical response to ivacaftor with lung clearance index in cystic fibrosis patients with a G551D-CFTR mutation and preserved spirometry: a randomised controlled trial.* Lancet Respir Med, 2013. 1(8): p. 630-8.

[51] Linnane, B., et al., *The findings of a clinical surveillance bronchoalveolar lavage programme in pre-school patients with cystic fibrosis.* Pediatr Pulmonol, 2014.

[52] Kerem, E., et al., *Pulmonary function and clinical course in patients with cystic fibrosis after pulmonary colonization with Pseudomonas aeruginosa.* J Pediatr, 1990. 116(5): p. 714-9.

[53] Rosenfeld, M., et al., *Baseline characteristics and factors associated with nutritional and pulmonary status at enrollment in the cystic fibrosis EPIC observational cohort.* Pediatr Pulmonol, 2010. 45(9): p. 934-44.

[54] Pamukcu, A., A. Bush, and R. Buchdahl, *Effects of pseudomonas aeruginosa colonization on lung function and anthropometric variables in children with cystic fibrosis.* Pediatr Pulmonol, 1995. 19(1): p. 10-5.

[55] Konstan, M.W., et al., *Risk factors for rate of decline in FEV1 in adults with cystic fibrosis.* J Cyst Fibros, 2012. 11(5): p. 405-11.

[56] Pentz, A., et al., *The impact of chronic pseudomonal infection on pulmonary function testing in individuals with cystic fibrosis in Pretoria, South Africa.* S Afr Med J, 2014. 104(3): p. 191-4.

[57] Lillquist, Y.P., E. Cho, and A.G. Davidson, *Economic effects of an eradication protocol for first appearance of Pseudomonas aeruginosa in cystic fibrosis patients: 1995 vs. 2009.* J Cyst Fibros, 2011. 10(3): p. 175-80.

[58] Nixon, G.M., et al., *Early airway infection, inflammation, and lung function in cystic fibrosis.* Arch Dis Child, 2002. 87(4): p. 306-11.

[59] Hoffman, L.R., et al., *Selection for Staphylococcus aureus small-colony variants due to growth in the presence of Pseudomonas aeruginosa.* Proc Natl Acad Sci U S A, 2006. 103(52): p. 19890-5.

[60] Besier, S., et al., *Prevalence and clinical significance of Staphylococcus aureus small-colony variants in cystic fibrosis lung disease.* J Clin Microbiol, 2007. 45(1): p. 168-72.

[61] Burns, J.L., et al., *Microbiology of sputum from patients at cystic fibrosis centers in the United States.* Clin Infect Dis, 1998. 27(1): p. 158-63.

[62] Ren, C.L., et al., *Presence of methicillin resistant Staphylococcus aureus in respiratory cultures from cystic fibrosis patients is associated with lower lung function.* Pediatr Pulmonol, 2007. 42(6): p. 513-8.

[63] Hubert, D., et al., *Association between Staphylococcus aureus alone or combined with Pseudomonas aeruginosa and the clinical condition of patients with cystic fibrosis.* J Cyst Fibros, 2013. 12(5): p. 497-503.

[64] Ratjen, F., et al., *Effect of continuous antistaphylococcal therapy on the rate of P. aeruginosa acquisition in patients with cystic fibrosis.* Pediatr Pulmonol, 2001. 31(1): p. 13-6.

[65] Smyth, A.R. and S. Walters, *Prophylactic anti-staphylococcal antibiotics for cystic fibrosis.* Cochrane Database Syst Rev, 2014. 11: p. CD001912.

[66] Ledson, M.J., et al., *Outcome of Burkholderia cepacia colonisation in an adult cystic fibrosis centre.* Thorax, 2002. 57(2): p. 142-5.

[67] Courtney, J.M., et al., *Clinical outcome of Burkholderia cepacia complex infection in cystic fibrosis adults.* J Cyst Fibros, 2004. 3(2): p. 93-8.

[68] Jones, A.M., et al., *Burkholderia cenocepacia and Burkholderia multivorans: influence on survival in cystic fibrosis.* Thorax, 2004. 59(11): p. 948-51.

[69] Murray, S., et al., *Impact of burkholderia infection on lung transplantation in cystic fibro*sis. Am J Respir Crit Care Med, 2008. 178(4): p. 363-71.

[70] Regan, K.H. and J. Bhatt, *Eradication therapy for Burkholderia cepacia complex in people with cystic fibrosis.* Cochrane Database Syst Rev, 2014. 10: p. CD009876.

[71] Bryant, J.M., et al., *Whole-genome sequencing to identify transmission of Mycobacterium abscessus between patients with cystic fibrosis: a retrospective cohort study.* Lancet, 2013. 381(9877): p. 1551-60.

[72] Qvist, T., et al., *Shifting paradigms of nontuberculous mycobacteria in cystic fibrosis.* Respir Res, 2014. 15: p. 41.

[73] Catherinot, E., et al., *Mycobacterium avium and Mycobacterium abscessus complex target distinct cystic fibrosis patient subpopulations.* J Cyst Fibros, 2013. 12(1): p. 74-80.

[74] Qvist, T., et al., *Epidemiology of nontuberculous mycobacteria among patients with cystic fibrosis in Scandinavia.* J Cyst Fibros, 2015. 14(1): p. 46-52.

[75] Olivier, K.N., et al., *Nontuberculous mycobacteria. II: nested-cohort study of impact on cystic fibrosis lung disease.* Am J Respir Crit Care Med, 2003. 167(6): p. 835-40.

[76] Coolen, N., et al., *Reduced risk of nontuberculous mycobacteria in cystic fibrosis adults receiving long-term azithromycin.* J Cyst Fibros, 2015.

[77] Lobo, L.J., et al., *Lung transplant outcomes in cystic fibrosis patients with pre-operative Mycobacterium abscessus respiratory infections.* Clin Transplant, 2013. 27(4): p. 523-9.

[78] McMahon, M.A., et al., *Radiological abnormalities associated with Aspergillus colonization in a cystic fibrosis population.* Eur J Radiol, 2012. 81(3): p. e197-202.

[79] Fillaux, J., et al., *Assessment of Aspergillus sensitization or persistent carriage as a factor in lung function impairment in cystic fibrosis patients*. Scand J Infect Dis, 2012. 44(11): p. 842-7.

[80] Waters, V., et al., *Chronic Stenotrophomonas maltophilia infection and mortality or lung transplantation in cystic fibrosis patients*. J Cyst Fibros, 2013. 12(5): p. 482-6.

[81] Amin, R. and V. Waters, *Antibiotic treatment for Stenotrophomonas maltophilia in people with cystic fibrosis*. Cochrane Database Syst Rev, 2014. 4: p. CD009249.

[82] Gungor, O., et al., *Frequency of fungi in respiratory samples from Turkish cystic fibrosis patients*. Mycoses, 2013. 56(2): p. 123-9.

[83] Chotirmall, S.H., et al., *Sputum Candida albicans presages FEV(1) decline and hospital-treated exacerbations in cystic fibrosis*. Chest, 2010. 138(5): p. 1186-95.

[84] Elphick, H.E. and G. Mallory, *Oxygen therapy for cystic fibrosis*. Cochrane Database Syst Rev, 2013. 7: p. CD003884.

[85] Martin, C., et al., *Prognostic value of six minute walk test in cystic fibrosis adults*. Respir Med, 2013. 107(12): p. 1881-7.

[86] Belkin, R.A., et al., *Risk factors for death of patients with cystic fibrosis awaiting lung transplantation*. Am J Respir Crit Care Med, 2006. 173(6): p. 659-66.

[87] Young, A.C., et al., *Randomised placebo controlled trial of non-invasive ventilation for hypercapnia in cystic fibrosis*. Thorax, 2008. 63(1): p. 72-7.

[88] Texereau, J., et al., *Determinants of mortality for adults with cystic fibrosis admitted in Intensive Care Unit: a multicenter study*. Respir Res, 2006. 7: p. 14.

[89] Efrati, O., et al., *Outcome of patients with cystic fibrosis admitted to the intensive care unit: is invasive mechanical ventilation a risk factor for death in patients waiting lung transplantation?* Heart Lung, 2010. 39(2): p. 153-9.

[90] Berlinski, A., et al., *Invasive mechanical ventilation for acute respiratory failure in children with cystic fibrosis: outcome analysis and case-control study*. Pediatr Pulmonol, 2002. 34(4): p. 297-303.

[91] Steinkamp, G. and B. Wiedemann, *Relationship between nutritional status and lung function in cystic fibrosis: cross sectional and longitudinal analyses from the German CF quality assurance (CFQA) project*. Thorax, 2002. 57(7): p. 596-601.

[92] Gozdzik, J., et al., *Relationship between nutritional status and pulmonary function in adult cystic fibrosis patients*. J Physiol Pharmacol, 2008. 59 Suppl 6: p. 253-60.

[93] McCarthy, C., et al., *The CF-ABLE score: a novel clinical prediction rule for prognosis in patients with cystic fibrosis*. Chest, 2013. 143(5): p. 1358-64.

[94] Steinkamp, G., et al., *[Stabilization of lung function in cystic fibrosis during long-term tube feeding via a percutaneous endoscopic gastrostomy]*. Pneumologie, 1990. 44(10): p. 1151-3.

[95] Steinkamp, G. and H. von der Hardt, *Improvement of nutritional status and lung function after long-term nocturnal gastrostomy feedings in cystic fibrosis.* J Pediatr, 1994. 124(2): p. 244-9.

[96] Stephenson, A.L., et al., *Longitudinal trends in nutritional status and the relation between lung function and BMI in cystic fibrosis: a population-based cohort study.* Am J Clin Nutr, 2013. 97(4): p. 872-7.

[97] Donovan, D.S., Jr., et al., *Bone mass and vitamin D deficiency in adults with advanced cystic fibrosis lung disease.* Am J Respir Crit Care Med, 1998. 157(6 Pt 1): p. 1892-9.

[98] Tschopp, O., et al., *Osteoporosis before lung transplantation: association with low body mass index, but not with underlying disease.* Am J Transplant, 2002. 2(2): p. 167-72.

[99] Putman, M.S., et al., *Trends in bone mineral density in young adults with cystic fibrosis over a 15year period.* J Cyst Fibros, 2015.

[100] Conwell, L.S. and A.B. Chang, *Bisphosphonates for osteoporosis in people with cystic fibrosis.* Cochrane Database Syst Rev, 2014. 3: p. CD002010.

[101] Sly, P.D., et al., *Risk factors for bronchiectasis in children with cystic fibrosis.* N Engl J Med, 2013. 368(21): p. 1963-70.

[102] McElvaney, O.J., et al., *The effect of the decoy molecule PA401 on CXCL8 levels in bronchoalveolar lavage fluid of patients with cystic fibrosis.* Mol Immunol, 2015. 63(2): p. 550-8.

[103] Colombo, C., et al., *Cytokine levels in sputum of cystic fibrosis patients before and after antibiotic therapy.* Pediatr Pulmonol, 2005. 40(1): p. 15-21.

[104] Bodini, A., et al., *Biomarkers of neutrophilic inflammation in exhaled air of cystic fibrosis children with bacterial airway infections.* Pediatr Pulmonol, 2005. 40(6): p. 494-9.

[105] Karpati, F., F.L. Hjelte, and B. Wretlind, *TNF-alpha and IL-8 in consecutive sputum samples from cystic fibrosis patients during antibiotic treatment.* Scand J Infect Dis, 2000. 32(1): p. 75-9.

[106] Dakin, C.J., et al., *Relationship between sputum inflammatory markers, lung function, and lung pathology on high-resolution computed tomography in children with cystic fibrosis.* Pediatr Pulmonol, 2002. 33(6): p. 475-82.

[107] Bhalla, M., et al., *Cystic fibrosis: scoring system with thin-section CT.* Radiology, 1991. 179(3): p. 783-8.

[108] Reeves, E.P., et al., *The involvement of glycosaminoglycans in airway disease associated with cystic fibrosis.* ScientificWorldJournal, 2011. 11: p. 959-71.

[109] Bergin, D.A., et al., *Airway inflammatory markers in individuals with cystic fibrosis and non-cystic fibrosis bronchiectasis.* J Inflamm Res, 2013. 6: p. 1-11.

[110] Linnane, S.J., et al., *Total sputum nitrate plus nitrite is raised during acute pulmonary infection in cystic fibrosis.* Am J Respir Crit Care Med, 1998. 158(1): p. 207-12.

[111] Anil, N., et al., *Induced sputum nitrites correlate with FEV1 in children with cystic fibrosis.* Acta Paediatr, 2010. 99(5): p. 711-4.

[112] Laguna, T.A., et al., *Sputum club cell protein concentration is associated with pulmonary exacerbation in cystic fibrosis.* J Cyst Fibros, 2014.

[113] Naudin, C., et al., *Human cysteine cathepsins are not reliable markers of infection by Pseudomonas aeruginosa in cystic fibrosis.* PLoS One, 2011. 6(9): p. e25577.

[114] Schulz, B.L., et al., *Glycosylation of sputum mucins is altered in cystic fibrosis patients.* Glycobiology, 2007. 17(7): p. 698-712.

[115] Liou, T.G., et al., *Sputum biomarkers and the prediction of clinical outcomes in patients with cystic fibrosis.* PLoS One, 2012. 7(8): p. e42748.

[116] Gray, R.D., et al., *Sputum and serum calprotectin are useful biomarkers during CF exacerbation.* J Cyst Fibros, 2010. 9(3): p. 193-8.

[117] Golden, B.E., et al., *Calprotectin as a marker of inflammation in cystic fibrosis.* Arch Dis Child, 1996. 74(2): p. 136-9.

[118] Moffitt, K.L., et al., *Inflammatory and immunological biomarkers are not related to survival in adults with Cystic Fibrosis.* J Cyst Fibros, 2014. 13(1): p. 63-8.

[119] Nick, J.A., et al., *Blood mRNA biomarkers for detection of treatment response in acute pulmonary exacerbations of cystic fibrosis.* Thorax, 2013. 68(10): p. 929-37.

[120] Schultz, H., et al., *BPI-ANCA of pediatric cystic fibrosis patients can impair BPI-mediated killing of E. coli DH5alpha in vitro.* Pediatr Pulmonol, 2004. 37(2): p. 158-64.

[121] Dorlochter, L., et al., *Anti-neutrophil cytoplasmatic antibodies and lung disease in cystic fibrosis.* J Cyst Fibros, 2004. 3(3): p. 179-83.

[122] Lindberg, U., et al., *BPI-ANCA and long-term prognosis among 46 adult CF patients: a prospective 10-year follow-up study.* Clin Dev Immunol, 2012. 2012: p. 370107.

[123] McKone, E.F., et al., *Association of sweat chloride concentration at time of diagnosis and CFTR genotype with mortality and cystic fibrosis phenotype.* J Cyst Fibros, 2015.

[124] Rowe, S.M., et al., *Optimizing nasal potential difference analysis for CFTR modulator development: assessment of ivacaftor in CF subjects with the G551D-CFTR mutation.* PLoS One, 2013. 8(7): p. e66955.

[125] Judge, E.P., et al., *Pulmonary abnormalities on high-resolution CT demonstrate more rapid decline than FEV1 in adults with cystic fibrosis.* Chest, 2006. 130(5): p. 1424-32.

[126] Mott, L.S., et al., *Progression of early structural lung disease in young children with cystic fibrosis assessed using CT.* Thorax, 2012. 67(6): p. 509-16.

[127] Dodd, J.D., et al., *Thin-section CT in patients with cystic fibrosis: correlation with peak exercise capacity and body mass index.* Radiology, 2006. 240(1): p. 236-45.

[128] Bannier, E., et al., *Hyperpolarized 3He MR for sensitive imaging of ventilation function and treatment efficiency in young cystic fibrosis patients with normal lung function.* Radiology, 2010. 255(1): p. 225-32.

[129] O'Connell, O.J., et al., *Radiologic imaging in cystic fibrosis: cumulative effective dose and changing trends over 2 decades.* Chest, 2012. 141(6): p. 1575-83.

[130] Brasfield, D., et al., *The chest roentgenogram in cystic fibrosis: a new scoring system.* Pediatrics, 1979. 63(1): p. 24-9.

[131] Taussig, L.M., et al., *A new prognostic score and clinical evaluation system for cystic fibrosis.* J Pediatr, 1973. 82(3): p. 380-90.

[132] Holzer, F.J., A. Olinsky, and P.D. Phelan, *Variability of airways hyper-reactivity and allergy in cystic fibrosis.* Arch Dis Child, 1981. 56(6): p. 455-9.

[133] Sawyer, S.M., et al., *Critical evaluation of three chest radiograph scores in cystic fibrosis.* Thorax, 1994. 49(9): p. 863-6.

[134] Brody, A.S., et al., *High-resolution computed tomography in young patients with cystic fibrosis: distribution of abnormalities and correlation with pulmonary function tests.* J Pediatr, 2004. 145(1): p. 32-8.

[135] Wainwright, C.E., et al., *Effect of bronchoalveolar lavage-directed therapy on Pseudomonas aeruginosa infection and structural lung injury in children with cystic fibrosis: a randomized trial.* JAMA, 2011. 306(2): p. 163-71.

[136] Pereira, F.F., et al., *Correlation between Bhalla score and spirometry in children and adolescents with cystic fibrosis.* Rev Assoc Med Bras, 2014. 60(3): p. 216-21.

[137] Shah, R.M., et al., *High-resolution CT in the acute exacerbation of cystic fibrosis: evaluation of acute findings, reversibility of those findings, and clinical correlation.* AJR Am J Roentgenol, 1997. 169(2): p. 375-80.

[138] Eshed, I., et al., *Bronchiectasis: correlation of high-resolution CT findings with health-related quality of life.* Clin Radiol, 2007. 62(2): p. 152-9.

[139] Shwachman, H. and L.L. Kulczycki, *Long-term study of one hundred five patients with cystic fibrosis; studies made over a five- to fourteen-year period.* AMA J Dis Child, 1958. 96(1): p. 6-15.

[140] Stollar, F., et al., *Shwachman-Kulczycki score still useful to monitor cystic fibrosis severity.* Clinics (Sao Paulo), 2011. 66(6): p. 979-83.

[141] Conway, S.P., et al., *The chest radiograph in cystic fibrosis: a new scoring system compared with the Chrispin-Norman and Brasfield scores.* Thorax, 1994. 49(9): p. 860-2.

[142] Chrispin, A.R. and A.P. Norman, *The systematic evaluation of the chest radiograph in cystic fibrosis.* Pediatr Radiol, 1974. 2(2): p. 101-5.

[143] Nathanson, I., et al., *Ultrafast computerized tomography of the chest in cystic fibrosis: a new scoring system*. Pediatr Pulmonol, 1991. 11(1): p. 81-6.

[144] Hayllar, K.M., et al., *A prognostic model for the prediction of survival in cystic fibrosis*. Thorax, 1997. 52(4): p. 313-7.

[145] Liou, T.G., et al., *Predictive 5-year survivorship model of cystic fibrosis*. Am J Epidemiol, 2001. 153(4): p. 345-52.

[146] Quon, B.S., et al., *Prevalence of Symptoms of Depression and Anxiety in Adults With Cystic Fibrosis Based on the PHQ-9 and GAD-7 Screening Questionnaires*. Psychosomatics, 2014.

[147] Quittner, A.L., et al., *Prevalence of depression and anxiety in patients with cystic fibrosis and parent caregivers: results of The International Depression Epidemiological Study across nine countries*. Thorax, 2014. 69(12): p. 1090-7.

[148] Fidika, A., M. Herle, and L. Goldbeck, *Symptoms of depression impact the course of lung function in adolescents and adults with cystic fibrosis*. BMC Pulm Med, 2014. 14: p. 205.

[149] Hilliard, M.E., et al., *Medication Beliefs Mediate Between Depressive Symptoms and Medication Adherence in Cystic Fibrosis*. Health Psychol, 2014.

[150] Schechter, M.S., et al., *Association of socioeconomic status with the use of chronic therapies and healthcare utilization in children with cystic fibrosis*. J Pediatr, 2009. 155(5): p. 634-9 e1-4.

[151] O'Connor, G.T., et al., *Median household income and mortality rate in cystic fibrosis*. Pediatrics, 2003. 111(4 Pt 1): p. e333-9.

[152] O'Connor, G.T., et al., *Case-mix adjustment for evaluation of mortality in cystic fibrosis*. Pediatr Pulmonol, 2002. 33(2): p. 99-105.

[153] Lavie, M., et al., Several siblings with Cystic Fibrosis as a risk factor for poor outcome. Respir Med, 2015. 109(1): p. 74-8.

[154] Collaco, J.M., et al., Interactions between secondhand smoke and genes that affect cystic fibrosis lung disease. JAMA, 2008. 299(4): p. 417-24.

8

In vivo Gene Correction of Cystic Fibrosis

Michael Sebastian Daniel Kormann

Abstract

The cystic fibrosis transmembrane conductance regulator (CFTR) gene was cloned over two decades ago and a vast number of pre-clinical and clinical studies have been performed since that time. Despite this progress, a true "cure" for the disease has not been achieved, partly because the lung is a major barrier for intruders, making it exceedingly difficult for new pharmaceutical formulations to penetrate target cells. Safety-engineered viral vectors, such as adeno-associated viral vectors (AAVs) or integrase-defective lentiviruses, have been used with moderate success in temporarily supplementing the expression of critical proteins. However, stability and safety concerns often dampen the effects of these approaches. With emerging technologies, such as modified messenger (mRNA) and new genome editing strategies, scientists are now exploring the possibility of not only supplementing defective proteins, but instead, correcting the genetic defects at their source. This chapter will highlight the theoretical possibilities and primary data in pre-clinical models supporting the efforts toward *in vivo* gene correction of cystic fibrosis (CF).

Keywords: Cystic fibrosis (CF), gene correction, messenger RNA (mRNA), zinc finger nuclease (ZFN), transcription activator-like effector nuclease (TALEN), clustered regularly interspaced short palindromic repeats (CRISPR), CRISPR/Cas9, dimeric CRISPR RNA-guided *Fok*I

1. Introduction

Cystic fibrosis (CF) is the most prevalent life-shortening autosomal recessive disorder in Caucasian populations [1]. Occurring in 1 out of every 3,500 newborns in the United States, and 1 out of every 2,000–3,000 in the European Union, CF affects more than 70,000 individuals worldwide [2]. Chronic lung disease is the major factor contributing to morbidity and mortality among CF patients, as abnormal airway secretions and chronic endobronchial infection lead to progressive airway obstruction. In addition to the respiratory tract, the disease may also affect the pancreas, liver, kidneys, intestine, and reproductive system [3].

Disease severity varies greatly among those with CF, depending largely upon the degree to which the lungs are affected. However, eventual deterioration of the lungs leading to airway obstruction and death is inevitable, and for many years the average CF patient was not expected to reach adulthood [2]. Over the course of the past three decades, advancements in modern medicine have allowed physicians to postpone debilitating changes to the lungs, slowing the progression of disease and allowing many individuals with CF to live well into their 50s or 60s. Despite these advances in current therapy, the median age of survival remains only 33.4 years [2], emphasizing the need for novel therapeutic approaches to further improve patient outcomes in CF.

2. The pathophysiology of cystic fibrosis

Cystic fibrosis is the direct result of a mutation in both alleles of *CFTR*. This gene is responsible for encoding the CFTR protein, a chloride ion channel anchored in the plasma membrane of lung cells, pancreatic cells, sweat and other exocrine glands. Functionally, CFTR is important for the production and movement of sweat, digestive fluids, and mucus across the membrane, where mutations in the encoding gene may result in impaired anion secretion and hyper-absorption of sodium across epithelia [4–6].

Over 1500 different mutations have been described in the CFTR gene, each leading to different defects in the CFTR protein itself [7]. In the most common mutation, the deletion of phenylalanine (F) from position 508 (ΔF508), improper protein folding results in the degradation of CFTR by the cell, which limits the amount of CFTR that reaches the epithelial cell surface. ΔF508-CFTR accounts for approximately 70% of CF cases worldwide and 90% of those occurring in the United States [7].

Alternative mutations in CFTR may result in truncation of the protein via premature stop codons, prevention of proper processing, folding, or trafficking to the plasma membrane, or interference with the chloride channel's ion transport ability, leading to poor gating or conductance [8]. A patient's specific CFTR gene mutation often dictates the severity of his or her disease, as well as the availability of drugs designed to target their particular protein defect.

In addition to mutations within *CFTR* itself, polymorphisms in other genes may also modify disease severity in patients with CF [9,10]. For instance, genetic variation in the gene encoding transforming growth factor β1 (*TGFβ1*) has been associated with more severe pulmonary phenotypes predictive of poorer long-term outcomes [9]. Polymorphisms in the histone-deacetylase-dependent transcriptional co-regulator, *IFRD1*, have also been shown to modulate the pathogenesis of CF lung disease through the regulation of neutrophil effector function [10,11].

Traditional management strategies for CF typically involve the use of antibiotics to treat infection as well as agents or mechanical devices to improve mucus clearance and prevent damage to the lungs. Non-CFTR ion channel agents, for instance, are small molecules designed to normalize the transport of sodium and chloride by targeting non-CFTR ion channels expressed by epithelial cells. Osmotic agents, or inhaled hypertonic solutions, have also been employed to restore airway surface liquid by drawing liquid out of the airway epithelium and into the mucus [12].

In more recent years, the characterization of *CFTR* mutations and genetic modifiers have provided numerous targets for the development of novel therapies aimed at treating the underlying cause, rather than symptoms, of the disease. These agents are designed to directly compensate for *CFTR* mutations in one of three main ways:

- Overcoming the specific functional defect in the patient's CFTR protein (Figure 1),
- Supplementing the cell with a functional copy of the CFTR protein (Figure 2), or
- Repairing the *CFTR* gene mutation at its source (Figure 3).

3. Targeting functional defects in CFTR Protein: Small molecule CFTR modulators

A number of small molecules have been designed to overcome the functional defects in CFTR protein caused by upstream gene mutations (Figure 1). These CFTR modulators can be classified into three families according to the specific functional defect that they target: premature stop codon suppressors, correctors, and potentiators [13].

Premature stop codon suppressors, otherwise known as production correctors or read-through agents, encourage the cell to overlook any premature stop codons transcribed within the *CFTR* mRNA (Figure 1A). They instruct cellular ribosomes to read-through these premature termination codons as the mRNA is being translated into protein. This encourages the production of full-length CFTR. Several *CFTR* mutations interfere with proper protein processing, resulting in misfolded CFTR that is degraded by the cell. **Correctors** focus on improving the processing and transport of CFTR protein to the cell surface (Figure 1B). By ensuring that CFTR is processed and folded correctly, the protein can be trafficked to the plasma membrane where it functions. Additional *CFTR* mutations allow this chloride ion channel to arrive at the plasma membrane, but cause defects in its gating or conductance ability. **Potentiators** work on these defects, to enhance opening of the channel or increasing the flow of chloride ions (Figure 1C) [13].

Lumacaftor (VX-809, Vertex Pharmaceuticals), for instance, is a CFTR corrector that increases trafficking of ΔF508-CFTR to the epithelial cell surface [14]. Lumacaftor has also been used in combination with ivacaftor (VX-770, Vertex Pharmaceuticals, trade name Kalydeco), a CFTR potentiator that improves the transport of chloride through CFTR channels rendered dysfunctional by G551D or R560T missense mutations. By binding to the channels and inducing

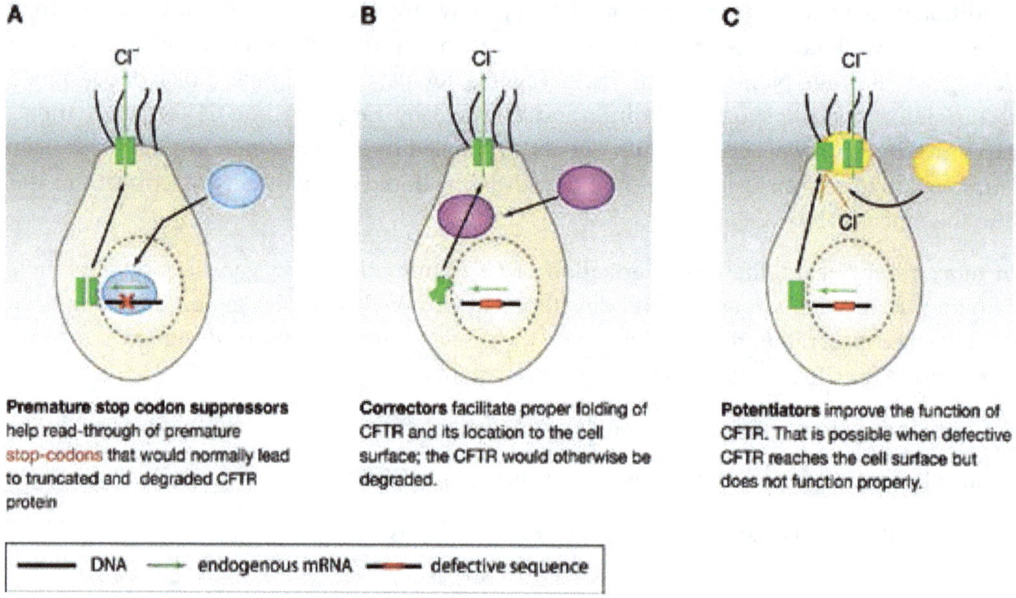

Figure 1. Small molecule CFTR modulators target functional defects within the CFTR protein. Three types of CFTR modulators have been developed: premature stop codon suppressors **(A)**, correctors **(B)**, and potentiators **(C)**. These small molecules act by targeting the transcription, translation, protein processing, membrane trafficking, and ion transport functionality of the CFTR protein, respectively.

a non-conventional mode of gating, ivacaftor increases the probability that the chloride channel is open [14]. Another small molecule CFTR modulator, ataluren (PTC124, PTC Therapeutics, trade name Translarna in the EU), is a production corrector that makes ribosomes less sensitive to G542X or W1282X nonsense mutations [15]. Overcoming these premature stop codons allows the synthesis of full-length, functional CFTR. Together, these small molecule modulators focus on addressing the functional defects in a patient's own CFTR protein.

Gene therapy: Gene supplementation and transcript supplementation therapy

Instead of addressing the functional deficit in a patient's endogenous CFTR, another approach involves supplementing the cell with an exogenous, functional copy of the protein (Figure 2). This can occur in one of several ways: through gene, transcript, or protein replacement therapy. By delivering a functional copy of the *CFTR*, subsequent mRNA transcript, or protein itself, the cell may regain enough CFTR function to halt the progression of disease. Protein replacement strategies have met limited success, as the therapeutic protein is often metabolized before it can enter the target tissue. Gene and transcript therapy approaches, however, continue to be investigated. Unlike CFTR modulators, these approaches have the potential to be used for all CF patients, regardless of the type of mutation they carry.

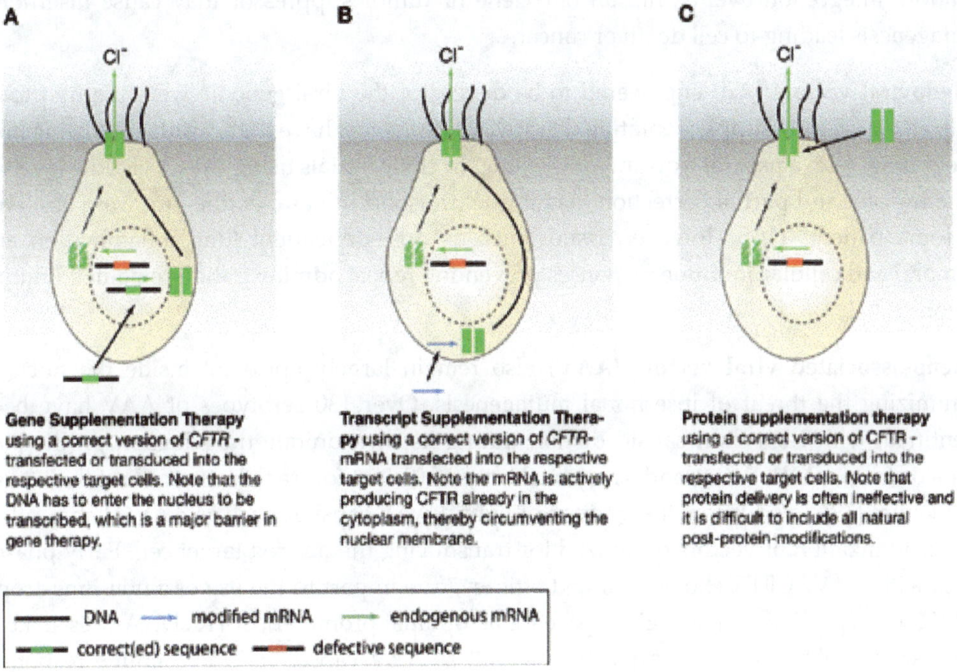

Figure 2. Gene, transcript, and protein replacement therapy supplement cells with a functional copy of the CFTR protein. Supplementing the cell with functional *CFTR* cDNA **(A)**, mRNA transcripts **(B)**, or CFTR protein **(C)** is another method of overcoming the genetic defects underlying Cystic Fibrosis.

4.1. Gene supplementation therapy

The two main forms of gene supplementation therapy are defined by the vehicle used to deliver functional cDNA to the cell: this consists of either viral or non-viral vectors (Figure 2A).

Non-viral vectors are typically comprised of plasmid DNA (pDNA) complexed with carrier molecules, such as cationic lipids or polymers. By binding to the negatively charged pDNA, these molecules either condense or encapsulate the DNA, forming lipoplexes or polyplexes that are then thought to be endocytosed by the cell [16]. In the absence of non-human, viral protein components, it is believed that non-viral vectors may incite minimal immune activation and increase the opportunity for repeat administration. However, even pDNA expression is often limited by CpG motifs that induce strong immune responses through innate immune receptors, such as Toll-like receptor 9 (TLR9) [17]. In addition, non-viral vectors are typically much less efficient than viral vectors at transfecting slowly dividing mammalian cells. This is due to the fact that viruses have evolved efficient strategies for improving cell entry, endosomal escape, cytoplasmic trafficking, and nuclear uptake, all of which make them naturally skilled vehicles for delivering therapeutic cDNA to the cell nucleus [16].

Viral vectors have been designed to harness these evolutionary advantages, while removing components of the viral genome that may cause harm. The ideal viral vector should be replication defective, non-immunogenic, and avoid integrating into actively transcribed genes. Random integration events into an oncogene or tumor suppressor may cause insertional mutagenesis leading to cell death or cancer.

Adenoviral vectors (Ad) engineered to be devoid of the viral genome were the first to be utilized for CF gene supplementation therapy. These vectors have the advantage of being non-integrating, with a natural tropism for the lung. In clinical trials using Ad-CFTR, low levels of gene transfer and partial correction of chloride transport in nasal epithelium were observed in some patients [16]. However, issues such as dose-dependent lung inflammation and humoral and cellular immune responses preventing repeat administration remained limiting factors.

Adeno-associated viral vectors (AAV) also remain largely episomal inside the nucleus, minimizing the threat of insertional mutagenesis. Over 130 serotypes of AAV have been identified, with each viral capsid demonstrating its own unique transduction profile [18]. Capsids from AAV1, 5, 6, 8, and 9 may be the most efficient for transducing cells of the airway epithelium [19]. In addition, the creation of hybrid AAV capsids, such as AAV6.2, may allow the customization of vectors optimized for transducing the desired target cell. Early phase I trials with AAV2.CFTR showed limited efficacy, due in part to the use of a non-lung-tropic AAV2 serotype, limited packaging space for an optimal promoter (*CFTR* cDNA uses 4.7kb of the vector's ~5kb packaging capacity), as well as AAV capsid-specific immune responses limiting repeat administration [16]. Strategies aimed at minimizing adaptive immunity to AAV vectors or reducing the need for repeat administration continue within the field. Removing CpG motifs from AAV vectors or designing hybrid AAV capsids has been shown to reduce innate and adaptive immune responses following intramuscular delivery [20,21]. Targeting AAV delivery to progenitor cells in mouse lung also shows promise as a means of avoiding lung cell turnover and circumventing the need for redelivery [22].

Lentiviral vectors based on recombinant human (HIV), simian (SIV), feline (FIV), and equine (EIV) immunodeficiency viruses have also been investigated for gene replacement therapy [16]. Lentiviral vectors are pseudotyped with the envelope proteins from various viruses to increase tissue tropism. The vesicular stomatitis virus G (VSV-G) envelope glycoprotein has most commonly been incorporated, although the F and HN proteins from murine parainfluenza virus type 1, or Sendai virus (SeV), may improve airway transduction. Studies with SeV-pseudotyped lentiviral vectors have accommodated repeat administration to murine airways in pre-clinical studies [23]. Should repeat administration also be feasible in human subjects, the two major remaining limitations to lentiviral use include safety concerns over genomic integration and scale-up of vector production. The concern over vector integration came to the forefront in 2003, when the integration of a retroviral vector used to treat X-linked severe combined immunodeficiency (X-SCID) triggered unexpected activation of a proto-oncogene leading to leukemia in nearly half of the trial's participants [24,25].

4.2. Transcript supplementation therapy

In recent years, transcript supplementation therapy has been introduced as an alternative to gene replacement therapy (Figure 2B). As mRNA transcripts are not capable of integrating into the chromosome, the threat of insertional mutagenesis is completely void. Following uptake via receptor-mediated endocytosis and lysosomal trafficking, mRNA also completely avoids the rate-limiting step of nuclear entry, being translated rapidly and efficiently directly in the cytoplasm [26]. With its naturally short half-life, mRNA transcripts are particularly useful for applications where short bursts of protein expression are desired. However, the addition of chemical modifications mimicking endogenous mRNA modification schemes has increased expression and stability, while decreasing immune responses. One major benefit to the use of chemically modified mRNA is the ability to readminister the vector as necessary.

The use of mRNA itself has long been appealing as an alternative to gene-based delivery vehicles. Unfortunately, for many years researchers were unable to use *in vitro* transcribed mRNAs to upregulate protein expression *in vivo*, as these transcripts were immediately recognized and destroyed by the immune system following injection [27]. Recent work has shown that by completely substituting uridine with pseudouridine during mRNA synthesis, the binding affinity of mRNA to innate immune receptors can be reduced, making systemic *in vivo* application possible [28,29]. More recent work has shown that partial substitution of combinations of various nucleotide modifications, more closely mimicking those observed in endogenous transcripts, can yield mRNA transcripts with further increased stability, specifically in murine lung [30,31]. This emphasizes that the design of mRNA may have substantially different effects in specific organs *in vivo* compared with *in vitro* use.

In one recent study, transcript therapy with chemically modified *surfactant protein B (SP-B)* mRNA exhibited success in achieving therapeutic levels of protein expression in a murine model of SP-B deficiency [30]. Repeated intratracheal administration of modified *Foxp3* mRNA to murine lung was also shown to alleviate asthma symptoms in two different models of experimental asthma [31]. Both of these models demonstrate the efficacy of nucleotide modified mRNA in achieving therapeutic levels of protein expression in the lung following repeated, *in vivo* delivery. As a vehicle for delivery, modified mRNA may present a safer alternative to viral and non-viral DNA-based approaches, as immune activation can be efficiently prevented and the possibility of genomic integration is eliminated. Importantly, however, due to the short half-life of mRNA, the benefits of modified mRNA transcripts may be better utilized outside of direct transcript supplementation.

5. Repairing the *CFTR* mutation: Gene correction with genome-editing nucleases

With residual limitations in optimizing gene and transcript supplementation therapies for CF lung disease, a new field has begun to emerge: aiming to correct, rather than supplement, the defective gene. Compared to gene or transcript replacement approaches, "gene correction" aims to replace the defective portion of the CFTR gene with a normal allele at its natural chromosomal location (Figure 3). The repair of a mutant gene directly at its original locus has two major advantages. Most importantly, the corrected gene remains under control of its endogenous promoter, hence assuring life-long expression and native regulation in the cell. Moreover, depending on the delivery vehicle(s) used, gene correction has the potential to avoid the involvement of foreign DNA, thus reducing the risk of insertional mutagenesis.

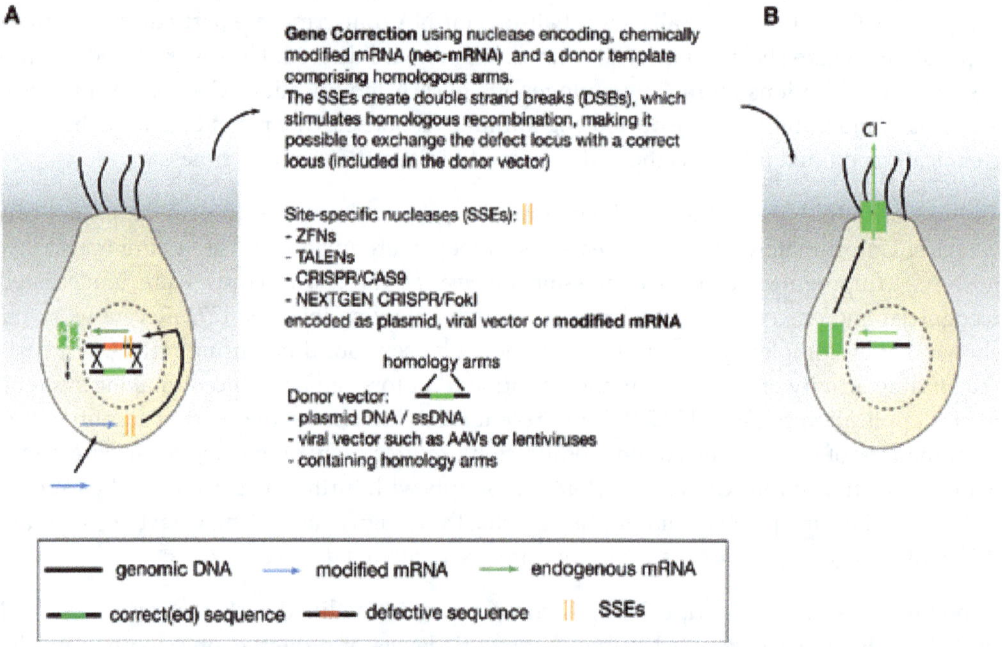

Figure 3. Gene correction approaches aim to repair the *CFTR* gene mutation directly at the endogenous chromosomal locus. The use of mRNA-encoded site-specific nucleases (SSE) can introduce double-strand breaks (DSB) near the genetic defect(s). If a donor vector with corrected sequence is also delivered to the cell, it can be utilized as a template for homologous repair (HR) as the cell works to repair the DSB (**A**). Successful homology-directed repair (HDR) will result in a corrected chromosomal locus, even after the SSE and donor template delivery vehicles are no longer expressed (**B**).

Several lines of investigation into viable gene correction approaches have been pursued. These involve the use of genome-editing nucleases, such as ZFNs, TALENs, or CRISPR-based systems, to take advantage of the cell's natural damage repair pathways. In this strategy, delivery of a site-specific-endonuclease (SSE) or SSE pair elicits a double-strand break (DSB) in the defective gene near the site of an unwanted mutation or sequence, initiating cellular repair mechanisms including homologous recombination (HR) and non-homologous end-joining (NHEJ).

NHEJ, an error-prone process, can be utilized to initiate mutations that essentially disrupt or knock out an undesirable gene. As NHEJ repairs the DSB by ligating the broken strands together, this process commonly results in small insertions or deletions of base pairs, known as indels. The generation of indels at the repair site can cause frame-shift mutations that prevent the protein from being properly transcribed and translated. This concept was demonstrated in 2008, when investigators utilized ZFNs and NHEJ to disrupt the HIV co-receptor, *CCR5*, rendering human CD4$^+$ T cells more difficult for the HIV virus to transfect [32]. Through this mechanism, multiple nuclease pairs can also be utilized to create two DSBs, where NHEJ may completely cut out large segments of unwanted genomic sequence [33,34].

Alternatively, a donor template can be delivered to the cell in addition to the nuclease(s), and used as a guide for directing HR, in a process referred to as homology-directed repair (HDR). In HDR, an extra-chromosomal donor fragment or "repair template" contains regions of significant homology up- and downstream of the DSB site. In between the homology arms, the repair template houses the desired, corrected sequence. Once the nuclease has cleaved, the regions of homology will be used as a template for rebuilding the site. As a result, the mutation-free sequence housed between homology arms is incorporated into the chromosome (Figure 3).

In cases where the patient is homozygous for the target allele, the uncleaved copy of the allele may be favored as a template for HR, decreasing efficiency. As such, it is important to provide the repair template in excess, to ensure that the target cell favors the repair template over the sister chromatid. It is also important to note that even when a repair template is provided in excess for HR, SSE binding and cleavage can also occur at off-target sites, which may initiate NHEJ. In the case of an off-target cutting event, NHEJ can cause unexpected mutations that may be harmful to the cell. As a result, potential off-target binding sites of the SSE should be predicted *in silico* and subsequently sequenced to monitor for deleterious off-target effects. Overall, HDR can be utilized to correct individual point mutations, as well as to insert larger fragments, such as complete copies of functional cDNA, into desired sites. To date, gene correction has been achieved *in vitro, ex vivo,* as well as directly in murine liver and lung [35–37].

Each of the available nuclease technologies utilizes a different method for recognizing specific sites and initiating DSB cleavage. In the following section, we will discuss the various mechanisms of action, as well as the pros and cons of each technology. It is important to note that in order to be safe for use in a clinical setting, nuclease technology must meet the following criteria:

- Minimal off-target activity:
    - High binding specificity
    - Transient nuclease expression
- High cleavage efficiency
- Delivery to the cell using vectors that minimize insertional mutagenesis risk

5.1. Zinc finger nucleases

Zinc fingers are a common DNA-binding protein that can be found in nearly half of all transcription factors in the human genome [38]. These naturally abundant proteins can be re-engineered to recognize and bind specific target sequences. ZFN technology takes advantage of this by attaching a DNA-cleaving nuclease to the zinc finger-binding domain. The result is a site-specific binding protein that can cleave a strand of DNA at a precise location.

ZFNs utilize the non-specific DNA cleavage domain from the *Fok*I restriction endonuclease to confer their cleavage activity [39]. Their design traditionally incorporates the wild-type *Fok*I cleavage domain; however, more recent studies have utilized variants with improved cleavage activity or specificity [40–42]. Functioning as a dimer, the *Fok*I domain requires two ZFN constructs, working together as a pair: one ZFN binds to a sequence immediately upstream of the intended cut site, while the other targets sequence immediately downstream of the cut site on the complementary strand (Figure 4A). This alignment places the C-terminal nucleases at a desired distance apart across the cut site, where they dimerize and create a DSB. Proper spacing of binding and cleavage domains is critical for optimal DSB induction.

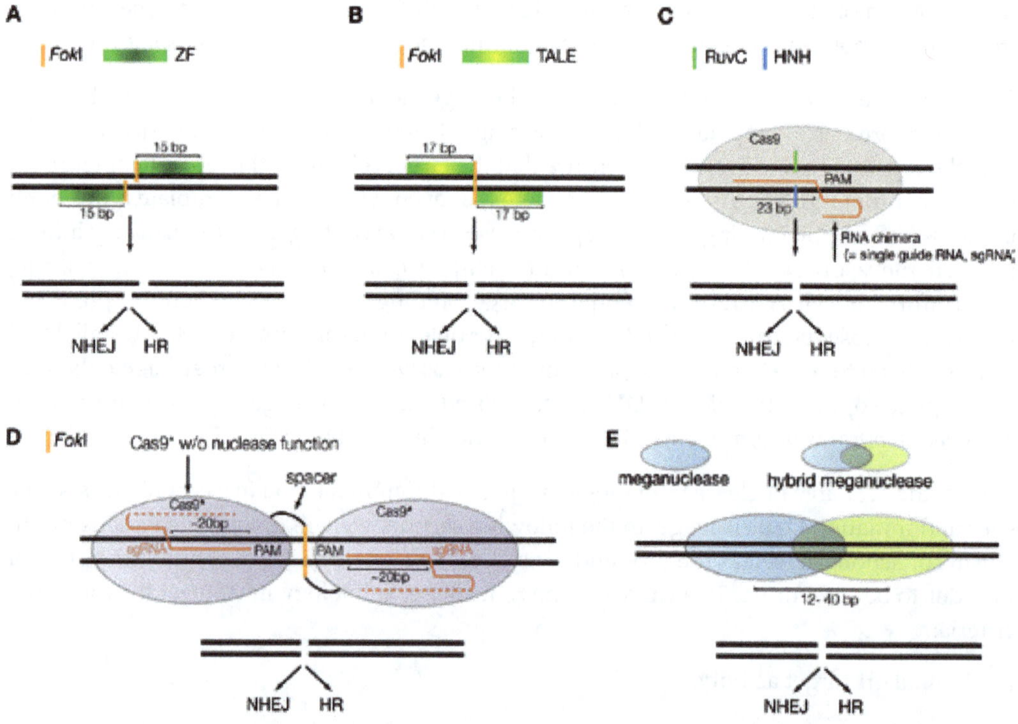

Figure 4. Genome-editing nucleases: Mechanisms of action. An overview of the mechanisms of DNA binding and cleavage used by ZFNs (**A**), TALENs (**B**), CRISPR/Cas9 (**C**), the dimeric CRISPR RNA-guided *Fok*I system (**D**), and meganucleases (**E**). PAM, protospacer adjacent motif; sgRNA, single guide RNA; RuvC, nuclease domain in Cas9 that cleaves the non-target strand of DNA; HNH, nuclease domain in Cas9 that cleaves the target strand of DNA.

Numerous evidence has supported the use of ZFNs for targeted gene editing in multiple species, including mice, rats, rabbits, pigs, plants, and zebrafish [38]. The use of this platform has also extended to the manipulation of stem cell populations *ex vivo*. In one seminal study, ZFNs facilitated targeted disruption of *CCR5*, a co-receptor involved in HIV entry [32]. By introducing the *CCR5*-Δ32 mutation into *ex vivo* expanded CD4$^+$ T cells, followed by engraftment into HIV-1 infected mice, these target cells no longer expressed functional CCR5 entry receptors, making them more resistant to infection. Further studies utilized a dual strategy to target both of the HIV entry co-receptors, CCR5 and CXCR4 [43]. The use of ZFNs was also successfully demonstrated *in vivo* in murine liver, to correct a model of hemophilia B, or factor IX (FIX) deficiency [36].

Despite this, ZFNs are not without their limitations. First, they are relatively difficult to engineer and expensive to purchase commercially, leaving them inaccessible to the majority of investigators. Secondly, not all sequences can be targeted by ZFNs, restricting their use in certain applications. And lastly, the specificity of ZFN pairs is not 100%, resulting in the potential for off-target cleavage events and related damage to occur. In the event of low specificity, off-target DSB induction may overwhelm cellular repair machinery leading to chromosomal rearrangements and/or cell death. These instances may also support random integration of donor DNA into undesirable locations, which has the potential to interfere with tumor suppressors, proto-oncogenes, or other actively transcribed genes [24,25].

5.2. Transcription activator-like effector nucleases

Transcription activator-like effector (TAL effector, or TALE) proteins are secreted by *Xanthomonas* bacteria upon infecting various species of plant. They function by binding to promoter sequences in the host to upregulate plant genes that are beneficial to bacterial infection. Similar to the concept of ZFNs, TALENs are built by fusing the DNA binding domain of a TAL effector to a DNA cleavage domain with nuclease activity [44–47]. The DNA binding domain consists of multiple repeats of a 33-34 amino acid sequence, where all but the 12th and 13th amino acids are highly conserved. By selecting a combination of repeat segments with the appropriate variable regions (Repeat Variable Diresidues, or RVDs), specific DNA binding domains can be engineered.

TALENs utilize the same non-specific DNA cleavage domain from the *Fok*I endonuclease to confer cleavage activity. As a result, this strategy also requires two TALENs to work together as a pair, binding non-palindromic sequences on complementary strands of DNA. Proper positioning of the DNA binding and cleavage domains around the cute site allows the *Fok*I endonuclease domains to dimerize and produce a site-specific DSB (Figure 4B) [48,49].

Compared with ZFNs, TALENs can cleave a broader, more comprehensive range of DNA sequences. In addition, they tend to be more accurate, reducing the potential for off-target cleavage events. Furthermore, as a result of the fast ligation-based automatable solid-phase high-throughput (FLASH) system reported in 2012, large-scale assembly of TALENs has also become a more efficient and cost-effective alternative [50].

5.3. CRISPR/Cas9

In 2012, the use of a novel genome-editing tool was described in human cell culture [51]. In bacteria and archaea, clustered regularly interspaced short palindromic repeats (CRISPR) work together with Cas genes to form a prokaryotic adaptive immune system that protects against foreign genetic elements such as plasmids or phages. Upon detecting viral DNA, for instance, this system converts segments of the foreign DNA into CRISPR RNAs (crRNA); the crRNA then combines with a trans-activating crRNA (tracrRNA). The crRNA–tracrRNA combination then guides a Cas9 DNA nuclease to a specific location within the viral DNA, called the protospacer, where a DSB is induced.

Investigators discovered that by designing a new crRNA and combining it with the tracrRNA, a "single-guide RNA" (sgRNA) could be produced that would direct the Cas9 nuclease activity to any desired location. Studies have shown that delivery of two components, the Cas9 nuclease and a corresponding sgRNA (containing both the crRNA and tracrRNA), were sufficient to elicit cleavage in a desired gene [52–55]. Hence, by retargeting the crRNA portion of the sgRNA, a site-specific genome-editing tool could be developed (Figure 4C).

Unlike ZFN and TALEN strategies, the nuclease cleavage domain in the CRISPR/Cas9 system is not fused to the DNA binding domain: instead, these are delivered to the cell in two separate components (Figure 4C). As a result of this design, only a single DNA binding domain has to be created. As this single protein-binding domain is significantly shorter than those required for TALEN or ZFN designs, CRISPR/Cas9 components are significantly easier and more cost effective to synthesize, making this technology more widely available to the research community at large. Despite lower costs and greater accessibility, the functional activity of CRISPR/Cas systems appears to be equal to or greater than their ZFN and TALEN counterparts.

As the CRISPR/Cas9 system is a relatively new genome engineering technology, it will be important for the field to thoroughly study any potential shortcomings. For instance, since a relatively short DNA binding domain and cleavage site are utilized, the risk of low specificity and potential off-target recognition may be greater [56].

5.4. Dimeric CRISPR RNA-guided *Fok*I nucleases

In an effort to reduce the risk of unwanted off-target mutations associated with monomeric CRISPR/Cas9 nucleases, a modified dimeric version has now been developed [57]. Where the monomeric Cas9 nuclease is recruited by one sgRNA of only ~100 nucleotides in length (with 17–20 nucleotides of complementarity to the target), dimerization offers an attractive strategy for improving the binding specificity of the Cas9 system (Figure 4D).

In this approach, a wild-type *Fok*I nuclease domain is fused to a catalytically inactive Cas9 (dCas9) protein. Two such *Fok*I-dCas9 fusions are recruited by two corresponding guide RNAs, where both are required to bind their respective target sites in order for *Fok*I dimerization and DSB induction to occur (Figure 4D). An appropriately designed spacer and protospacer adjacent motif (PAM) are also critical for driving efficient cleavage. Overall, this RNA-guided *Fok*I nuclease (RFN) strategy has been shown to elicit robust genome editing efficiencies while reducing known off-target mutations to undetectable levels [57].

5.5. Meganucleases

Meganucleases are another form of endonuclease utilized for genome editing approaches. They are unique in that their DNA recognition and cleavage functions are naturally combined in a single domain. There are five classes available, where I-SceI, I-CreI, and I-DmoI are perhaps the most widely used. Consisting of a large recognition site of 12 to 40 base pairs, meganucleases also offer high specificity and precision; however, historically, they were only capable of tolerating minor variations in their recognition site sequence, decreasing the probability of an available meganuclease for each desired application. In recent years, investigators have begun customizing meganucleases to expand their targeting repertoire. Two main approaches have been taken: modifying the specificity of existing meganucleases, and/or developing chimeric meganucleases with new recognition sites. In the latter approach, by fusing the DNA-binding domains of two different meganucleases, functional heterodimers can be designed for optimal efficacy and specificity (Figure 4E).

6. The best vehicle for the job

In genome editing, the identification of components capable of eliciting HDR is only half the battle. Efficiently delivering those components to the target cell can be an equally important hurdle to overcome. Unlike gene and transcript replacement therapies, where the goal is to achieve stable, long-term expression of a supplemental protein, gene editing has the advantage of requiring only short-term expression of the foreign components in the cell. Once these components have been expressed, induced a DSB, and triggered HDR, their presence is no longer necessary. In fact, in the attempt to minimize unwanted off-target cleavage activity and prolonged DSB induction, the ideal nuclease-delivery vehicle should only be transiently expressed.

Additionally, without the need for integration to promote stable expression, non-integrating delivery vehicles are also preferable, to minimize the risk of insertional mutagenesis. Delivery vehicles must also be capable of transducing target cells efficiently, to facilitate gene correction in enough cells to overcome the initial defect. To summarize, since transient expression of the nuclease is sufficient for stable modification of the genome, the ideal nuclease delivery vehicle should be:

- Short-lived,
- Non-integrating, and
- Able to enter target cells efficiently.

A variety of vectors have been utilized to deliver genome-editing reagents to the cell. Initial *in vivo* studies have included AAV viral vectors as well as integrase-defective lentiviruses. Using AAV-encoded ZFNs, for instance, Li and colleagues demonstrated direct *in vivo* gene correction using HDR in a murine model of FIX deficiency [36]. Despite these successes, early *in vivo* strategies have not fulfilled two of the critical components for nuclease delivery vehicles: transience and lack of potential integration. In addition, with respect to translation of these approaches to CF airway disease, none of these strategies reported targeting cells in the lung.

Due to its short half-life and inability to integrate into the genome, modified mRNA is gaining interest as an ideal vector for site-specific nuclease delivery: one that would address two of the main outstanding issues previously discussed. Transient expression of mRNA-encoded nucleases would also minimize the long-term threat of off-target events associated with the use of stably expressing, and possibly integrating viral vectors.

7. Gene correction in the lung

In a recent study, nuclease-encoding chemically modified mRNA (nec-mRNA) was described as a novel vehicle for delivering genome-editing components directly to the lung [37]. Using a murine model of SP-B deficiency, nec-mRNA-encoded ZFNs were able to demonstrate the first report of life-prolonging gene correction specifically within lung tissue.

In the transgenic mouse model of SP-B deficiency, SP-B cDNA is under the control of a Tetracycline-inducible promoter [58]. Administration of doxycycline allows SP-B to be expressed at wild-type levels. If doxycycline is removed, SP-B expression drops and mice begin to exhibit phenotypic changes similar to those seen in humans with the disease: thickened alveolar walls, heavy cellular infiltration, increased macrophages and neutrophils, interstitial edema, congestion, augmented cytokines in the lavage, a significant drop in lung function, and acute onset of respiratory distress leading to death within days [59,60].

In order to demonstrate the value of nec-mRNA for lung-based genome-editing applications, this report utilized HDR to insert a constitutive CAG promoter immediately upstream of the SP-B cDNA. The resulting doxycycline-independent expression was able to significantly prolong the life of treated mice [37].

While this study was not performed in a humanized mouse model, the approach was able to demonstrate that extra-chromosomal nec-mRNA is capable of transducing airway epithelial cells, expressing genome-editing reagents, and achieving HDR rates sufficient for therapeutic levels of protein expression. Main findings from the study include:

i. mRNA modification schemes can be customized to optimize expression and minimize immunity.

ii. Intratracheal delivery of nec-mRNA is able to target airway epithelial cells.

iii. Complexing nec-mRNA to chitosan-coated nanoparticles can increase transduction efficiency in the lung.

iv. nec-mRNA expression is transient in comparison to AAV-encoded ZFNs.

v. nec-mRNA-mediated ZFN delivery can facilitate HDR rates comparable to AAV-encoded ZFNs.

8. Hurdles to success: Limitations to gene correction for cystic fibrosis

The lung has evolved with natural defense mechanisms against foreign pathogens. As such, a number of intracellular and extracellular barriers must be overcome in order to target new technologies to the lung [61]. In addition to this, the lungs of CF patients are even more difficult to target, owing to the increased airway mucus (sputum) lining the lungs. Especially in more progressed CF patients, thickened mucus linings have proven prohibitive in several gene replacement therapy approaches. Hida and colleagues reported that expectorated sputum from CF patients effectively traps and slows the diffusion of both Ad and AAV viral vectors [62]. For instance, where the sputum penetration of muco-inert nanoparticles is reduced by only 40-fold compared with pure water, that of Ad and AAV particles is slowed by 3,000-fold and 12,000-fold, respectively. Poor penetration of mucus layers may be a major component preventing effective viral gene replacement therapy or the use of viral vectors to deliver genome-editing components for CF.

Limits to stable expression of functional CFTR also play an important role. For gene replacement therapy approaches, this may include immune responses against the vector capsid, the inability to re-administer, as well as turnover of CFTR-expressing lung cells. For gene correction approaches, transient expression of nucleases does not destabilize the downstream effects of HDR. However, lung cell turnover continues to be an issue, making the possibility of re-administration important.

The levels of CFTR expression required to halt the progression of CF lung disease remain largely unknown, as well as the cell types most suited as targets. While airway epithelial cells are generally considered to be the ideal target, airway histology and entry receptor expression patterns may impact the ability of this cell type to be transduced. The absence of adenoviral entry receptors on the apical surface of airway epithelium, for instance, is one of the major reasons that adenoviral gene therapy vectors are no longer pursued. Furthermore, turnover of these terminally differentiated cells will eventually require therapeutics to be redelivered to new target cells.

In addition to the most relevant cell type, another question remains: is it preferable to obtain low levels of CFTR in a high percentage of cells, or high levels of CFTR in only ~10% of cells? Gene replacement and correction approaches are more likely to attain the latter, although it remains unknown whether this will be sufficient to show therapeutic effect. One recent study has shown that restoration of normal mucus transport rates in cultured CF human airway epithelial cells required at least 25% of surface epithelial cells to be targeted by CFTR gene replacement therapy [63]. Whether this figure will translate to clinical benefit in an *in vivo* setting remains to be seen.

9. Supplemental strategies and future directions

Due to the limitations of targeting the lung, it remains unclear whether novel replacement and correction approaches will find success for Cystic Fibrosis lung disease. Efforts to overcome these barriers remain the subject of further investigation.

As one recent study demonstrated, combining nec-mRNA with chitosan-coated poly(lactide-co-glycolide) nanoparticles may be one viable method for overcoming the CF sputum barrier to lung cell targeting [37,64]. Recent progress in the development of mucus penetrating nanoparticles (MPP) may provide an opportunity to further overcome this barrier [65]. Drug-loaded MPPs with non-adhesive coatings have been shown to penetrate mucus layers at rates nearly as fast as pure water. These developments may allow the penetration of delivery vehicles to airway epithelium, without reducing the protective function of the mucus itself. Furthermore, adjuvant regimens of N-acetylcysteine (NAC) with or without recombinant human DNase (rhDNase) were used to increase diffusivity of nanocomplexed, non-viral gene delivery vectors through sputum layers [66]. This strategy was able to increase gene expression by ~12-fold, making it another potential avenue for improving targeting in the lungs of CF patients. Complexes of pDNA or mRNA with GL67:DOPE:DMPE-PEG5000 (GL67) liposomes have also been described as a potential avenue for augmenting non-viral respiratory gene transfer [67]. Overall, developments in nanoparticle technology combined with advancements in aerosol-delivery devices may hold promise for the field.

Route of administration may be an important consideration as well, especially given the tendency for inhaled therapeutics to be entrapped in the mucus layer. Intratracheal high-pressure spraying approaches have been effective in targeting airway epithelial cells in pre-clinical models [30,31,37], although efficiency is likely to decrease in the face of CF sputum. Preliminary evidence supports the claim that intravenous routes of administration may also target airway cells efficiently, while avoiding the barriers to a direct airway approach.

The continued development of humanized animal models of CF, including mouse, pig, and ferret models, will further our ability to investigate novel therapeutic strategies [68,69]. An early mouse model, *CFTR*^{tm1UNC}, knocked out murine *CFTR* through a stop codon in exon 10; however, these mice showed a drastic drop in survival rates due to severe intestinal obstruction [70,71]. To overcome lethal intestinal defects, the mice were then 'gut-corrected' with a human *CFTR* construct driven by an intestinal-specific FABP promoter [72]. Studies in the FABP-hCFTR/*Cftr*^{tm1UNC} gut-corrected model have demonstrated that the human CFTR protein is indeed functional in mice. Using this or other models as a foundation, it may be possible to introduce a transgenic construct containing a mutated human *CFTR* driven by a lung-specific promoter. Creating humanized mice expressing the *CFTR*-ΔF508 mutation, for instance, may offer an excellent tool for studying gene correction using nucleases and repair templates designed for direct translation to the clinic.

In addition to the development of novel animal models, the identification of human lung stem cell populations has offered new hope for overcoming the issue of lung cell turnover [73]. If genome-editing vehicles could be efficiently targeted to lung stem cell populations, such as bronchioalveolar stem cells (BASCs) [74], Clara cells [75], or alveolar type II (ATII) progenitors [76], HDR in these self-renewing populations could support indefinite CFTR production.

Engineering strategies to minimize the risk of off-target cleavage and donor integration will also continue to be an important area of development. Along these lines, it will be critical to more thoroughly define standardized parameters for measuring off-target effects. State-of-the-art techniques that can be used for measuring outcome parameters will also aid in assessing overall efficacy. Combining efforts to overcome these barriers to lung targeting, cell turnover, proper animal models, and off-target effects will enable the field to make continued progress toward a novel gene correction strategy for the treatment of Cystic Fibrosis.

10. Conclusion

Over two decades since the cloning of the CFTR gene, numerous strategies have been investigated to identify clinically relevant genetic variants, target cells of the airway, and overcome deleterious mutations. Rather than masking symptoms of the disease, novel therapies strive to address the underlying genetic cause of the Cystic Fibrosis phenotype. Agents have approached this goal with varying strategies, including attempts to overcome the patient's functional CFTR defects, supplement their cells with a functional copy of the protein, or directly repair genomic mutations at their source. Innovations in viral and non-viral delivery vehicles and methods for overcoming barriers to lung targeting have allowed for promising progress in recent years. Coupled with novel genome-editing reagents, such as ZFNs, TALENs, and the CRISPR/Cas9 system, the promise of a novel therapeutic approach is becoming an increasingly attainable goal within the field. Further advancement in minimizing off-target activity, increasing the efficiency of site-specific cleavage, and optimizing robust, transient, non-integrating nuclease delivery vehicles will bring us closer to achieving stable modification of the genome in the race toward *in vivo* gene correction of Cystic Fibrosis.

Author details

Michael Sebastian Daniel Kormann

Address all correspondence to: kormann.michael@gmail.com

University Children's Clinic Department of Pediatrics I, Pediatric Infectiology & Immunology, Translational Genomics and Gene Therapy in Pediatrics, University of Tübingen, Tübingen, Germany

References

[1] Tobias ES, Connor M, Ferguson-Smith M. Essential Medical Genetics. John Wiley & Sons; 2011.

[2] WHO | Genes and human disease. WHO. n.d. http://www.who.int/genomics/public/geneticdiseases/en/index2.html (accessed February 16, 2015).

[3] O'Sullivan BP, Freedman SD. Cystic fibrosis. Lancet. 2009;373:1891–904. DOI:10.1016/S0140-6736(09)60327–5.

[4] Stutts MJ, Canessa CM, Olsen JC, Hamrick M, Cohn JA, Rossier BC, et al. CFTR as a cAMP-dependent regulator of sodium channels. Science. 1995;269:847–50.

[5] Mall M, Hipper A, Greger R, Kunzelmann K. Wild type but not deltaF508 CFTR inhibits Na+ conductance when coexpressed in Xenopus oocytes. FEBS Letters. 1996;381:47–52.

[6] Matsui H, Grubb BR, Tarran R, Randell SH, Gatzy JT, Davis CW, et al. Evidence for periciliary liquid layer depletion, not abnormal ion composition, in the pathogenesis of cystic fibrosis airways disease. Cell. 1998;95:1005–15.

[7] Bobadilla JL, Macek M, Fine JP, Farrell PM. Cystic fibrosis: a worldwide analysis of CFTR mutations--correlation with incidence data and application to screening. Human Mutation. 2002;19:575–606. DOI:10.1002/humu.10041.

[8] Rowe SM, Miller S, Sorscher EJ. Cystic fibrosis. The New England Journal of Medicine. 2005;352:1992–2001. DOI:10.1056/NEJMra043184.

[9] Drumm ML, Konstan MW, Schluchter MD, Handler A, Pace R, Zou F, et al. Genetic modifiers of lung disease in cystic fibrosis. The New England Journal of Medicine. 2005;353:1443–53. DOI:10.1056/NEJMoa051469.

[10] Gu Y, Harley ITW, Henderson LB, Aronow BJ, Vietor I, Huber LA, et al. Identification of IFRD1 as a modifier gene for cystic fibrosis lung disease. Nature. 2009;458:1039–42. DOI:10.1038/nature07811.

[11] Hector A, Kormann M, Kammermeier J, Burdi S, Marcos V, Rieber N, et al. Expression and regulation of interferon-related development regulator-1 in cystic fibrosis neutrophils. American Journal of Respiratory Cell and Molecular Biology. 2013;48:71–7. DOI:10.1165/rcmb.2012-0061OC.

[12] Anderson P. Emerging therapies in cystic fibrosis. Therapeutic Advances in Respiratory Disease. 2010;4:177–85. DOI:10.1177/1753465810371107.

[13] Rogan MP, Stoltz DA, Hornick DB. Cystic fibrosis transmembrane conductance regulator intracellular processing, trafficking, and opportunities for mutation-specific treatment. Chest. 2011;139:1480–90. DOI:10.1378/chest.10-2077.

[14] Boyle MP, Bell SC, Konstan MW, McColley SA, Rowe SM, Rietschel E, et al. A CFTR corrector (lumacaftor) and a CFTR potentiator (ivacaftor) for treatment of patients with cystic fibrosis who have a phe508del CFTR mutation: a phase 2 randomised controlled trial. The Lancet Respiratory Medicine. 2014;2:527–38. DOI:10.1016/S2213-2600(14)70132-8.

[15] Kerem E, Konstan MW, De Boeck K, Accurso FJ, Sermet-Gaudelus I, Wilschanski M, et al. Ataluren for the treatment of nonsense-mutation cystic fibrosis: a randomised, double-blind, placebo-controlled phase 3 trial. The Lancet Respiratory Medicine. 2014;2:539–47. DOI:10.1016/S2213-2600(14)70100-6.

[16] Griesenbach U, Alton EWFW. Moving forward: cystic fibrosis gene therapy. Human Molecular Genetics. 2013;22:R52–8. DOI:10.1093/hmg/ddt372.

[17] Zhou R, Norton JE, Zhang N, Dean DA. Electroporation-mediated transfer of plasmids to the lung results in reduced TLR9 signaling and inflammation. Gene Therapy. 2007;14:775–80. DOI:10.1038/sj.gt.3302936.

[18] Gao G, Vandenberghe LH, Wilson JM. New recombinant serotypes of AAV vectors. Current Gene Therapy. 2005;5:285–97.

[19] Limberis MP, Vandenberghe LH, Zhang L, Pickles RJ, Wilson JM. Transduction efficiencies of novel AAV vectors in mouse airway epithelium in vivo and human ciliated airway epithelium in vitro. Molecular Therapy: The Journal of the American Society of Gene Therapy. 2009;17:294–301. DOI:10.1038/mt.2008.261.

[20] Faust SM, Bell P, Cutler BJ, Ashley SN, Zhu Y, Rabinowitz JE, et al. CpG-depleted adeno-associated virus vectors evade immune detection. The Journal of Clinical Investigation. 2013;123:2994–3001. DOI:10.1172/JCI68205.

[21] Mays LE, Wang L, Tenney R, Bell P, Nam H-J, Lin J, et al. Mapping the structural determinants responsible for enhanced T cell activation to the immunogenic adeno-associated virus capsid from isolate rhesus 32.33. Journal of Virology. 2013;87:9473–85. DOI:10.1128/JVI.00596-13.

[22] Liu X, Luo M, Guo C, Yan Z, Wang Y, Lei-Butters DCM, et al. Analysis of adeno-associated virus progenitor cell transduction in mouse lung. Molecular Therapy: The Journal of the American Society of Gene Therapy. 2009;17:285–93. DOI:10.1038/mt.2008.248.

[23] Mitomo K, Griesenbach U, Inoue M, Somerton L, Meng C, Akiba E, et al. Toward gene therapy for cystic fibrosis using a lentivirus pseudotyped with Sendai virus envelopes. Molecular Therapy: The Journal of the American Society of Gene Therapy. 2010;18:1173–82. DOI:10.1038/mt.2010.13.

[24] Hacein-Bey-Abina S, von Kalle C, Schmidt M, Le Deist F, Wulffraat N, McIntyre E, et al. A serious adverse event after successful gene therapy for X-linked severe combined immunodeficiency. The New England Journal of Medicine. 2003;348:255–6. DOI:10.1056/NEJM200301163480314.

[25] Hacein-Bey-Abina S, Von Kalle C, Schmidt M, McCormack MP, Wulffraat N, Leboulch P, et al. LMO2-associated clonal T cell proliferation in two patients after gene therapy for SCID-X1. Science. 2003;302:415–9. DOI:10.1126/science.1088547.

[26] Lorenz C, Fotin-Mleczek M, Roth G, Becker C, Dam TC, Verdurmen WPR, et al. Protein expression from exogenous mRNA: uptake by receptor-mediated endocytosis and trafficking via the lysosomal pathway. RNA Biology. 2011;8:627–36. DOI: 10.4161/rna.8.4.15394.

[27] Kariko K, Muramatsu H, Ludwig J, Weissman D. Generating the optimal mRNA for therapy: HPLC purification eliminates immune activation and improves translation

of nucleoside-modified, protein-encoding mRNA. Nucleic Acids Research. 2011;39:e142. DOI:10.1093/nar/gkr695.

[28] Kariko K, Muramatsu H, Welsh FA, Ludwig J, Kato H, Akira S, et al. Incorporation of pseudouridine into mRNA yields superior nonimmunogenic vector with increased translational capacity and biological stability. Molecular Therapy. 2008;16:1833–40. DOI:10.1038/mt.2008.200.

[29] Kariko K, Muramatsu H, Keller JM, Weissman D. Increased erythropoiesis in mice injected with submicrogram quantities of pseudouridine-containing mRNA encoding erythropoietin. Molecular Therapy. 2012;20:948–53. DOI:10.1038/mt.2012.7.

[30] Kormann MS, Hasenpusch G, Aneja MK, Nica G, Flemmer AW, Herber-Jonat S, et al. Expression of therapeutic proteins after delivery of chemically modified mRNA in mice. Nature Biotechnology. 2011;29:154–7. DOI:10.1038/nbt.1733.

[31] Mays LE, Ammon-Treiber S, Mothes B, Alkhaled M, Rottenberger J, Muller-Hermelink ES, et al. Modified Foxp3 mRNA protects against asthma through an IL-10-dependent mechanism. The Journal of Clinical Investigation. 2013;123:1216–28. DOI: 10.1172/JCI65351.

[32] Perez EE, Wang J, Miller JC, Jouvenot Y, Kim KA, Liu O, et al. Establishment of HIV-1 resistance in CD4+ T cells by genome editing using zinc-finger nucleases. Nature Biotechnology. 2008;26:808–16. DOI:10.1038/nbt1410.

[33] Mali P, Yang L, Esvelt KM, Aach J, Guell M, DiCarlo JE, et al. RNA-guided human genome engineering via Cas9. Science. 2013;339:823–6. DOI:10.1126/science.1232033.

[34] Cong L, Ran FA, Cox D, Lin S, Barretto R, Habib N, et al. Multiplex genome engineering using CRISPR/Cas systems. Science. 2013;339:819–23. DOI:10.1126/science.1231143.

[35] Cox DBT, Platt RJ, Zhang F. Therapeutic genome editing: prospects and challenges. Nature Medicine. 2015;21:121–31. DOI:10.1038/nm.3793.

[36] Li H, Haurigot V, Doyon Y, Li T, Wong SY, Bhagwat AS, et al. In vivo genome editing restores haemostasis in a mouse model of haemophilia. Nature. 2011;475:217–21. DOI:10.1038/nature10177.

[37] Dewerth A, Mays L, Mahiny A, et al. In vivo genome editing using nuclease-encoding mRNA corrects SP-B deficiency. Nature Biotechnology. 2015. Manuscript accepted.

[38] Segal DJ. Bacteria herald a new era of gene editing. eLife. 2013;2:e00563. DOI:10.7554/eLife.00563.

[39] Urnov FD, Rebar EJ, Holmes MC, Zhang HS, Gregory PD. Genome editing with engineered zinc finger nucleases. Nature Reviews Genetics. 2010;11:636–46. DOI: 10.1038/nrg2842.

[40] Doyon Y, Vo TD, Mendel MC, Greenberg SG, Wang J, Xia DF, et al. Enhancing zinc-finger-nuclease activity with improved obligate heterodimeric architectures. Nature Methods. 2011;8:74–9. DOI:10.1038/nmeth.1539.

[41] Szczepek M, Brondani V, Büchel J, Serrano L, Segal DJ, Cathomen T. Structure-based redesign of the dimerization interface reduces the toxicity of zinc-finger nucleases. Nature Biotechnology. 2007;25:786–93. DOI:10.1038/nbt1317.

[42] Guo J, Gaj T, Barbas CF. Directed evolution of an enhanced and highly efficient FokI cleavage domain for zinc finger nucleases. Journal of Molecular Biology. 2010;400:96–107. DOI:10.1016/j.jmb.2010.04.060.

[43] Didigu CA, Wilen CB, Wang J, Duong J, Secreto AJ, Danet-Desnoyers GA, et al. Simultaneous zinc-finger nuclease editing of the HIV coreceptors ccr5 and cxcr4 protects CD4+ T cells from HIV-1 infection. Blood. 2014;123:61–9. DOI:10.1182/blood-2013-08-521229.

[44] Rusk N. TALEs for the masses. Nature Methods. 2011;8:197.

[45] Miller JC, Tan S, Qiao G, Barlow KA, Wang J, Xia DF, et al. A TALE nuclease architecture for efficient genome editing. Nature Biotechnology. 2011;29:143–8. DOI: 10.1038/nbt.1755.

[46] Boch J. TALEs of genome targeting. Nature Biotechnology. 2011;29:135–6. DOI: 10.1038/nbt.1767.

[47] Zhang F, Cong L, Lodato S, Kosuri S, Church GM, Arlotta P. Efficient construction of sequence-specific TAL effectors for modulating mammalian transcription. Nature Biotechnology. 2011;29:149–53. DOI:10.1038/nbt.1775.

[48] Mussolino C, Cathomen T. TALE nucleases: tailored genome engineering made easy. Current Opinion in Biotechnology. 2012;23:644–50. DOI:10.1016/j.copbio.2012.01.013.

[49] Bedell VM, Wang Y, Campbell JM, Poshusta TL, Starker CG, Krug RG, et al. In vivo genome editing using a high-efficiency TALEN system. Nature. 2012;491:114–8. DOI: 10.1038/nature11537.

[50] Reyon D, Tsai SQ, Khayter C, Foden JA, Sander JD, Joung JK. FLASH assembly of TALENs for high-throughput genome editing. Nature Biotechnology. 2012;30:460–5. DOI:10.1038/nbt.2170.

[51] Jinek M, Chylinski K, Fonfara I, Hauer M, Doudna JA, Charpentier E. A programmable dual-RNA-guided DNA endonuclease in adaptive bacterial immunity. Science (New York, NY). 2012;337:816–21. DOI:10.1126/science.1225829.

[52] Jinek M, East A, Cheng A, Lin S, Ma E, Doudna J. RNA-programmed genome editing in human cells. eLife. 2013;2:e00471. DOI:10.7554/eLife.00471.

[53] Cho SW, Kim S, Kim JM, Kim J-S. Targeted genome engineering in human cells with the Cas9 RNA-guided endonuclease. Nature Biotechnology. 2013;31:230–2. DOI: 10.1038/nbt.2507.

[54] Hwang WY, Fu Y, Reyon D, Maeder ML, Tsai SQ, Sander JD, et al. Efficient genome editing in zebrafish using a CRISPR-Cas system. Nature Biotechnology. 2013;31:227–9. DOI:10.1038/nbt.2501.

[55] Barrangou R. RNA-mediated programmable DNA cleavage. Nature Biotechnology. 2012;30:836–8. DOI:10.1038/nbt.2357.

[56] Lin Y, Cradick TJ, Brown MT, Deshmukh H, Ranjan P, Sarode N, et al. CRISPR/Cas9 systems have off-target activity with insertions or deletions between target DNA and guide RNA sequences. Nucleic Acids Research. 2014;42:7473–85. DOI:10.1093/nar/gku402.

[57] Tsai SQ, Wyvekens N, Khayter C, Foden JA, Thapar V, Reyon D, et al. Dimeric CRISPR RNA-guided FokI nucleases for highly specific genome editing. Nature Biotechnology. 2014;32:569–76. DOI:10.1038/nbt.2908.

[58] Schultze N, Burki Y, Lang Y, Certa U, Bluethmann H. Efficient control of gene expression by single step integration of the tetracycline system in transgenic mice. Nature Biotechnology. 1996;14:499–503. DOI:10.1038/nbt0496-499.

[59] Nogee LM. Alterations in SP-B and SP-C expression in neonatal lung disease. The Annual Review of Physiology. 2004;66:601–23. DOI:10.1146/annurev.physiol.66.032102.134711.

[60] Clark JC, Wert SE, Bachurski CJ, Stahlman MT, Stripp BR, Weaver TE, et al. Targeted disruption of the surfactant protein B gene disrupts surfactant homeostasis, causing respiratory failure in newborn mice. Proceedings of the National Academy of Sciences of the United States of America. 1995;92:7794–8.

[61] Ruge CA, Kirch J, Lehr C-M. Pulmonary drug delivery: from generating aerosols to overcoming biological barriers-therapeutic possibilities and technological challenges. The Lancet Respiratory Medicine. 2013;1:402–13. DOI:10.1016/S2213-2600(13)70072–9.

[62] Hida K, Lai SK, Suk JS, Won SY, Boyle MP, Hanes J. Common gene therapy viral vectors do not efficiently penetrate sputum from cystic fibrosis patients. PloS One. 2011;6:e19919. DOI:10.1371/journal.pone.0019919.

[63] Zhang L, Button B, Gabriel SE, Burkett S, Yan Y, Skiadopoulos MH, et al. CFTR delivery to 25% of surface epithelial cells restores normal rates of mucus transport to human cystic fibrosis airway epithelium. PLoS Biology. 2009;7:e1000155. DOI: 10.1371/journal.pbio.1000155.

[64] Nafee N, Taetz S, Schneider M, Schaefer UF, Lehr CM. Chitosan-coated PLGA nanoparticles for DNA/RNA delivery: effect of the formulation parameters on complexa-

tion and transfection of antisense oligonucleotides. Nanomedicine: Nanotechnology, Biology, and Medicine. 2007;3:173–83. DOI:10.1016/j.nano.2007.03.006.

[65] Ensign LM, Schneider C, Suk JS, Cone R, Hanes J. Mucus penetrating nanoparticles: biophysical tool and method of drug and gene delivery. Advanced Materials (Deerfield Beach, FL). 2012;24:3887–94.

[66] Suk JS, Boylan NJ, Trehan K, Tang BC, Schneider CS, Lin J-MG, et al. N-acetylcysteine enhances cystic fibrosis sputum penetration and airway gene transfer by highly compacted DNA nanoparticles. Molecular Therapy: The Journal of the American Society of Gene Therapy. 2011;19:1981–9. DOI:10.1038/mt.2011.160.

[67] Andries O, De Filette M, Rejman J, De Smedt SC, Demeester J, Van Poucke M, et al. Comparison of the gene transfer efficiency of mRNA/GL67 and pDNA/GL67 complexes in respiratory cells. Molecular Pharmaceutics. 2012;9:2136–45. DOI:10.1021/mp200604h.

[68] Yan Z, Stewart ZA, Sinn PL, Olsen JC, Hu J, McCray PB, et al. Ferret and pig models of cystic fibrosis: prospects and promise for gene therapy. Human Gene Therapy Clinical Development. 2015. DOI:10.1089/humc.2014.154.

[69] Olivier AK, Gibson-Corley KN, Meyerholz DK. Animal models of cystic fibrosis: gastrointestinal, pancreatic and hepatobiliary disease and pathophysiology. American Journal of Physiology Gastrointestinal and Liver Physiology. 2015:ajpgi.00146.2014. DOI:10.1152/ajpgi.00146.2014.

[70] Snouwaert JN, Brigman KK, Latour AM, Malouf NN, Boucher RC, Smithies O, et al. An animal model for cystic fibrosis made by gene targeting. Science (New York, NY). 1992;257:1083–8.

[71] Clarke LL, Grubb BR, Gabriel SE, Smithies O, Koller BH, Boucher RC. Defective epithelial chloride transport in a gene-targeted mouse model of cystic fibrosis. Science (New York, NY). 1992;257:1125–8.

[72] Zhou L, Dey CR, Wert SE, DuVall MD, Frizzell RA, Whitsett JA. Correction of lethal intestinal defect in a mouse model of cystic fibrosis by human CFTR. Science (New York, NY). 1994;266:1705–8.

[73] Kajstura J, Rota M, Hall SR, Hosoda T, D'Amario D, Sanada F, et al. Evidence for human lung stem cells. The New England Journal of Medicine. 2011;364:1795–806. DOI:10.1056/NEJMoa1101324.

[74] Kim CFB, Jackson EL, Woolfenden AE, Lawrence S, Babar I, Vogel S, et al. Identification of bronchioalveolar stem cells in normal lung and lung cancer. Cell. 2005;121:823–35. DOI:10.1016/j.cell.2005.03.032.

[75] Hong KU, Reynolds SD, Giangreco A, Hurley CM, Stripp BR. Clara cell secretory protein-expressing cells of the airway neuroepithelial body microenvironment include a label-retaining subset and are critical for epithelial renewal after progenitor

cell depletion. American Journal of Respiratory Cell and Molecular Biology. 2001;24:671–81. DOI:10.1165/ajrcmb.24.6.4498.

[76] Fujino N, Kubo H, Suzuki T, Ota C, Hegab AE, He M, et al. Isolation of alveolar epithelial type II progenitor cells from adult human lungs. Laboratory Investigation; a Journal of Technical Methods and Pathology. 2011;91:363–78. DOI:10.1038/labinvest.2010.187.

9

Therapy for Cystic Fibrosis Caused by Nonsense Mutations

Roberto Gambari, Giulia Breveglieri, Francesca Salvatori, Alessia Finotti and Monica Borgatti

Abstract

Nonsense mutations cover about 10% of cystic fibrosis (CF) patients and generate premature termination codons (PTCs) leading to premature translational termination and causing the synthesis of truncated non-functional or partially functional CFTR (cystic fibrosis transmembrane conductance regulator) protein. The read-through approach is the suppression of translation terminations at PTCs and it has been developed as a therapeutic strategy to restore full-length protein using aminoglycoside antibiotics or PTC124. Phenotypic consequences of PTCs can be exacerbated by the nonsense-mediated mRNA decay (NMD) pathway, which detects and degrades mRNA containing PTC. Therefore, modulation of NMD is also of interest as a potential target for suppression therapy. Not all PTCs are susceptible to the read-through treatment alone, especially where the nonsense mutations are combined with other CFTR mutations. For example, many CF patients present the highly frequent F508del CF mutation, causing an alteration of the cell membrane positioning of the CFTR channel. Pharmacological correctors that rescue the trafficking of F508del CFTR may overcome this defect. A combined administration of correctors/potentiators, read-through molecules, and/or NMD inhibitors, depending on the genotype of the CF patients, could be the basis for the design of a personalized therapeutic approach.

Keywords: Cystic fibrosis, PTCs, read-through, NMD inhibitors, correctors, potentiators

1. Introduction

1.1. Classes of mutation in cystic fibrosis

The CFTR protein is a cAMP-regulated chloride channel that resides in the apical membrane of epithelial cells of different organs such as the intestines, lung, pancreas, and sweat glands. However, the main pathologic symptom of cystic fibrosis (CF) is respiratory disease with recurring infections, inflammation, and obstructions that induce progressive lung damage and possible respiratory difficulties [1].

More than 1,900 different CFTR mutations have been reported so far and can be generally categorized into five classes (Table 1). Approximately 40% of CFTR mutations belong to class I. Nonsense mutations cover 10% of CF patients, but in some populations specific nonsense mutations can occur in up to 50% of CF subjects. For example, G542X mutation, the most common CFTR nonsense mutation, has been found in 2% of Caucasian CF patients. The most frequent mutation of class II is the F508del mutation (a deletion of the phenylalanine residue at position 508) found in 75% of CF patients. While for class III, the G551D mutation has been found in approximately 4% of CF patients. Class I-III mutations determine an important defect in CFTR function and cause a severe CF phenotype, while mutations belonging to Classes IV-V permit a residual CFTR protein function and induce a milder CF phenotype. There is general consensus on the fact that in order to ameliorate the CF phenotype, the restoration of at least 5–35% of normal CFTR function is necessary [1-4].

Class	I	II	III	IV	V
Types of mutations	Nonsense; Frame shift	Missense	Missense	Missense	Missense
Defect on CFTR	No expression	No correct localization to cell membrane	No chloride channel function	Reduced chloride channel conductance	Reduced expression
Examples	G542, W1282X	F508del	G551D	R117H; R334W	A445E
Possible pharmacological therapy	Read-through	Correctors	Potentiators	Potentiators	Potentiators

Table 1. Principal classes of CF mutations and therapeutic intervention.

1.2. PTCs and NMD mechanism

Premature termination codons (PTCs) lead to premature translational termination resulting in absent functional proteins. Different inherited and acquired diseases can be attributable to PTCs, such as cystic fibrosis, Duchenne muscular dystrophy (DMD), mucopolysaccharidosis, spinal muscular atrophy (SMA) type I and type II, X-linked nephrogenic diabetes insipidus, rhinitis pigmentosa X-linked, nephropathic cystinosis, and β-thalassemia [5].

PTCs are responsible for about 10% of CF cases worldwide, but are particularly common in Ashkenazi Jews (40% of Israeli CF patients) [6]. The translation of PCT-containing mRNAs leads to the formation of truncated CFTR, in most cases lacking in its function [7].

During molecular evolution, a mechanism to eliminate these aberrant mRNAs containing PTCs has been developed, known as nonsense-mediated mRNA decay (NMD). This process of quality control is observed in all eukaryotic organisms and has an important role in the regulation of many cellular functions. Its physiological substrates act in a wide range of processes such as transcription, DNA repair, cell growth, intracellular transport, and NMD itself. Through this process, the mRNA levels containing PTCs are reduced but not completely eliminated, inducing a reduced level of proteins, which are synthesized in a truncated form [5].

In mammals the NMD process operates by the recognition of a premature stop codon. It is observed that the ability of PTCs in inducing NMD depends on its location with respect to the sequence downstream and associated proteins [8]. The NMD process often occurs in mammalian cells after the splicing of pre-mRNA and, in most cases, is controlled by the exon junction complex (EJC). This complex consists of at least 10 proteins binding to regions consisting of 20–24 nucleotides upstream of the exon-exon junction and including UPF2 and UPF3 proteins.

According to the currently proposed models of the NMD mechanism, for the majority of mRNAs, the stop codons that are localized more than 50–55 nucleotides upstream of an exon-exon junction are recognized as premature, since the EJC is found downstream to the stop codon. The EJC is recognized by UPF2 and UPF3 and ribosomes start to translate the mRNA until reaching the PTC. The termination of the translation is triggered by the recognition of PTCs by eRF1 and eRF3, release factors recruited by ribosomes. These proteins then recruit the NMD key factor UPF1, which in turn binds to the SMG1 kinase. These four proteins (eRF1, eRF3, UPF1, SMG1) constitute the SURF complex, responsible for ribosome blocking. When the PTC is upstream of this EJC, UPF1 at the termination site may interact with UPF2 (associated with EJC) causing the phosphorylation of UPF1 by SMG1 and the dissociation of release factors (eRF1 and eRF3). The phosphorylated UPF1 recruits additional factors (SMG5, SMG6, and SMG7) triggering NMD. Once the NMD is stimulated, target transcripts are degraded by 5′ and 3′ exonucleases [5].

2. PTCs and NMD mechanism as targets for CF therapy

2.1. The read-through approach in CF

With the aim of overcoming the effects of the presence of PTCs in CF, several drugs were studied, such as aminoglycoside antibiotics and PTC124 (PTC Therapeutics), and found to be able to incorporate a random amino acid at the PTC position of mRNAs. This induces a ribosomal read-through of the premature, but not of the natural termination codons, restoring CFTR function in CF patients [9-10]. These treatments may provide a means of restoring clinically relevant levels of protein function in patients carrying PTCs in the mutated gene, and introduce new hope for the development of a pharmacologic approach for the cure of several important genetic diseases, including CF [9-10].

2.1.1. *Aminoglycosides*

Aminoglycoside antibiotics selectively bind to ribosomes (at decoding aminoacyl site, A-site) and cause the insertion of a near cognate amino-acyl tRNA into this ribosomal A site, allowing ribosome read-through at PTC and production of a full-length protein [11].

Previous studies have shown that a variety of aminoglycosides are able to suppress CFTR nonsense mutations and restore functional CFTR protein levels not only in mouse models, but also in human clinical trials [1,12-16].

Gentamicin and amikacin are able to suppress the common G542X nonsense mutation in a transgenic CF mouse model, restoring approximately 20–30% of full-length CFTR protein, suggesting these compounds as read-through molecules to treat CF patients carrying PTCs [1]. In particular, the CFTR nonsense transgenic mouse model carrying a human CFTR cDNA with G542X nonsense mutation was used to screen the read-through activity of different aminoglycosides [1,12]. Five to thirty-four mg/kg of gentamicin was administered by daily subcutaneous injections for 14 days and found to induce a 22% increase of the wild-type CFTR function. Similar results were observed with amikacin, used at 15–170 mg/kg, while tobramycin was much less efficient than these two aminoglycosides in rescuing CFTR function [1,12,13].

In humans, Wilschanski et al. [1,14] reported a study where 0.9 mgs of gentamicin were administered daily via nasal drops for 14 days in nine CF patients. The data obtained demonstrated a significant improvement in chloride conductance by nasal potential difference (PD) measurements. Full-length CFTR protein was also detected in the nasal epithelia of treated CF patients. On the contrary, patients homozygous for the F508del mutation, used as a control group, did not show improvements in the CFTR function or restoration of CFTR protein [14].

Clancy et al. [15] reported a study where 2.5 mg/kg of gentamicin was administered intravenously every 8 hours for one week to 10 CF patients. They reported a three-fold increased incidence of nasal PD readings in the direction of chloride secretion in treated PTC subjects relative to CF controls. Airway chloride secretion was also stronger, with a high level of chloride secretion not detected in the control subjects, while sweat chloride measurements were not increased. In recent studies [1, 16], two different groups (11 CF patients with nonsense mutations and 18 CF patients without nonsense mutations) were treated with 3.6 mg of gentamicin or tobramycin daily by a nasal spray device for 28 days. The results indicated no improvement in chloride ion transport or CFTR localization using these two aminoglycosides. The authors underlined that nasally administered aminoglycosides did not produce detectable improvement in CFTR function because the CF subjects were heterozygous for different CFTR mutations [16]. This suggests that not all premature stop mutations are susceptible to the read-through treatment alone in order to ameliorate the phenotype of CF patients carrying nonsense mutations. When the read-through approach is combined with the use of potentiators/correctors of CFTR, however, the clinical outcome may be much more positive and this strategy could delineate a personalized therapeutic approach based on the CF genotype of patients [16].

A recent study using tobramycin was performed in yeast models with modulated NMD by UPF1 deletion [17]. Yeast strains were transformed with the Renilla/Firefly dual-luciferase reporter plasmids carrying either nonsense (UAG, UGA, UAA) or sense (CAG, CGA, CAA) codon between the luciferase genes. Tobramycin, a aminoglycoside antibiotic normally used to treat *Pseudomonas aeruginosa* pulmonary infection in CF patients, exhibited read-through ability on PTCs preferentially in the absence of NMD mechanism. These findings could be an explanation of the lower activity of tobramycin in restoring CFTR synthesis observed in mouse models and human clinical trials, while the data indicate possible combined treatment of tobramycin in the presence of NMD inhibitors.

Most of the novel aminoglycoside molecules have been synthetized with the major aim of optimizing their antibacterial activity, and not with the objective of obtaining the highest possible read-through action on PTCs. Current clinical studies investigating this class of molecules were performed using only commercially available aminoglycosides, such as gentamicin, amikacin, and tobramycin [14-18]. The general conclusion of these studies is that tobramycin presented a low efficiency as PTC suppressors, while gentamicin was efficient but toxic [14-18]. Alternative options to gentamicin could be amikacin [13] or paromomycin [19], two aminoglycosides with lower cellular toxicity, but not yet studied in human clinical trials as read-through molecules.

A future goal should be the design and synthesis of new aminoglycosides with high read-through activity and low toxicity. Baasov et al. [18] reported the synthesis of a series of new derivatives of paromomycin proposed as read-through molecules in vitro. In particular NB30, a pseudo-trisaccharide derivative, had higher read-through activity compared to paromomycin and gentamicin and reduced toxicity [20, 21]. Another derivate, NB124, presented a more efficient read-through activity than gentamycin. It restored full-length CFTR expression and chloride transport in Fischer rat thyroid cells stably transduced with a CFTR-G542XcDNA transgene and 7% of wild-type CFTR function in primary human bronchial epithelial CF cells with G542X/delF508 genotype [22].

These studies suggest that the reduction of the efficiency of translation termination, such as in the case of induction of ribosomal read-through, is a potential strategy for developing treatments of genetic diseases caused by PTCs. It is known that aminoglycosides cause toxic side effects that do not seem directly associated with their ability to suppress PTC. Monitoring the read-through efficiency of aminoglycosides with low toxic side effects is required and the synthesis of novel aminoglycoside derivatives exhibiting better parameters of administration to the patient, as well as availability and lower toxicity in vivo, is of interest to the research community.

2.1.2. PTC124

PTC124 (3-(5-(2-fluorophenyl)-1,2,4-oxadiazol-3-yl)-benzoic acid), also known as Ataluren, is a small non-aminoglycoside molecule that has been suggested to allow PTC read-through even though its target has yet to be identified [23]. It is an orally available and non-toxic small molecule, identified by HTS and is the first drug in its class. PTC124 appears to allow cellular machinery to read-through premature stop codons in mRNA, enabling the translation process to produce full-length, functional proteins [24]. In a transgenic mouse model carrying CFTR with nonsense mutations, 0.9 mg/ml of PTC124 was administered orally for 14–21 days. The results reported a partial CFTR expression at the apical surface of intestinal tissues and a restoration of normal CFTR function up to 24% with dose given in a liquid diet or 29% with at dose of 15–60 mg/kg daily by subcutaneous injections [1,25].

PTC124 was studied in two different Phase II human clinical trials with modest results in terms of efficacy [26-27]. In one study [26], PTC124 was orally administered to 23 CF patients carrying nonsense mutations. They were treated with 16 mg/kg daily of PTC124 for 14 days, then after 14 days without treatment, with a dose of 40 mg/kg daily for further 14 days. An improvement of chloride conductance was observed by nasal potential difference measurements after the two treatments, where approximately half of the patients showed measurements within the normal range [1,26]. Another Phase II trial was conducted with a similar treatment schedule for 12 weeks in 19 CF patients carrying nonsense mutations [27]. An increased nasal chloride transport in approximately 60% of treated patients was reported. CFTR function was restored more efficiently with increased time of treatment [1, 27]. PTC124 has also been examined in 30 pediatric CF patients with nonsense mutations [1, 28]. PTC124 was administered in two 14-day cycles as described earlier. Approximately 50% of the treated patients partially restored CFTR-mediated nasal epithelial chloride transport and full-length CFTR protein at the apical membrane of nasal epithelial cells, with only mild or no adverse effects.

Despite these successes in Phase II trials [11,27,28], PTC124 did not significantly improve the primary end-point in large Phase III clinical trials. A study [29], enrolling patients from 36 sites in 11 countries in North America and Europe, showed no improvement in the primary endpoint (forced expiratory volume in the first second, $FEV_1\%$) as predicted. It did however demonstrate conservation of lung function compared to placebo in a predefined subset of subjects who were not treated with the inhaled antibiotic tobramycin, known to influence the efficacy of PTC124 [29,30].

The development of novel small molecules having efficient read-through activity on PTCs and restoring CFTR function with low toxicity should be considered as a major issue in CF research. The CF read-through therapy clinical trials indicate that both gentamicin and PTC124 are able to restore CFTR protein in a fraction of CF patients with PTCs. Longer-term studies will be required to determine whether the therapeutic effects found in patients upon short-term treatment can be realized, and if sufficient CFTR can be rescued to reduce pathological respiratory aspects of CF [1]. The NMD inhibitors studied may lead to the discovery of biomolecules to be employed in combination with read-through correctors, in order to achieve clinically relevant results.

2.2. NMD inhibitors in CF

PTCs located >50–55 nucleotides upstream of an exon-exon junction can be minimized by NMD in order to detect and degrade mRNA containing PTC and minimize the negative consequences of nonsense mutations [5]. This should be carefully considered in the context of the development of read-through approach for restoring CFTR function. NMD is a cellular mechanism, aimed to detect and degrade PTC containing mRNA [31-34] and as part of an mRNA surveillance system, it has a crucial role in preventing accumulation of aberrant transcripts and their translation [32,34]. Down-modulation of NMD is an important therapeutic goal, in order to (a) maintain mRNA levels suitable for read-through correction and (b) restore sufficient full-length protein expression levels. The major molecular consequences of nonsense mutations are the promotion of premature translational termination and NMD. These two features are strictly associated.

The efficiency of restoration of correct translation using read-through molecules, with respect to modulation of NMD is still an unresolved problem. Differences in NMD efficiency of CFTR transcripts carrying the W1282X mutation among different epithelial cell lines have been reported [35], and in some CF cells the NMD of all transcripts was efficient and in others NMD was less efficient. Down regulation of NMD in cells carrying the W1282X mutation was reported to increase the level of CFTR nonsense transcripts and enhanced the CFTR chloride channel activity in response to gentamicin [9].

Data published to date indicate that the efficiency of PTC read-through is low [10], probably due to degradation of PTC-mRNA by NMD mechanism, depleting substrates available for read-through correction. Modulation of NMD, aimed to increase CFTR mRNA available to PTC read-through, could be another important therapeutic goal [9]. A possible strategy to modulate NMD mechanism may be based on novel molecules acting as NMD inhibitors. These molecules should not affect physiological substrates of NMD mechanism.

Recently Wang et al. [36] have demonstrated that a modest depletion (80% of the activity of untreated cells) of UPF1 or UPF2 through shRNA could suppress NMD activity without affecting the proliferation or survival of cells. This suggests that pharmacologic NMD inhibition could be proposed as a therapeutic approach with limited toxicity or side effects. In particular, the same group identified NMD inhibitors (called NMDIs) acting against targeting SMG7-UPF1 complex obtained from a virtual library screening, with various chemical backbones and acting at nanomolar concentration [37]. It was demonstrated that the combination of a read-through drug and NMDIs increased protein expression and relative biological functions of a PTC-mutated p53. These novel data are promising, as previous pharmacologic inhibitors, useful in investigating the NMD mechanism, have been found to be toxic, did not synergize with read-through molecules and had an unknown mechanism of action [38,39].

Amlexanox, a drug used for over 30 years orally or topically to treat asthma and aphthous ulcers [40,41], has also been identified [42] as a potent NMD inhibitor. Amlexanox is not citotoxic, does not inhibit general translation, and does not affect natural NMD substrate expression. This drug presents a dual activity of interest in CF research, that is, induction of an increased level of PTC mRNA, and induction of efficient expression of full-length and functional CFTR protein. The novelty of amlexanox is the ability to both inhibit NMD and facilitate PTC read-through, in contrast to other read-through molecules that present only read-through activity strongly influenced by the identity of the PTC and its nucleotide environment [43]. Amlexanox in combination with PTC124 induces an increase of CFTR channel activity in cells with heterozygous genotype for nonsense mutations [43].

The clinical use of these molecules may be possible after further studies relative to the short- and long-term effects of potent NMD inhibition as the combination of a read-through approach with pharmacologic NMD inhibition is an appealing therapeutic strategy for CF patients carrying nonsense mutations.

2.3. Treatment of CF heterozygous patients for nonsense mutations

Clancy's group [16] nasally administered aminoglycosides did not produce detectable changes in CFTR function in subjects heterozygous for a variety of stop codon mutations within CFTR, suggesting the need to perform a combined therapy based on the most potent suppressors of nonsense mutations co-delivered with CFTR potentiators and/or correctors [16]. Many CF patients heterozygous for premature stop mutations carry a genotype with F508del. Initial results of a Phase II trial of VX-809, a lead F508del CFTR corrector developed by Vertex Pharmaceuticals (Cambridge, Massachusetts, USA), established that systemic administration of the compound for 4 weeks modestly improved sweat chloride at the highest dose tested compared with placebo [44]. VX-809 is reported to normalize the gating of corrected F508del-CFTR but has no direct potentiating action suggesting that one straightforward approach could be the co-administration with a potentiator of CFTR channel gating [11,44,45]. If CF patients have nonsense mutations together with F508del, a cocktail of potentiators of CFTR channel gating, CFTR correctors, and read-through molecules could be proposed as a therapeutic strategy.

Xue X et al. [22] reported a novel synthetic aminoglycoside based on NB124 that efficiently restored CFTR function in primary human bronchial epithelial (HBE) CF cells carrying PTC (G542X/delF508). The efficacy of NB124 was further enhanced by addition of the oral CFTR potentiator Ivacaftor (VX-770) to airway cells expressing CFTR PTCs [22]. Ivacaftor exhibited excellent activity and pharmacokinetic properties, providing the opportunity to treat the underlying cause of CF in combination with CFTR correctors and read-through molecules, depending on the CFTR mutations [46].

Many new compounds are expected to be proposed in the future for the potentiation and correction of CFTR. One example is 4,6,4'-trimethylangelicin (TMA), a psoralen-related compound, which obtained the orphan drug designation from the EMA and is already in clinical use for psoriasis. Tamanini et al. [47] demonstrated that TMA, at nanomolar concentrations, inhibited the expression of the IL-8 gene in bronchial epithelial cells in which the inflammatory response has been challenged with *P. aeruginosa*. The acute addition (15 minutes treatment) of 250 nM TMA potentiated FSK-stimulated chloride secretion in airway cell monolayers expressing wild type CFTR or in CF cells in which F508del CFTR was already rescued to the apical membrane by overexpressing the interacting protein NHERF1. More recently, the same group [48] found that long pre-incubation with nanomolar concentrations of TMA was able to effectively restore both F508del CFTR-dependent chloride secretion and F508del CFTR cell surface expression in both primary or secondary airway cell monolayers homozygous for F508del mutation. These results indicate that TMA, besides its anti-inflammatory and potentiator activities, also displays corrector properties, suggesting that this compound (or more effective analogues) could be a potential candidate for combination therapies with read-through molecules.

Other CFTR potentiator and/or corrector molecules with different mechanisms of action have been recently reported in literature [11]. These include the cyanoquinoline CoPo-22 [49], the inhibitor Hsp90 co-chaperone Aha1 [50], phosphodiesterase type V (PDE5) inhibitors [51-53], the isoflavones genistein, and curcumin [54]. Additional studies concerning their mechanism of action and toxicity are required before clinical testing, and combination with read-through molecules can be considered.

3. Conclusions

More than 1,900 different CFTR mutations have been reported in CF patients, 10% being nonsense mutations and 75% represented by the most frequent CF F508del mutation [1,11]. In order to ameliorate the CF phenotype, restoration of at least 5–35% of normal CFTR function is required [2-4]. Several CFTR modulator therapies have been investigated in vitro and in late phase clinical trials, including CFTR potentiators, correctors, and PTC read-through molecules [1,2-5,9-16,21-30,37-39,42,45]. To achieve substantial clinical benefit in CF, a combined administration of two correctors with synergistic action [55,56] or a corrector with a potentiator that counteracts distinct conformational defects in trafficking and activation of F508del CFTR [57, 58] are required.

Current open clinical trials, excluding studies with unknown status, are being conducted on Ivacaftor and PTC124 (Table 2).

Ivacaftor alone is not sufficient to efficiently alter CFTR activity in patients with CF homozygous for F508del [59]. The difficulty in achieving higher levels of correction is due to the fact that the F508del mutation induces multiple conformational defects in the mutant protein.

In current clinical trials (Table 2) Ivacaftor is being tested in combination with CFTR correctors such as Lumacaftor (VX-809, Vertex Pharmaceuticals, Cambridge, Massachusetts, USA) and VX-661 (Vertex Pharmaceuticals) in order to correct the protein misfolding and increase the CFTR localization to the cell surface.

VX-809 is selective for F508del CFTR and enhances chloride secretion to 15% of that found in non-CF human bronchial cells [45,48,55]. Preclinical research [45,60] and known effects of the F508 deletion on gating in addition to cellular processing [56-58] support the combination strategy of VX-809 (or VX-661, an alternate CFTR corrector to VX-809) with Ivacaftor in current human clinical trials (Table 2).

Alternatively, dual-acting molecules (such as TMA [47,48], aminoarylthiazole [61], and cyanoquinoline [49,62] derivatives) that both correct F508del CFTR and potentiate the F508del CFTR-dependent chloride permeability has been proposed, avoiding multiple combined administration.

Molecule	Title of Study	ClinicalTrials.gov Identifier
Ivacaftor(VX770; Kalydeco)	Ivacaftor (Kalydeco) and Insulin in Cystic Fibrosis (CF)	NCT02039986
	Short Term Effects of Ivacaftor in Non-G551D Cystic Fibrosis Patients	NCT01784419
	Ivacaftor in French Patients with Cystic Fibrosis and a G551D Mutation (IVACAFTOR1)	NCT02194881
	A Phase 3 Study to Evaluate the Efficacy and Safety of Ivacaftor and VX-661 in Combination with Ivacaftor in Subjects Aged 12 Years and Older with Cystic Fibrosis, Heterozygous for the F508del-CFTR Mutation	NCT02392234
	A Phase 3 Study of VX-661 in Combination with Ivacaftor in Subjects Aged 12 Years and Older with Cystic Fibrosis, Who Have One F508del-CFTR Mutation and a Second Mutation that Has Been Demonstrated to Be Clinically Responsive to Ivacaftor	NCT02412111
	Study to Evaluate Lumacaftor and Ivacaftor Combination Therapy in Subjects 12 Years and Older with Advanced Lung Disease (Phase III)	NCT02390219
	Airway Infection, Inflammatory Markers and Exercise Capacity in Patients with Cystic Fibrosis and at Least One G551D Mutation Taking VX-770 (Ivacaftor) (Phase IV)	NCT01937325
	A Randomized, Double-Blind, Placebo-Controlled, Parallel-Group Study to Evaluate the Efficacy and Safety of VX-661 in Combination with Ivacaftor (Phase III)	NCT02347657
	(Study: Vertex IIS) Does Ivacaftor Alter Wild Type CFTR-Open Probability in the Sweat Gland Secretory Coil?	NCT02310789
Ataluren(PTC124)	Study of Ataluren in Nonsense Mutation Cystic Fibrosis (ACT CF), Phase III	NCT02139306
N91115	Study of N91115 in Patients with Cystic Fibrosis Homozygous F508del-CFTR Mutation (SNO4) (Phase I)	NCT02275936
Glycerol Phenylbutyrate	Glycerol Phenylbutyrate Corrector Therapy For CF (GPBA)	NCT02323100
FDL169	FTIH – Single and Repeat Oral Doses of FDL169 in Healthy Volunteers (Phase I)	NCT02359357

Table 2. Current open clinical trials on CFTR modulators (source ClinicalTrials.gov).

Other ongoing human clinical trials are investigating novel CFTR modulators on F508del such as N91115, glycerol phenylbutyrate, FDL169 (Table 2). N91115 is currently in Phase I. In next Phase II this molecule will be studied in addition to Lumacaftor/Ivacaftor.

The combination of CFTR potentiators and correctors could result in effective therapies in a large proportion of patients with CF (Table 2).

Other CFTR modulator classes include molecules with read-through activity, such as PTC124 currently in Phase III clinical study. Based on efficacy in vitro and in animal models [10,25,63], PTC124 was studied in a series of conflicting Phase II trials [26-28,63]. A long-term study has demonstrated no improvement in FEV1 % predicted, the primary endpoint. Conversely a small effect on lung function was demonstrated in a predefined subset of individuals untreated with inhaled antibiotics that can modify the efficiency of PTC124 [29,63]. So further clinical studies for this compound should be necessary to demonstrate its activity in CF as read-through therapeutic approach also in combination with NMD inhibitors or potentiators/correctors as reported in studies in vitro [22,43].

Results to date suggest, in the case of nonsense mutations, efficient and therapeutic restoration of a functional CFTR channel may be possible drugs administered in combination.

In conclusion, it is essential to stratify CF patients with the aim of creating a personalized therapy based on the use of a combination of drugs targeted at specific classes of mutations. This approach represents an appealing therapeutic strategy and should be the subject of further investigation.

Acknowledgements

This work was supported by contributions from Fondazione Cariparo (Cassa di Risparmio di Padova e Rovigo) to RG, Italian Cystic Fibrosis Research Foundation (FFC#2/2010 and FFC#1/2012) to M.B and (FFC#17/2010 and FFC#8/2014) to RG.

Our thanks to Dr. Amanda J Neville MSB for her comments and corrections of the English text.

Author details

Roberto Gambari[1,2], Giulia Breveglieri[1,2], Francesca Salvatori[1,2], Alessia Finotti[1] and Monica Borgatti[1*]

*Address all correspondence to: monica.borgatti@unife.it

1 Department of Life Sciences and Biotechnology, Biochemistry and Molecular Biology Section, University of Ferrara, Ferrara, Italy

2 Biotechnology Center, University of Ferrara, Ferrara, Italy

References

[1] Keeling KM, Wang D, Conard SE, Bedwell DM. Suppression of premature termination codons as a therapeutic approach. Critical Reviews in Biochemistry and Molecular Biology. 2012;47:444-463. DOI: 10.3109/10409238.2012.694846.

[2] Kerem E. Pharmacologic therapy for stop mutations: how much CFTR activity is enough? Current Opinion in Pulmonary Medicine. 2004;10:547-552.

[3] Zhang L, Button B, Gabriel SE, Burkett S, Yan Y, Skiadopoulos MH, Dang Yl, Vogel LN, Mckay T, Mengos A, Boucher RC, Collins PL, Pickles RJ. CFTR delivery to 25% of surface epithelial cells restores normal rates of mucus transport to human cystic fibrosis airway epithelium. PLoS Biology. 2009;7:e1000155. DOI: 10.1371/journal.pbio.1000155.

[4] Amaral MD. Processing of CFTR: traversing the cellular maze--how much CFTR needs to go through to avoid cystic fibrosis? Pediatric Pulmonology. 2005;39:479-491.

[5] Linde L, Kerem B. Introducing sense into nonsense in treatments of human genetic diseases. Trends Genetics. 2008;24:552-563. DOI: 10.1016/j.tig.2008.08.010.

[6] Bobadilla JL, Macek M Jr, Fine JP, Farrell PM. Cystic fibrosis: a worldwide analysis of CFTR mutations--correlation with incidence data and application to screening. Human Mutation. 2002;19:575-606.

[7] Nicholson P, Yepiskoposyan H, Metze S, Zamudio Orozco R, Kleinschmidt N, Mühlemann O. Nonsense-mediated mRNA decay in human cell: mechanistic insights, functions beyond quality control and double-life of NMD factors. Cellular and Molecular Life Sciences 2010;67:677-700. DOI: 10.1007/s00018-009-0177-1.

[8] Behm-Ansmant I, Kashima I, Rehwinkel J, Saulière J, Wittkop N, Izaurralde E. mRNA quality control: an ancient machinery recognizes and degrades mRNAs with nonsense codons. FEBS Letters. 2007;58:2845-2853.

[9] Linde L, Boelz S, Nissim-Rafinia M, Oren YS, Wilschanski M, Yaacov Y, Virgilis D, Neu-Yilik G, Kulozik AE, Kerem E, Kerem B. Nonsense-mediated mRNA decay affects nonsense transcript levels and governs response of cystic fibrosis patients to gentamicin. The Journal of Clinical Investigation. 2007;1173:683-692.

[10] Welch EM, Barton ER, Zhuo J, Tomizawa Y, Friesen WJ, Trifillis P, Paushkin S, Patel M, Trotta CR, Hwang S, Wilde RG, Karp G, Takasugi J, Chen G, Jones S, Ren H, Moon YC, Corson D, Turpoff AA, Campbell JA, Conn MM, Khan A, Almstead NG, Hedrick J, Mollin A, Risher N, Weetall M, Yeh S, Branstrom AA, Colacino JM, Babiak J, Ju WD, Hirawat S, Northcutt VJ, Miller LL, Spatrick P, He F, Kawana M, Feng H, Jacobson A, Peltz SW, Sweeney HL. PTC124 targets genetic disorders caused by nonsense mutations. Nature. 2007;447:87-91.

[11] Ikpa PT, Bijvelds MJ, de Jonge HR. Cystic fibrosis: toward personalized therapies. The International Journal of Biochemistry & Cell Biology. 2014;52:192-200. DOI: 10.1016/j.biocel.2014.02.008.

[12] Du M, Jones JR, Lanier J, Keeling KM, Lindsey JR, Tousson A, Bebok Z, Whitsett JA, Dey CR, Colledge WH, Evans MJ, Sorscher EJ, Bedwell DM. Aminoglycoside suppression of a premature stop mutation in a Cftr-/- mouse carrying a human CFTR-G542X transgene. Journal of Molecular Medicine. 2002;80:595-604.

[13] Du M, Keeling KM, Fan L, Liu X, Kovacs T, Sorscher E, Bedwell DM. Clinical doses of amikacin provide more effective suppression of the human CFTR-G542X stop mutation than gentamicin in a transgenic CF mouse model. Journal of Molecular Medicine. 2006;84:573-582.

[14] Wilschanski M, Yahav Y, Yaacov Y, Blau H, Bentur L, Rivlin J, Aviram M, Bdolah-Abram T, Bebok Z, Shushi L, Kerem B, Kerem E. Gentamicin-induced correction of CFTR function in patients with cystic fibrosis and CFTR stop mutations. The New England Journal Medicine. 2003;349:1433-1441.

[15] Clancy JP, Bebok Z, Ruiz F, King C, Jones J, Walker L, Greer H, Hong J, Wing L, Macaluso M, Lyrene R, Sorscher EJ, Bedwell DM. Evidence that systemic gentamicin suppresses premature stop mutations in patients with cystic fibrosis. American Journal Respiratory and Critical Care Medicine. 2001;163:1683-1692.

[16] Clancy JP, Rowe SM, Bebok Z, Aitken ML, Gibson R, Zeitlin P, Berclaz P, Moss R, Knowles MR, Oster RA, Mayer-Hamblett N, Ramsey B. No detectable improvements in cystic fibrosis transmembrane conductance regulator by nasal aminoglycosides in patients with cystic fibrosis with stop mutations. American Journal of Respiratory Cell and Molecular Biology. 2007;37:57-66.

[17] Altamura N, Castaldo R, Finotti A, Breveglieri G, Salvatori F, Zuccato C, Gambari R, Panin GC, Borgatti M. Tobramycin is a suppressor of premature termination codons. Journal of Cystic Fibrosis. 2013;12:806-811. DOI: 10.1016/j.jcf.2013.02.007.

[18] Hainrichson M, Nudelman I, Baasov T. Designer aminoglycosides: the race to develop improved antibiotics and compounds for the treatment of human genetic diseases. Organic & Biomolecular Chemistry. 2008;6:227-239. DOI: 10.1039/b712690p.

[19] Howard MT, Anderson CB, Fass U, Khatri S, Gesteland RF, Atkins JF, Flanigan KM. Readthrough of dystrophin stop codon mutations induced by aminoglycosides. Annals of Neurology. 2004;55:422-426.

[20] Nudelman I, Rebibo-Sabbah A, Shallom-Shezifi D, Hainrichson M, Stahl I, Ben-Yosef T, Baasov T. Redesign of aminoglycosides for treatment of human genetic diseases caused by premature stop mutations. Bioorganic & Medicinal Chemistry Letters. 2006;16:6310-6315.

[21] Rebibo-Sabbah A, Nudelman I, Ahmed ZM, Baasov T, Ben-Yosef T. In vitro and ex vivo suppression by aminoglycosides of PCDH15 nonsense mutations underlying type 1 Usher syndrome. Human Genetics. 2007;122:373-381.

[22] Xue X, Mutyam V, Tang L, Biswas S, Du M, Jackson LA, Dai Y, Belakhov V, Shalev M, Chen F, Schacht J, J Bridges R, Baasov T, Hong J, Bedwell DM, Rowe SM. Synthetic aminoglycosides efficiently suppress cystic fibrosis transmembrane conductance regulator nonsense mutations and are enhanced by ivacaftor. American Journal of Respiratory Cell and Molecular Biology. 2014;50:805-816. DOI: 10.1165/rcmb.2013-0282OC.

[23] Lentini L, Melfi R, Di Leonardo A, Spinello A, Barone G, Pace A, Palumbo Piccionello A, Pibiri I. Toward a rationale for the PTC124 (Ataluren) promoted readthrough of premature stop codons: a computational approach and GFP-reporter cell-based assay. Molecular Pharmaceutics. 2014;11:653-664. DOI: 10.1021/mp400230s.

[24] Ryan NJ. Ataluren: first global approval. Drugs. 2014;74:1709-1714. DOI: 10.1007/s40265-014-0287-4.

[25] Du M, Liu X, Welch EM, Hirawat S, Peltz SW, Bedwell DM. PTC124 is an orally bioavailable compound that promotes suppression of the human CFTR-G542X nonsense allele in a CF mouse model. Proceedings of the National Academy of Sciences of the United States of America. 2008;105:2064-2069. DOI: 10.1073/pnas.0711795105.

[26] Kerem E, Hirawat S, Armoni S, Yaakov Y, Shoseyov D, Cohen M, Nissimrafinia M, Blau H, Rivlin J, Aviram M, Elfring GL, Northcutt VJ, Miller LL, Kerem B, Wilschanski M. Effectiveness of PTC124 treatment of cystic fibrosis caused by nonsense mutations: a prospective phase II trial. Lancet. 2008;372:719-727. DOI: 10.1016/S0140-6736(08)61168-X.

[27] Wilschanski M, Miller LL, Shoseyov D, Blau H, Rivlin J, Aviram M, Cohen M, Armoni S, Yaakov Y, Pugatch T, Cohen-Cymberknoh M, Miller NL, Reha A, Northcutt VJ, Hirawat S, Donnelly K, Elfring GL, Ajayi T, Kerem E. Chronic ataluren (PTC124) treatment of nonsense mutation cystic fibrosis. The European Respiratory Journal. 2011;38:59-69. DOI: 10.1183/09031936.00120910.

[28] Sermet-Gaudelus I, Boeck KD, Casimir GJ, Vermeulen F, Leal T, Mogenet A, Roussel D, Fritsch J, Hanssens L, Hirawat S, Miller NL, Constantine S, Reha A, Ajayi T, Elfring GL, Miller LL. Ataluren (PTC124) induces cystic fibrosis transmembrane conductance regulator protein expression and activity in children with nonsense mutation cystic fibrosis. American Journal Respiratory and Critical Care Medicine 2010;182:1262-1272. DOI: 10.1164/Rccm.201001-0137oc.

[29] Kerem E, Konstan MW, De Boeck K, Accurso FJ, Sermet-Gaudelus I, Wilschanski M, Elborn JS, Melotti P, Bronsveld I, Fajac I, Malfroot A, Rosenbluth DB, Walker PA, McColley SA, Knoop C, Quattrucci S, Rietschel E, Zeitlin PL, Barth J, Elfring GL, Welch EM, Branstrom A, Spiegel RJ, Peltz SW, Ajayi T, Rowe SM. Cystic Fibrosis Ataluren Study Group. Ataluren for the treatment of nonsense-mutation cystic fibro-

sis: a randomised, double-blind, placebo-controlled phase 3 trial. The Lancet Respiratory Medicine. 2014; 2:539-547. DOI: 10.1016/S2213-2600(14)70100-6.

[30] Bell SC, De Boeck K, Amaral MD. New pharmacological approaches for cystic fibrosis: promises, progress, pitfalls. Pharmacology & Therapeutics. 2015;145:19-34. DOI: 10.1016/j.pharmthera.2014.06.005.

[31] Bhuvanagiri M, Schlitter AM, Hentze MW et al. NMD: RNA biology meets human genetic medicine. The Biochemical Journal. 2010;430:365-377. DOI: 10.1042/BJ20100699.

[32] Khajavi M, Inoue K, Lupski JR. Nonsense-mediated mRNA decay modulates clinical outcome of genetic disease. European Journal of Human Genetics 2006;14:1074-1081.

[33] Nicholson P, Yepiskoposyan H, Metze S, Zamudio Orozco R, Kleinschmidt N, Mühlemann O. Nonsense-mediated mRNA decay in human cells: mechanistic insights, functions beyond quality control and the double-life of NMD factors. Cellular and Molecular Life Sciences. 2010;67:677-700. DOI: 10.1007/s00018-009-0177-1.

[34] Stalder L, Muhlemann O. The meaning of nonsense. Trends in Cell Biology 2008;18:315-321. DOI: 10.1016/j.tcb.2008.04.005.

[35] Linde L, Boelz S, Neu-Yilik G, Kulozik AE, Kerem B. The efficiency of nonsense-mediated mRNA decay is an inherent character and varies among different cells. European Journal of Human Genetics. 2007;15:1156-1162.

[36] Wang D, Zavadil J, Martin L, Parisi F, Friedman E, Levy D, Harding H, Ron D, Gardner LB. Inhibition of nonsense-mediated RNA decay by the tumor microenvironment promotes tumorigenesis. Molecular and Cellular Biology 2011;31:3670-3680. DOI: 10.1128/MCB.05704-11.

[37] Martin L, Grigoryan A, Wang D, Wang J, Breda L(1), Rivella S, Cardozo T, Gardner LB. Identification and characterization of small molecules that inhibit nonsense-mediated RNA decay and suppress nonsense p53 mutations. Cancer Research. 2014;74:3104-3113. DOI: 10.1158/0008-5472.CAN-13-2235.

[38] Keeling KM, Wang D, Dai Y, Murugesan S, Chenna B, Clark J, Belakhov V, Kandasamy J, Velu SE, Baasov T, Bedwell DM. Attenuation of nonsense-mediated mRNA decay enhances in vivo nonsense suppression. PLoS ONE 2013;8:e60478. DOI: 10.1371/journal.pone.0060478.

[39] Durand S, Cougot N, Mahuteau-Betzer F, Nguyen CH, Grierson DS, Bertrand E, Tazi J, Lejeune F. Inhibition of nonsense-mediated mRNA decay (NMD) by a new chemical molecule reveals the dynamic of NMD factors in P-bodies. The Journal of Cell Biology 2007;178:1145-1160.

[40] Saijo T, Kuriki H, Ashida Y, Makino H, Maki Y. Mechanism of the action of amoxanox (AA-673), an orally active antiallergic agent. International Archives of Allergy and Applied Immunology 1985;78:43-50.

[41] Meng W, Dong Y, Liu J, Wang Z, Zhong X, Chen R, Zhou H, Lin M, Jiang L, Gao F, Xu T, Chen Q, Zeng X. A clinical evaluation of amlexanox oral adhesive pellicles in the treatment of recurrent aphthous stomatitis and comparison with amlexanox oral tablets: a randomized, placebo controlled, blinded, multicenter clinical trial. Trials 2009;10:30. DOI: 10.1186/1745-6215-10-30.

[42] Gonzalez-Hilarion S, Beghyn T, Jia J, Debreuck N, Berte G, Mamchaoui K, Mouly V, Gruenert DC, Déprez B, Lejeune F. Rescue of nonsense mutations by amlexanox in human cells. Orphanet Journal of Rare Diseases 2012;7:58. DOI: 10.1186/1750-1172-7-58.

[43] Bidou L, Hatin I, Perez N, Allamand V, Panthier JJ, Rousset JP. Premature stop codons involved in muscular dystrophies show a broad spectrum of readthrough efficiencies in response to gentamicin treatment. Gene Therapy. 2004;11:619-627.

[44] Sloane PA, Rowe SM. Cystic fibrosis transmembrane conductance regulator protein repair as a therapeutic strategy in cystic fibrosis. Current Opinion in Pulmonary Medicine. 2010;16:591-597. DOI: 10.1097/MCP.0b013e32833f1d00.

[45] Van Goor F, Hadida S, Grootenhuis PD, Burton B, Stack JH, Straley KS, Decker CJ, Miller M, McCartney J, Olson ER, Wine JJ, Frizzell RA, Ashlock M, Negulescu PA. Correction of the F508del-CFTR protein processing defect in vitro by the investigationaldrug VX-809. Proceedings of the National Academy of Sciences of the United States of America. 2011;108:18843–18848. DOI: 10.1073/pnas.1105787108.

[46] Hadida S, Van Goor F, Zhou J, Arumugam V, McCartney J, Hazlewood A, Decker C, Negulescu P, Grootenhuis PD. Discovery of N-(2,4-di-tert-butyl-5-hydroxyphenyl)-4-oxo-1,4-dihydroquinoline-3-carboxamide (VX-770, ivacaftor), a potent and orally bioavailable CFTR potentiator. Journal of Medicinal Chemistry. 2014;57:9776-9795. DOI: 10.1021/jm5012808.

[47] Tamanini A, Borgatti M, Finotti A, Piccagli L, Bezzerri V, Favia M, Guerra L, Lampronti I, Bianchi N, Dall'Acqua F, Vedaldi D, Salvador A, Fabbri E, Mancini I, Nicolis E, Casavola V, Cabrini G, Gambari R. Trimethylangelicin reduces IL-8 transcription and potentiates CFTR function. American Journal of Physiology. Lung Cellular and Molecular Physiology. 2011;300:L380-90. DOI: 10.1152/ajplung.00129.2010.

[48] Favia M, Mancini MT, Bezzerri V, Guerra L, Laselva O, Abbattiscianni AC, Debellis L, Reshkin SJ, Gambari R, Cabrini G, Casavola V. Trimethylangelicin promotes the functional rescue of mutant F508del CFTR protein in cystic fibrosis airway cells. American Journal of Physiology. Lung Cellular and Molecular Physiology. 2014;307:L48-61. DOI: 10.1152/ajplung.00305.2013.

[49] Phuan PW, Yang B, Knapp JM, Wood AB, Lukacs GL, Kurth MJ, Verkman AS. Cyanoquinolines with independent corrector and potentiator activities restore DeltaPhe508-cystic fibrosis transmembrane conductance regulator chloride channel

function in cystic fibrosis. Molecular Pharmacology. 2011;80:683-693. DOI: 10.1124/mol.111.073056.

[50] Koulov AV, LaPointe P, Lu B, Razvi A, Coppinger J, Dong MQ, Matteson J, Laister R, Arrowsmith C, Yates JR 3rd, Balch WE. Biological and structural basis for Aha1 regulation of Hsp90 ATPase activity in maintaining proteostasis in the human disease cystic fibrosis. Molecular Biology of the Cell. 2010;21:871-884. DOI: 10.1091/mbc.E09-12-1017.

[51] Dhooghe B, Noel S, Bouzin C, Behets-Wydemans G, Leal T. Correction of chloride transport and mislocalization of CFTR protein by vardenafil in the gastrointestinal tract of cystic fibrosis mice. PLoS One. 2013;8:e77314. DOI: 10.1371/journal.pone.0077314.

[52] Leier G, Bangel-Ruland N, Sobczak K, Knieper Y, Weber WM. Sildenafil acts as potentiator and corrector of CFTR but might be not suitable for the treatment of CF lung disease. Cellular Physiology and Biochemistry: International Journal of Experimental Cellular Physiology, Biochemistry, and Pharmacology. 2012;29:775-790. DOI: 10.1159/000265129.

[53] Noel S, Dhooghe B, Leal T. PDE5 inhibitors as potential tools in the treatment of cystic fibrosis. Frontiers in Pharmacology 2012;3:167.

[54] Sohma Y, Yu YC, Hwang TC. Curcumin and genistein: the combined effects on disease-associated CFTR mutants and their clinical implications. Current Pharmaceutical Design. 2013;19:3521-3528.

[55] Ren HY, Grove DE, De La Rosa O, Houck SA, Sopha P, Van Goor F, Hoffman BJ, Cyr DM. VX-809 corrects folding defects in cystic fibrosis transmembrane conductance regulator protein through action on membrane-spanning domain 1. Molecular Biology of the Cell. 2013;24:3016-3024. DOI: 10.1091/mbc.E13-05-0240.

[56] Holleran JP, Glover ML, Peters KW, Bertrand CA, Watkins SC, Jarvik JW, Frizzell RA. Pharmacological rescue of the mutant cystic fibrosis transmembrane conductance regulator (CFTR) detected by use of a novel fluorescence platform. Molecular Medicine. 2012;18: 685-696. DOI: 10.2119/molmed.2012.00001.

[57] Okiyoneda T, Veit G, Dekkers JF, Bagdany M, Soya N, Xu H, Roldan A, Verkman AS, Kurth M, Simon A, Hegedus T, Beekman JM, Lukacs GL. Mechanism-based corrector combination restores DeltaF508- CFTR folding and function. Nature Chemical Biology. 2013;9:444-454. DOI: 10.1038/nchembio.1253.

[58] Verkman AS, Galietta LJ. Chloride channels as drug targets. Nature Reviews. Drug Discovery. 2009;8:153-171. DOI: 10.1038/nrd2780.

[59] Flume PA, Liou TG, Borowitz DS, Li H, Yen K, Ordoñez CL, Geller DE. VX 08-770-104 Study Group. Ivacaftor in subjects with cystic fibrosis who are homozygous for the F508del-CFTR mutation. Chest. 2012;142:718-724.

[60] Van Goor F, Hadida S, Grootenhuis PD, Burton B, Cao D, Neuberger T, Turnbull A, Singh A, Joubran J, Hazlewood A, Zhou J, McCartney J, Arumugam V, Decker C, Yang J, Young C, Olson ER, Wine JJ, Frizzell RA, Ashlock M, Negulescu P. Rescue of CF airway epithelial cell function in vitro by a CFTR potentiator, VX-770. Proceedings of the National Academy of Sciences of the United States of America. 2009;106:18825-18830. DOI: 10.1073/pnas.0904709106.

[61] Pedemonte N, Tomati V, Sondo E, Caci E, Millo E, Armirotti A, Damonte G, Zegarra-Moran O, Galietta LJ. Dual activity of aminoarylthiazoles on the trafficking and gating defects of the cystic fibrosis transmembrane conductance regulator chloride channel caused by cystic fibrosis mutations. The Journal of Biological Chemistry. 2011;286:15215-15226. DOI: 10.1074/jbc.M110.184267.

[62] Knapp JM, Wood AB, Phuan PW, Lodewyk MW, Tantillo DJ, Verkman AS, Kurth MJ. Structure-activity relationships of cyanoquinolines with corrector-potentiator activity in ΔF508 cystic fibrosis transmembrane conductance regulator protein. Journal of Medicinal Chemistry. 2012;55:1242-1251. DOI: 10.1021/jm201372q.

[63] Rowe SM, Borowitz DS, Burns JL, Clancy JP, Donaldson SH, Retsch-Bogart G, Sagel SD, Ramsey BW. Progress in cystic fibrosis and the CF Therapeutics Development Network. Thorax. 2012;67:882-890. DOI: 10.1136/thoraxjnl-2012-202550.

10

Cystic Fibrosis Related Diabetes

Paula Dyce, Gareth Huw Jones and
Martin J Walshaw

Abstract

Cystic fibrosis related diabetes (CFRD) is a common co-morbidity of cystic fibrosis. It is associated with diminishing lung function, poorer nutritional state, and a worse prognosis and its early diagnosis and treatment is important. In addition, the adverse pulmonary effects of CFRD may be present for up to 10 years prior to diagnosis.

Prevalence increases with age from 1 to 2% below 10 years of age, 20% of adolescents and 40-50% by adulthood, and up to 90% of adults with CF will have some degree of glucose intolerance by 40 years of age.

Although its pathophysiology is not well understood, the primary cause is thought to be the fatty infiltration of the pancreas leading to fibrosis and destruction of the pancreatic cells resulting in beta cell destruction and progressive insulin deficiency.

Oral glucose tolerance testing (OGTT) remains the method of choice for a diagnosis of type I, type II and gestational diabetes; it is less discriminating in CFRD where early glucose trends are important, and continuous glucose monitoring may prove a more useful diagnostic and management tool.

Diabetic complications occur in CFRD and annual screening for these is necessary. As life expectancy rises, diabetic complications may become more prevalent.

This chapter discusses the diagnosis and treatment of CFRD and touches on developments in research which will enhance the future management of this increasingly common and important manifestation of the CF condition.

Keywords: Cystic fibrosis related diabetes, Screening, Oral glucose tolerance testing, Continuous glucose monitoring, Cystic Fibrosis Related Diabetes

1. Introduction

Cystic Fibrosis Related Diabetes (CFRD) is a form of abnormal glucose handling (dysglycaemia) that is quite different to other forms of diabetes. It is uncommon in childhood, rarely occurring in those under 10 years of age, but its incidence rises inexorably as patients survive longer, affecting up to 50% of CF adults [1, 2].

The development of CFRD is associated with a significantly higher mortality rate [2, 3, 4], and has a deleterious impact on pulmonary function [5] with the degree of glucose intolerance being directly related to the decline in FEV1 [6]. Those with CFRD suffer more frequent infective exacerbations and have a higher burden of colonisation with pathogens such as *Pseudomonas aeruginosa* and *Burkholderia cepacia* as well as a poorer nutritional status – all of which are known to be associated with poorer outcomes [7].

However, dysglycaemia is a progressive phenomenon in many CF patients, and the associated increased morbidity occurs many years prior to a formal diagnosis of CFRD [8, 9, 10]. This has fuelled the debate as to how the diagnosis should be made – the current "gold standard" diagnostic test for diabetes mellitus (the oral glucose tolerance test, OGTT) [11] may not be appropriate in the CF population, since the optimal time to introduce treatment (currently limited exclusively to insulin-based therapies) may be at an earlier stage of dysglycaemia.

We will explore these issues as well as consider future developments in this emerging area of CF care.

2. Epidemiology, prevalence and incidence

Historically, CFRD was typically only seen in paediatric practice as a pre-terminal complication in those with advanced respiratory failure. It remains relatively rare in children under the age of 10 (2), affects less than 5% of individuals during their early teen years, but the incidence rises exponentially with age, occurring in approximately 20% of adolescents and up to 50% of individuals in their fourth decade. The average age of onset for CFRD is 18-21 years (12).

Furthermore, it is estimated that 70-90% of all adult CF patients will have some degree of glucose intolerance and therefore dysglycaemia is the commonest co-morbidity that complicates care in adult CF and its prevalence is likely to increase further as life expectancy continues to rise.

In addition to age, other factors associated with an increased incidence of CFRD are severity of CFTR mutation, poor pulmonary function, low BMI, pancreatic insufficiency, liver dysfunction, and corticosteroid use (5, 7, 13, 14).

3. Pathophysiology

The pathophysiology of CFRD is still poorly understood. CFTR may have a role in the cell signalling that contributes to both the timely release of and response to insulin and restoration of abnormal CFTR function.

However, although Ivacaftor (which corrects the underlying gene product defect in patients with a gating mutation) has reportedly led to normalisation of sugar handling in a single individual [15], it seems likely that the pathways directly involving CFTR are of only minor significance to overall glucose homeostasis.

CFRD involves a complex interplay between a state of relative insulin deficiency, particularly during the first phase response, and variable insulin resistance during infective exacerbations. Some level of dysglycaemia is detectable in most pancreatic-insufficient patients and the hallmark of CFRD is the presence of post-prandial glucose excursions that may be followed by spontaneous hypoglycaemic episodes.

Below we consider mechanisms that contribute to abnormal glucose handling in CF.

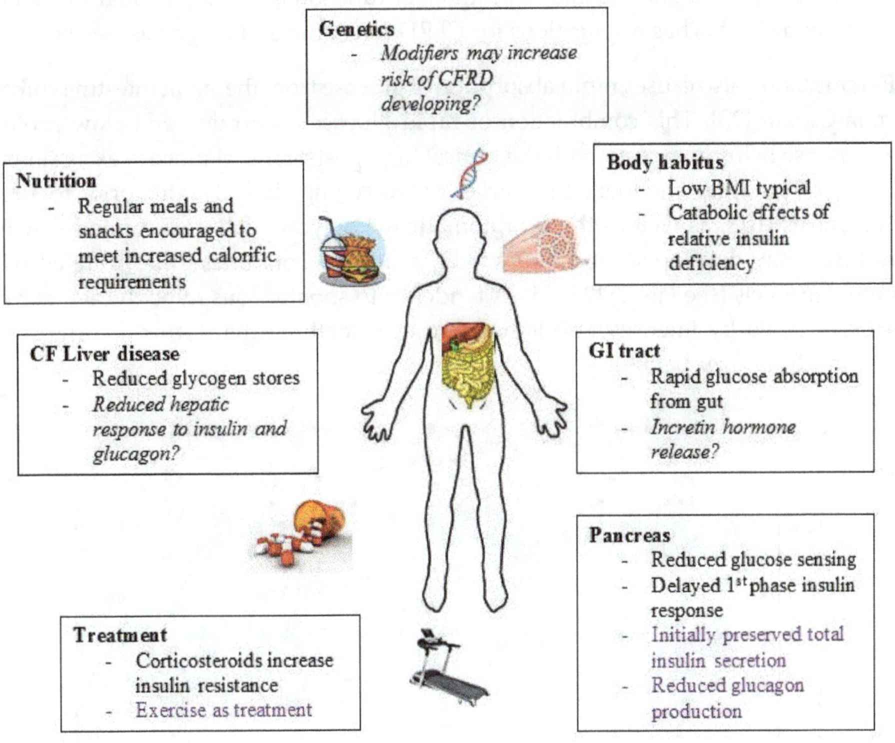

Figure 1. Factors influencing glucose handling in CF. *Italicised* – unclear role. Purple – factors pre-disposing to reactive hypoglycaemic episodes

3.1. Pancreatic responses in CF

The predominant mechanism underpinning dysglycaemia in CF patients is sluggish clearance of proteolytic enzymes from the pancreatic ducts causing progressive β-cell destruction that directly reduces insulin levels, as well as causing ischaemic damage and amyloid deposition [16], further impairing the ability of remaining islet cells to sense and respond to glucose levels appropriately [17]. It seems likely that the same mechanism might also prevent incretin hormones (e.g. GLP-1 and GIP) from evoking their physiological insulinogenic effect during the post-prandial period, although this is an area still under investigation (see below).

Loss of pancreatic endocrine function is a continuum in patients with CF with impaired release of both insulin and glucagon [18]. Those with significant pancreatic insufficiency (almost 90% of patients with CF use pancreatic enzyme supplements [5]) have deranged glucose handling even if not formally diabetic [17], typically displaying a slow and prolonged insulin response to stimulation [18, 19].

The initial abnormality seen in CF patients is a delayed first-phase insulin response combined with preserved total insulin secretion that occurs in response to various stimuli even in CF subjects with normal glucose tolerance [10, 18, 20, 21, 22, 23]. Even at this early stage, patient outcomes can be affected and the loss of pulmonary function is directly related to the degree of dysglycaemia [6]: this has implications for CFRD screening and diagnosis (see below).

The CFTR mutation also causes rapid absorption of glucose from the small intestine compared to the non-CF gut [23]. This combination of rapid glucose absorption and slow prolonged insulin response helps to explain both the typical high post-prandial glucose excursions seen in this group (Fig. 2) (an independent marker of worsening clinical status prior to a formal CFRD diagnosis [10]), as well as the symptomatic hypoglycaemia (often termed reactive or rebound) that may develop several hours later, as insulin continues to be secreted despite falling glucose levels (see Fig. 2) [24, 25]. A tendency to spontaneous hypoglycaemia may be further exacerbated by intense periods of exercise, something that forms a cornerstone of treatment in CF [11] (see below).

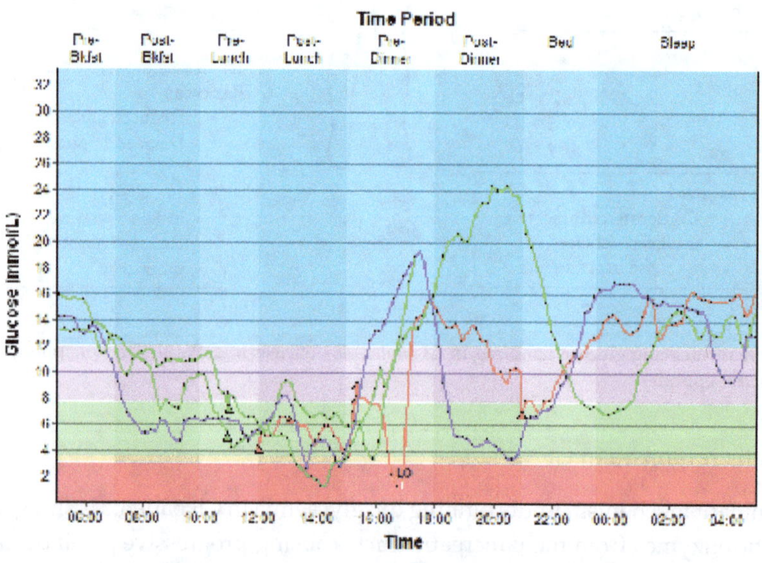

Figure 2. Continuous glucose monitoring showing a typical glucose profile seen in CFRD

As progressive damage to the pancreas accumulates, there is an associated loss of endocrine tissue such that over time patients become relatively insulinopaenic [26]. Although pancreatic β-cell mass may be significantly reduced in patients with CFRD [27, 28], absolute insulinopaenia and ketoacidosis, typical features of Type 1 Diabetes (T1DM) [29], do not occur even in the minority of patients with sufficient pancreatic damage to cause fasting hyperglycaemia. Indeed, the presence of true ketoacidosis is so rare in this population that its occurrence should stimulate investigation for the development of concurrent T1DM [11, 30, 31]. It is possible that the loss of α-cells as part of the indiscriminate pancreatic damage that occurs in CF results in relatively low glucagon levels, protecting against the development of ketosis as well as adding to the propensity for symptomatic hypoglycaemia [32].

3.2. Insulin sensitivity in CF

The role of insulin sensitivity in the development of CFRD is unclear: CFTR may have a theoretical role in cell signalling to increase glucose uptake by peripheral tissues but such responses are predominantly mediated through GLUT receptors. Insulin resistance increases during periods of acute illness [33] including pulmonary exacerbations which may frequently occur in those with an underlying suppurative lung condition. Hardin et al. [34] suggested that insulin sensitivity may be abnormal even in clinically stable CF patients, where on-going indolent infection may up-regulate inflammatory pathways, thereby inducing a degree of chronic insulin resistance.

However, despite these mechanisms, it is relatively rare for pancreatic-sufficient CF individuals, even when colonised with pathogens and suffering regular exacerbations, to develop significant dysglycaemia [35] and overall it has been shown that insulin resistance is not a major determinant of the development of diabetes in CF [36].

It is recognised that at times of high inflammatory stresses or concurrent glucocorticoid use – such as during a pulmonary exacerbation – insulin resistance may contribute to or unmask clinically relevant dysglycaemia in predisposed individuals [17, 30, 34] and extra glucose monitoring is therefore recommended during such periods [37] since initiation or escalation of treatment may be required [30]. As the nutritional aspects of CF care are increasingly well addressed particularly by the early institution of highly effective pancreatic enzyme supplementation, it is becoming increasingly common for patients with CF to have a raised BMI - indeed almost a quarter of patients in one recent series were reported to be overweight or obese [38]. It may be that in future, insulin resistance will play a larger role in the development of dysglycaemia in this population.

3.3. Other factors

Not all CF individuals with pancreatic insufficiency develop CFRD, raising the possibility that other genetic factors might play a part [39].

However, with few exceptions, antibodies associated with the development of T1DM have not been found in CFRD [40-42]. Genetic variation in the CAPN10 gene, which encodes Calpain-10, may be a common risk factor for the development of both CFRD and T2DM [43], explaining in part why CF individuals with a familial history of T2DM are at increased risk of developing CFRD themselves [35] despite a lack of insulin resistance.

It seems likely that genetic modifiers have a significant role in determining to what extent dysglycaemia complicates the clinical course of an individual with cystic fibrosis. [35].

Glucose handling may also be disturbed in individuals with CF-related liver disease, particularly in severe cases where the hepatic uptake and storage of glucose is diminished, potentially rendering treatment for hypoglycaemia with exogenous glucagon ineffective. Chronic kidney disease, which may develop in CF because of recurrent uroliathiasis/nephrocalcinosis, repeated exposure to nephrotoxic medications or indeed as a complication of CFRD itself, may also effect glucose regulation.

Although it is unclear how important this is for overall blood sugar control, severe renal failure may lead to an accumulation of exogenous insulin therapy causing an apparent improvement in diabetic control (if judged by insulin requirements) as well as predisposing to hypoglycaemic episodes.

Incretin hormones released from the bowel are a major determinant of pancreatic responses in the post-prandial period, causing significantly more insulin to be secreted compared to the presence of glucose alone – this so-called incretin effect is lost in T2DM and a range of treatments that target components of the diffuse endocrine system have revolutionised the treatment of this condition. Whilst it has been shown that enteroendocrine cells are present in the expected amounts in the bowels of both animal models and direct intestinal biopsies from children with CF [44, 45], the incretin effect itself has not been definitively investigated in a CF setting, with various small-scale studies showing conflicting results. Whether or not the incretin system is attenuated in CF, it is unclear whether augmenting its function pharmacologically would in any way improve the responses of a pathologically damaged pancreas.

Considering the mechanisms above, it is clear to see that although CFRD has a number of features in common with both T1DM and T2DM it is clearly significantly different to both – a comparison of CFRD with the more common forms of diabetes is shown in Table 1.

	CFRD	T1DM	T2DM
Insulin resistance	Variable	Minimal	Significant
Insulin deficiency	Relative	Absolute	Variable
Typical BMI	Low	Low	High
Complications	Pulmonary, weight loss, microvascular	Microvascular	Macrovascular
Treatment	Insulin	Insulin	Oral agents +/- insulin
Ketosis	Very rare	Common	Rare

Table 1. Comparison of CFRD with other forms of diabetes

4. Screening and diagnosis

Dysglycaemia is often detectable for several years prior to a formal diagnosis of CFRD, and early detection is important to prevent pulmonary function decline and weight loss developing [6, 8]. Timely intervention with appropriate treatment may have a profound impact on a patient's health and well-being. In the next section, we will discuss the various methods of screening for CFRD.

4.1. Diagnosis

The World Health Organisation, Diabetes UK, American Diabetes Association and UK CF Trust all consider that the formal diagnosis of CFRD should be based on responses to a standard 75 g oral glucose tolerance test (see Table 2) and recommend that it is carried out annually from late childhood. Given the impact of pulmonary decline in early CFRD, tighter thresholds were discussed, but currently the general diagnostic criteria are still applied to CF.

- 2-hr 75g OGTT plasma glucose result ≥11.1 mmol/l
- Fasting plasma glucose ≥7.0 mmol/l
- HBA1C ≥6.5% (A1C <6.5% does not rule out CFRD because this value is often spuriously low in CF.)
- Classical symptoms of diabetes (polyuria and polydipsia) in the presence of a casual glucose level ≥11.1 mmol/l

Table 2. Diagnostic criteria for CFRD (any of the following)

These criteria were originally established by consensus opinion in 1998 [3]. The previously used sub-categorisation of the diabetic response to recognise whether or not fasting hyperglycaemia was also present (often abbreviated as CFRD FH+ and CFRD FH-, respectively), is now considered to be obsolete since the differentiation adds little to management [46].

The OGTT was originally designed to detect individuals, predominantly with insulin resistance, who were most likely to benefit from intervention aimed at preventing the microvascular sequelae of dysglycaemia. Although these do occur in CFRD, they are relatively late phenomena, where pulmonary decline (leading to increased mortality) occurs much earlier.

Furthermore, OGTT responses are highly variable in the CF population, where insulin resistance waxes and wanes and glucose absorption alters depending on a variety of factors peculiar to this cohort [17]. An opportunistic annual screen for diabetes carried out when an individual with CF is well may poorly reflect their overall glucose handling.

Screening for diabetes based on the 2-hour glucose value alone has been shown to be of less use in the CF population [47]. Furthermore, the dose of glucose used to stress the endocrine function of the pancreas during an OGTT may be inadequate in CF, where individuals have high calorific requirements and may routinely ingest carbohydrate loads much higher than the 75 g bolus typically used in the diagnostic test.

Given these facts, as well as the typical insulin response profile seen in patients with CF, basing the diagnosis of, as well as screening for, CFRD by means of an OGTT, as is currently recommended [11], is clearly imperfect [48], leading to the conclusion that the under-diagnosis of clinically relevant dysglycemia is common.

Patients with CF may experience significant hyperglycaemic excursions shortly after eating, which then rapidly correct to the euglycaemic range as the delayed first-phase insulin response belatedly begins; this not only devalues diagnostic tests such as the OGTT (which uses the 2-hour glucose value to diagnose diabetes) but also means that measures of average glucose control, such as glycosylated haemoglobin levels (the HbA1c test), may be misleadingly normal or even low in this group and therefore of much less clinical relevance in CFRD than in other forms of diabetes [49]. One study from Denmark found only 16% of patients had elevated HbA1c values at the time CFRD was diagnosed [50]; others have found similar results [49]. The utility of HbA1c may be further devalued by the increased red cell turnover commonly seen in CF patients [49, 51]. As progressive decline in pancreatic endocrine function in the CF population is related to increased morbidity years before a formal diagnosis of CFRD is made by OGTT [8, 9, 10] and given that HbA1c is at best an unreliable marker of glucose handling [49], other methods of assessing clinically important dysglycaemia, such as 1-hour OGTT result, serial glucose monitoring or Continuous Glucose Monitoring (CGM), have now been advocated as better markers of clinically relevant dysglycaemia.

Elevation of 1-hour glucose level during an OGTT has been shown to be a better predictor of declining pulmonary function than a standard 2-hour result [9] as well as correlating better with other methods of diabetic screening [53]. Currently, the UK CF Trust advocates the use of both a standard 2-hour OGTT as well as a period of serial glucose monitoring (that entails checking levels before and 2-hours after meals and at bedtime for several days) to establish if clinically relevant hyperglycaemia requiring treatment is present [49].

For effective serial glucose monitoring to take place, patients must be empowered and educated with regards to the technique including timing, hand washing, correct sampling procedures as well as meter and strip management. Misleading results have been documented [54] due to poor technique, therefore patient-recorded measurements should be considered with a degree of caution, particularly one-off abnormal readings. Additionally, there is a risk that patients, fearful of a further increase in their treatment burden associated with being diagnosed with CFRD, will report lower glucose readings, fail to document high levels or simply fabricate results altogether.

However, a CGM system circumvents many of the inherent weaknesses associated with self-reported serial monitoring whilst enabling an accurate glucose profile to be established. Worn for a period of 3-5 days typically on the arm or abdomen, a CGM system consists of a transmitter with a flexible plastic sensor which sits just below the skin allowing regular measurement of interstitial glucose. Readings are sent wirelessly to a receiver automatically every minute without any user input, although an occasional finger-prick reading is required to calibrate readings against blood glucose levels.

The use of CGM has been validated in the CF population [55] whilst others have shown that it may be superior to other modes of screening for dysglycaemia [56]. The visual output obtained from a CGM can be a useful tool in highlighting sugar control issues with patients

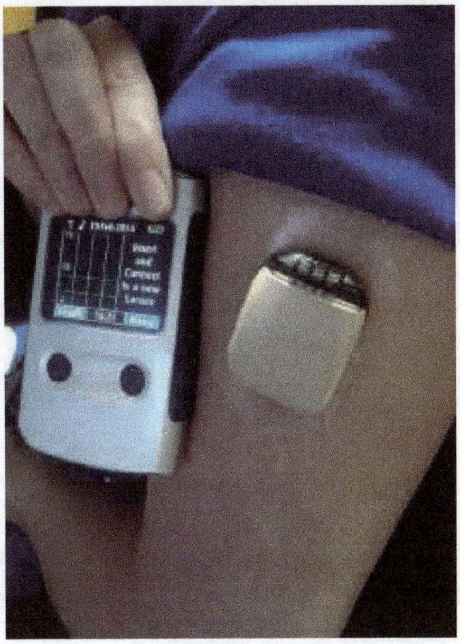

Figure 3. CGM in situ with separate base unit

and allow for highly individualised treatment regimens to be decided. A positive CGM result – that is a value of more than 7.87.8mmol/l for over 4.5% of the test – is associated with a worse prognosis in terms of CF-specific endpoints (i.e. pulmonary function and weight) as well as being a better predictor of future risk of development of CFRD than an OGTT [57], which has been shown to give unreliable results when used as a screening tool [58].

5. Clinical features, signs and symptoms

The biochemical and clinical detection and diagnosis of CFRD can be difficult, since symptoms of polyuria, polydipsia and weight loss only occur in one third of cases [8]. An unexplained decline in pulmonary function or difficulty maintaining or gaining weight should alert health care professionals to the possibility of underlying significant dysglycaemia, impaired glucose tolerance or even CFRD. Poor weight gain or weight loss can often be identified in the preceding 12 months prior to a diagnosis of CFRD [57].

6. Consequences of dysglycaemia in CF

Multiple studies and reviews of large registry datasets have demonstrated a clear link between dysglycaemia and poor outcomes in pulmonary health in CF [3, 5, 43], but the mechanism by which hyperglycaemia, often intermittent rather than sustained in this population, causes the observed decline in lung function is less clear. Plausible theories include direct pulmonary damage or suppression of various components of the immune system in the setting of hyperglycaemia leading to an increased risk of pulmonary infections which might also be more severe in nature [14], as has been demonstrated in other types of diabetes [44]. Insulin therapy has been shown to reduce sputum pathogen levels in CF patients [45]. It has also been hypothesised that the predominant factor in the decline in both respiratory function and nutritional status is a direct consequence of the altered protein metabolism experienced by CF patients who become relatively deficient in insulin therefore losing its important anabolic effects [14]. CFRD has been considered to be a risk factor for the development of distal intestinal obstruction syndrome in cystic fibrosis patients [59]; however, it is unclear how strong the association really is between these two conditions [60] or what causal mechanism might be involved.

6.1. Microvascular complications

Microvascular complications may develop in CFRD leading to the typical associated pathologies (retinopathy, nephropathy and neuropathy), any of which may significantly impact the on-going management of the condition, particularly the development of visual impairment, gastroparesis and renal failure.

Where glucose control has deteriorated to the point that fasting hyperglycaemia is present (a relatively rare occurrence in the CFRD population), a significant proportion will also have developed retinopathy and microalbuminaemia (16% and 14%, respectively) [61]. Almost half of all CFRD patients will display some degree of neuropathy, in most cases where the dysglycaemia has been present for over a decade [43].

Examples of autonomic dysfunction and gastroparesis have been reported [61], although the latter condition may be difficult to differentiate from the delayed gastric emptying that occurs in up to 50% of the CF population regardless of their glucose tolerance [43].

Overall, the prevalence of microvascular complications is less in CFRD than in other forms of diabetes, possibly due to the partially preserved endogenous insulin production and sensitivity leading to relatively short periods of hyperglycaemia.

6.2. Macrovascular complications

Although there is nothing to suggest dysglycaemia is not a significant risk factor for the development of macrovascular complications in individuals with CF, as it is in other populations, at present their occurrence very infrequently complicates the management of CFRD.

Although there are case reports of both coronary artery disease and strokes occurring in diabetic CF patients [62, 63], there is at present no evidence of excess mortality attributable to cardiovascular or cerebrovascular disease despite these patients often having co-existing dyslipidaemia.

Currently, the consequences of significant dysglycaemia are likely to manifest earlier and more profoundly in other ways, e.g. deteriorating lung function, but as the life expectancy of the general CF population continues to rise there is likely to be both a concurrent increase in the incidence of CFRD and ultimately macrovascular complications.

7. Treatment and management

Treatment of CFRD is currently exclusively limited to insulin therapy, since by the time CFRD is formally diagnosed the predominant issue is one of failure of insulin secretion. Evidence of improved outcomes with insulin therapy is established for those who have a positive OGTT with and without fasting hyperglycaemia [2, 39, 64]. It is also recommended that insulin is initiated in those patients that exhibit diabetic responses whilst suffering an infective exacerbation [11], which presumably reflects a group with poor pancreatic reserve, meaning that they are unable to respond adequately when peripheral insulin resistance increases due to higher levels of inflammation or treatment with corticosteroids. The UK CF Trust (2004) guidelines for the management of CFRD [11] have produced recommendations for instigation of treatment, which are as follows; Treatment should be considered:

- When impaired glucose tolerance on OGTT is associated with weight loss or deteriorating clinical condition
- When there are episodes of transient hyperglycaemia
- When a diabetic glucose tolerance on OGTT, but normal glucose monitoring, is associated with weight loss or deteriorating clinical condition

Definite indications for initiating treatment are:

- CF-related diabetes, that is, diabetic OGTT and/or regular hyperglycaemia
- Pregnancy with impaired glucose tolerance or diabetes

Better awareness and more aggressive management of CFRD have led to a considerable improvement in outcomes over the last 5 years including mortality [2]. As discussed above, the concept of truly normal glucose tolerance in the majority of adult CF patients, especially if pancreatic-insufficient, is a fallacy and all such patients could be reasonably considered in a 'pre-diabetic' state; however, the role of early treatment to prevent CFRD is less clear. Small studies have previously suggested only a trend towards improvement in various outcomes when CF patients with impaired glucose tolerance (IGT) received long-acting insulins [65].

As total insulin secretion is often preserved or only marginally decreased in non-diabetic CF patients, the use of insulin therapy in such a group may not be as efficacious and any benefits must be weighed against the increased treatment burden (which is considerable for the vast majority of CF patients) and the risk of hypoglycaemia.

However, there is now increasing evidence to support initiation of treatment in non-diabetic groups with improvement in pulmonary and other clinical outcomes seen after insulin treatment was started [64, 66, 67], particularly those with positive CGM results [57], although it is currently too early to know if such benefits are sustained long-term or will impact upon mortality rates.

The treatment of CFRD can prove challenging with treatment strategies having to constantly be changed due to the variability and disease progression of CF. There are many different variables associated with CF that have to be taken into consideration when managing CFRD.

7.1. Pharmacological treatments of CFRD

Whenever treatment for dysglycaemia in CF patients is initiated, the only modality with an established evidence base is insulin therapy. Biguinide therapy potentially offers anti-inflammatory activity as well as anti-diabetic effects and was shown to improve glucose control in 4 patients without significant side effects over a 10-year period [68]. However, given that insulin resistance is not the predominant abnormality in stable CF patients [36], coupled with concerns about an increased risk of hepatitis, lactic acidosis, weight loss and pancreatitis [69], metformin has not been widely used in this cohort.

A small study (n=12) using acarbose in a group of CF patients with IGT receiving inpatient antibiotics for a pulmonary exacerbation showed an improvement in glucose profile compared to placebo but also a very high incidence of GI side effects [70].

Secretagogues, such as the sulphonylureas, have been shown to be of little benefit in a CF setting whilst increasing the risk of symptomatic hypoglycaemia in this group [71].

Dietary modification can play a role in decreasing very high post-prandial glucose excursions in CF patients and Balzer et al. have suggested that adopting a low glycaemic index diet could be advantageous in CFRD [72]. As such, insulin remains the only recommended treatment for CFRD [11]; however, even the use of short-acting insulin in a bolus regime, attempting to control post-prandial glucose excursions, still risks symptomatic hypoglycaemia developing as endogenous hormone levels belatedly rise.

The incretin system is particularly important in the post-prandial handling of carbohydrate; therefore, agents that enhance its effects are of considerable interest in the management of CFRD, particularly as theoretically at least they have a much lower propensity to cause hypoglycaemia. However, the widespread use of these agents has not yet been investigated in a CF-specific setting, although initial small-scale use seems to have been well tolerated [73].

7.2. Insulin regimes for insulin therapy

Different types of insulin are available for use to treat CFRD. Their different modes of action need to be correlated with glucose profiles and individual requirements of the patient in order to manage glucose levels effectively.

The main categories of insulin are:

- Long-acting insulin analogues – Normally administered once daily with a duration of 18-24 hours, achieving a steady state after 2-3 days (e.g. insulin glargine; detemir or degludec).

- Intermediate insulin – Onset of action 2-3 hours with a duration of 16-35 hours (e.g. insulin isophane).
- Short-acting insulin – Onset of action 30-60 minutes and duration of up to 8 hours (e.g. soluble insulin).
- Rapid-acting insulin analogues – Onset of action 15 minutes and duration of action 2-5 hours (e.g. insulin aspart, lispro or glulisine).
- Pre- mix insulin – Onset of action 30-60 minutes duration up to 24 hours (e.g. biphasic isophane insulin).
- Pre-mix insulin analogue – Onset of action 15 minutes duration up to 24 hours (e.g. biphasic insulin aspart, lispro).

Typically, either a basal/bolus or a combination of both is used to treat CFRD [74].

Short acting rapid insulin before meals remains the insulin of choice for those without fasting hyperglycaemia.

Taking into account treatment burden, long lasting basal insulin needs to be considered and is frequently given [74].

Pre-mix insulin is used in some cases although with the variability in eating patterns this may prove detrimental.

7.3. Multidisciplinary approach to management

When diagnosing and managing patients with CFRD, it is of paramount importance that the multidisciplinary team have excellent knowledge relating to this complication. In ideal circumstances an endocrinologist with experience of CF will form part of the regular multidisciplinary team caring for patients, but in many centres the task of coordinating diabetic care will be delegated to a specialist nurse.

Communication is crucial to ensure patients are fully informed about the condition, particularly the differences between CFRD and other types of diabetes as patients may come with pre-conceived notions that could impact their engagement with treatment and on-going management, e.g. undertake wholly inappropriate calorie restriction.

Wherever possible, both the specialist CF dietician and clinical psychologist should be involved at the earliest opportunity to ensure the best possible expert care and management for the patient.

8. Screening for complications in CFRD

An important aspect of managing CFRD is effective screening for the development of complications. As such it is recommended that at least annually patients with CFRD have the following assessed:

- Clinical history - number of admissions with reasons
- Height, weight and BMI
- Pulmonary function
- Blood pressure
- Alcohol and smoking
- Hypoglycaemia – identify cause and optimise treatment
- Exercise
- Foot examination - pedal pulses, sensory and vibration check.
- Sexual dysfunction
- Frequency of distal intestinal obstruction syndrome (DIOS)
- Full dietetic review - Meals, snacks, enzymes, supplements, feeds.
- Insulin therapy
- Injection technique.
- Insulin site check
- Home blood glucose monitoring.
- Psychosocial support
- Urine sample for Microalbuminuria
- HbA1c
- Urea and electrolytes, creatinine clearance (selected cases)
- Lipid profile
- Retinopathy screening referral

Additionally, annual screening is an opportunity to identify educational gaps and discuss how the patient is coping with their CFRD.

9. The challenges of CFRD

The distinct glucose profile typically seen in CFRD presents clear challenges not only for establishing the diagnosis in the first place but also for managing the condition in general.

9.1. Dietary considerations

The primary aim of nutritional management in relation to CFRD is the achievement of a normal nutritional status [3]. CFRD has different and conflicting dietary recommendations from that of type 1 or type 2 diabetes. CFRD patients have up to 150% the calorific requirements of other diabetic patients and require a diet containing both high fat and protein levels.

Patients with CF require regular snacks in between meals in order to meet their increased metabolic requirements and often resort to consuming foodstuff that is high in refined sugars – such as so called 'energy drinks' – in order to maintain their weight, especially as it obviates the need to medicate with enzyme supplements [75].

Ingestion of products that contain even modest quantities of highly refined sugar can not only cause glucose excursions but may also precipitate a reactive hypoglycaemic episode – a phenomenon that can be seen during 7-15% of diagnostic OGTTs [24, 76].

The use of a diet rich in carbohydrates that have a low glycaemic index (GI) is encouraged in type 2 diabetics both to aid blood glucose control and weight reduction, however little robust evidence exists of benefit from a similar approach in a CFRD population and there are concerns that low GI diets might lead to inappropriate weight loss in this group [72].

Recommendations from American researchers have suggested that carbohydrate counting may have a role in CFRD [3] however in other countries this approach is reserved for T1DM alone, with the CF dietetic community in the United Kingdom favouring regular meals and snacks containing a mixture of both complex and refined carbohydrates be taken with or just after eating other foods [75]– an approach that anecdotally can reduce both the post-prandial glucose excursions as well as subsequent reactive hypoglycaemia occurring.

Dietary assessment is therefore an important part of the management of CFRD particularly to assess and modify refined sugar intake whilst ensuring overall calorific requirements and a healthy weight are maintained.

9.2. Exercise

Regular exercise forms an important cornerstone of the general management of CF and is widely advocated [46] although direct evidence that it specifically improves overall blood sugar control in CFRD is lacking [77] although there is an on-going trial exploring this currently [78] CFRD patients need to be aware of the risk of precipitating hypoglycaemia during exercise and should be educated about extra monitoring during times of exertion.

9.3. Liver disease

CF affects all of the major organs in the body including the liver and the prevalence of CFRD is higher in patients who have liver disease [79]. As discussed previously significant liver disease may lead to a reduction in hepatic glycogen stores, exacerbating the risk of symptomatic hypoglycaemia developing and potentially reducing the response to exogenous glucagon used to treat such episodes. In addition, although it may be difficult to quantify, CF-liver disease could lead to subtle impairments of hepatic insulin secretion and catabolism which may contribute to the overall dysglycaemia suffered by this group [79].

9.4. Hypoglycaemia

As mentioned elsewhere in this chapter hypoglycaemia is not uncommon in CFRD [24]. Furthermore, it has been demonstrated that hypoglycaemia awareness is also impaired as a result of frequent subclinical hypoglycaemic episodes and a diminished glucagon response [32]. Therefore, careful consideration must be given to when blood sugar monitoring is carried out as well as the timing, type and amount of insulin used for treatment.

9.5. Corticosteroids

Oral corticosteroids (e.g. prednisolone) are frequently used during pulmonary exacerbations in CF, and the concomitant elevation in blood glucose may necessitate a change in diabetes management in these patients. Patients may also require increased supervision and treatment during times of infection where blood glucose levels often fluctuate rapidly. There is evidence that CF patients with normoglycaemia exhibit diabetic glucose tolerance during pulmonary exacerbations [80]. This is likely to be due to the stress of infection and inflammation that unmasks the early alterations in glucose homeostasis [81]. Additionally, when infection subsides and patients stop corticosteroids, blood glucose can dramatically drop causing hypoglycaemia and careful support and advice is required during this time.

10. Future developments

There are a number of areas currently at a research stage that may be of benefit in the management of CFRD.

Many centres are moving away from a reliance on the standard 2-hour OGTT to diagnose CFRD, with the use of CGM becoming more widespread to detect clinically significant dysglycemia at an earlier stage.

A number of clinical trials are exploring the use of incretin based therapy in individuals with CF [82, 83] and such therapies theoretically offer an ideal combination of glucose lowering effects with a smaller risk of precipitating hypoglycaemia, especially as concerns about the risk of pancreatitis associated with these type of medications have somewhat lessened recently [84].

Ultimately novel experimental treatments being developed for other forms of diabetes such as stem cell implantation may be applicable to individuals with CFRD.

Author details

Paula Dyce, Gareth Huw Jones and Martin J Walshaw*

*Address all correspondence to: mwalshaw@doctors.org.uk

Adult CF Centre, Liverpool Heart & Chest Hospital, United Kingdom

References

[1] Van den Berg JM, Kouwenberg JM, Heijerman HG. Demographics of glucose metabolism in cystic fibrosis. *J Cyst Fibros*. 2009;8(4):276-9.

[2] Moran A, Dunitz J, Nathan B, Saeed A, Holme B, Thomas W. Cystic fibrosis-related diabetes: current trends in prevalence, incidence, and mortality. *Diabetes Care*. 2009;32(9):1626-31

[3] Moran A, Hardin D, Rodman D, Allen HF, Beall RJ, Borowitz D, et al. Diagnosis, screening and management of cystic fibrosis related diabetes mellitus: a consensus conference report. *Diabetes Res Clin Pract*. 1999;45(1):61-73.

[4] Bismuth E, Laborde K, Taupin P, Velho G, Ribault V, Jennane F, et al. Glucose tolerance and insulin secretion, morbidity, and death in patients with cystic fibrosis. *J Pediatr*. 2008;152(4):540-5, 5.e1.

[5] Koch C, Rainisio M, Madessani U, Harms HK, Hodson ME, Mastella G, et al. Presence of cystic fibrosis-related diabetes mellitus is tightly linked to poor lung function in patients with cystic fibrosis: data from the European Epidemiologic Registry of Cystic Fibrosis. *Pediatr Pulmonol*. 2001;32(5):343-50.

[6] Milla CE, Warwick WJ, Moran A. Trends in pulmonary function in patients with cystic fibrosis correlate with the degree of glucose intolerance at baseline. *Am J Respir Crit Care Med*. 2000;162(3 Pt 1):891-5.

[7] Marshall BC, Butler SM, Stoddard M, Moran AM, Liou TG, Morgan WJ. Epidemiology of cystic fibrosis-related diabetes. *J Pediatr*. 2005;146(5):681-7.

[8] Lanng S, Thorsteinsson B, Nerup J, Koch C. Influence of the development of diabetes mellitus on clinical status in patients with cystic fibrosis. *Eur J Pediatr*. 1992;151(9): 684-7.

[9] Brodsky J, Dougherty S, Makani R, Rubenstein RC, Kelly A. Elevation of 1-hour plasma glucose during oral glucose tolerance testing is associated with worse pulmonary function in cystic fibrosis. *Diabetes Care*. 2011;34(2):292-5.

[10] Costa M, Potvin S, Hammana I, Malet A, Berthiaume Y, Jeanneret A, et al. Increased glucose excursion in cystic fibrosis and its association with a worse clinical status. *J Cyst Fibros*. 2007;6(6):376-83.

[11] Cystic Fibrosis Trust: Management of Cystic Fibrosis Related Diabetes Clinical Care Guidelines (2004), CF Trust, Bromley.

[12] Moran A, Doherty L, Wang X, Thomas W. Abnormal glucose metabolism in cystic fibrosis. *J Pediatr*, 1998;133(1):10-17.

[13] Adler AI, Shine BS, Chamnan P, Haworth CS, Bilton D. Genetic determinants and epidemiology of cystic fibrosis–related diabetes: results from a British cohort of children and adults. *Diabetes Care*. 2008;31:1789–94.

[14] Solomon MP, Wilson DC, Corey M, Kalnins D, Zielenski J, Tsui LC, Pencharz P, Durie P, Sweezey NB. Glucose intolerance in children with cystic fibrosis. *J Pediatr*. 2003;142:128–132.

[15] Resolution of cystic fibrosis–related diabetes with Ivacaftor therapy. *Am J Resp Critic Care Med*. 2014;190(5):590-91.

[16] Couce M, O'Brien TD, Moran A, Roche PC, Butler PC. Diabetes mellitus in cystic fibrosis is characterized by islet amyloidosis. *J Clin Endocrinol Metab*. 1996;81(3):1267-72.

[17] Brennan AL, Geddes DM, Gyi KM, Baker EH. Clinical importance of cystic fibrosis-related diabetes. *J Cyst Fibros*. 2004;3(4):209-22.

[18] Moran A, Diem P, Klein DJ, Levitt MD, Robertson RP. Pancreatic endocrine function in cystic fibrosis. *J Pediatr*. 1991;118(5):715-23.

[19] Cucinotta D, De Luca F, Arrigo T, Di Benedetto A, Sferlazzas C, Gigante A, et al. First-phase insulin response to intravenous glucose in cystic fibrosis patients with different degrees of glucose tolerance. *J Pediatr Endocrinol*. 1994;7(1):13-7.

[20] Lippe BM, Sperling MA, Dooley RR. Pancreatic alpha and beta cell functions in cystic fibrosis. *J Pediatr*. 1977;90:751–55 [PubMed].

[21] Arrigo T, Cucinotta D, Conti Nibali S, Di Cesare E, Di Benedetto A, Magazzù G, De Luca F. Longitudinal evaluation of glucose tolerance and insulin secretion in non-diabetic children and adolescents with cystic fibrosis: results of a two-year follow-up. *Acta Paediatr*. 1993;82:249–53 [PubMed].

[22] Lanng S, Thorsteinsson B, Røder ME, Orskov C, Holst JJ, Nerup J, Koch C. Pancreas and gut hormone responses to oral glucose and intravenous glucagon in cystic fibrosis patients with normal, impaired, and diabetic glucose tolerance. *Acta Endocrinologica*. 1993;128:207–214 [PubMed].

[23] Frase LL, Strickland AD, Kachel GW, Krejs GJ. Enhanced glucose absorption in the jejunum of patients with cystic fibrosis. *Gastroenterology*. 1985;88(2):478-84.

[24] Battezzati A, Battezzati PM, Costantini D, et al. Spontaneous hypoglycemia in patients with cystic fibrosis. *Eur J Endocrinol*. 2007;156:369–76.

[25] Hartling SG, Garne S, Binder C, et al. Proinsulin, insulin, and C-peptide in cystic fibrosis after an oral glucose tolerance test. *Diabetes Res*. 1988;7:165–169.

[26] Lombardo F, De Luca F, Rosano M, Sferlazzas C, Lucanto C, Arrigo T, et al. Natural history of glucose tolerance, beta-cell function and peripheral insulin sensitivity in cystic fibrosis patients with fasting euglycemia. *Eur J Endocrinol*. 2003;149(1):53-9.

[27] Soejima K, Landing BH. Pancreatic islets in older patients with cystic fibrosis with and without diabetes mellitus: morphometric and immunocytologic studies. *Pediatr Pathol.* 1986;6(1):25-46.

[28] Löhr M, Goertchen P, Nizze H, Gould NS, Gould VE, Oberholzer M, et al. Cystic fibrosis associated islet changes may provide a basis for diabetes. An immunocytochemical and morphometrical study. *Virchows Arch A Pathol Anat Histopathol.* 1989;414(2):179-85.

[29] Swartz LM, Laffel LM. A teenage girl with cystic fibrosis-related diabetes, diabetic ketoacidosis, and cerebral edema. *Pediatr Diabetes.* 2008;9(4 Pt 2):426-30.

[30] Laguna TA, Nathan BM, Moran A. Managing diabetes in cystic fibrosis. *Diabetes Obes Metab.* 2010;12(10):858-64.

[31] Atlas AB, Finegold DN, Becker D, Trucco M, Kurland G. Diabetic ketoacidosis in cystic fibrosis. *Am J Dis Child.* 1992;146(12):1457-8.

[32] Drummond, R., Ross, E., Bicknell, S., Small, M. and Jones, G. Insulin therapy in patients with cystic fibrosis related diabetes mellitus: benefit, timing of initiation and hypoglycaemia. *Pract Diab Int.* 2011;28: 177–182. doi: 10.1002/pdi.1588.

[33] Yki-Jarvinen H, Sammalkorpi K, Koivisto VA, Nikkila EA. Severity, duration, and mechanisms of insulin resistance during acute infections. *J Clin Endocrinol Metab.* 1989;69(2):317–23.

[34] Hardin DS, Leblanc A, Marshall G, Seilheimer DK. Mechanisms of insulin resistance in cystic fibrosis. *Am J Physiol Endocrinol Metab.* 2001;281(5):E1022-8.

[35] Blackman SM, Hsu S, Vanscoy LL, Collaco M, Ritter SE, Naugton K, Cutting GR. Genetic modifiers play a substantial role in diabetes complicating cystic fibrosis. *J Clin Endocrinol Metabol.* 2009: 94(4):1302–1309.

[36] Mohan K, Miller H, Dyce P, Grainger R, Hughes R, Vora J, et al. Mechanisms of glucose intolerance in cystic fibrosis. *Diabet Med.* 2009;26(6):582-8.

[37] O'Riordan SM, Robinson PD, Donaghue KC, Moran A. Management of cystic fibrosis-related diabetes in children and adolescents. *Pediatr Diabetes.* 2009;10 Suppl 12:43-50.

[38] Hanna RM, Weiner DJ. Overweight and obesity in patients with cystic fibrosis: A center-based analysis. *Pediatr Pulmonol.* 2015;50:35–41. doi: 10.1002/ppul.23033

[39] Moran A. Cystic fibrosis-related diabetes: an approach to diagnosis and management. *Pediatr Diabetes.* 2000;1:41–8.

[40] Carrington M, Krueger LJ, Holsclaw DS Jr, Iannuzzi MC, Dean M, Mann D. Cystic fibrosis-related diabetes is associated with HLA DQB1 alleles encoding Asp-57- molecules. *J Clin Immunol.* 1994;14:353–58.

[41] Minicucci L, Cotellessa M, Pittaluga L, Minuto N, d'Annunzio G, Azanzini MA, Lorini R. Beta-cell autoantibodies and diabetes mellitus family history in cystic fibrosis. *J Pediatr Endocrinol Metab*. 2005;18:755–60.

[42] Nousia-Arvanitakis S, Galli-Tsinopoulou A, Dracoulacos D, Karamouzis M, Demitriadou A. Islet autoantibodies and insulin dependent diabetes mellitus in cystic fibrosis. *J Pediatr Endocrinol Metab*. 2000;13:319–24.

[43] Moran A, Becker D, Casella SJ, Gottleib PA, Kirkman MS, Marshall, BS, Slovis B. The CFRD consensus conference Committee: Epidemiology, pathophysiology, and prognostic implications of cystic fibrosis–related diabetes. *Diabetes Care*. 2010;33(12): 2677-83.

[44] Hjelte L, Flodstrom-Tullberg M, Nilsson A, Wierup N, Sundler F. Neuroendocrine characterization of the intestine of F508del CFTR mice. *J Cyst Fibros*. 2011 June;10 Suppl 1: S69:A270.

[45] Buchanan KD, Kerr JI, Johnston CF, Redmond AO, Craig BG. The diffuse endocrine system in cystic fibrosis. *Scand J Gastroenterol Suppl*. 1983;82:155-63.

[46] Moran A, Brunzell C, Cohen RC, et al., the CFRD Guidelines Committee. Clinical Care Guidelines for Cystic Fibrosis–Related Diabetes: A position statement of the American Diabetes Association and a clinical practice guideline of the Cystic Fibrosis Foundation, endorsed by the Pediatric Endocrine Society. *Diabetes Care*. 2010;33(12): 2697-2708. doi:10.2337/dc10-1768.

[47] Dobson L, Sheldon CD and Hattersley AT. Conventional measures underestimate glycaemia in cystic fibrosis patients. *Diabetic Med*. 2004;21:691–96. doi: 10.1111/j. 1464-5491.2004.01219.x

[48] Walshaw M. Routine OGTT screening for CFRD – no thanks. *J Royal Soc Med*. 2009;102(Suppl 1):40-44. doi:10.1258/jrsm.2009.s19009.

[49] Holl RW, Buck C, Babka C, Wolf A, Thon A. HbA1c is not recommended as a screening test for diabetes in cystic fibrosis. *Diabetes Care*. 2000;23(1):126.

[50] Lanng S, Hansen A, Thorsteinsson B, Nerup J, Koch C. Glucose tolerance in patients with cystic fibrosis: five year prospective study. *BMJ*. 1995;311(7006):655–59. doi: 10.1136/bmj.311.7006.655.

[51] Godbout A, Hammana I, Potvin S, Mainville D, Rakel A, Berthiaume Y, Rabasa-Lhoret R. No relationship between mean plasma glucose and glycated haemoglobin in patients with cystic fibrosis-related diabetes. *Diabetes Metabol*. 2008;34(6):568-73.

[52] Brennan AL, Gyi KM, Wood DM, Hodson ME, Geddes DM, Baker EH. Relationship between glycosylated haemoglobin and mean plasma glucose concentration in cystic fibrosis. *J Cyst Fibros*. 2006;5:27–31.pmid:16202666.

[53] Dyce P, Jones GH, Walshaw M. Comparison of continuous glucose monitoring (CGM) and oral glucose tolerance testing (OGTT) in the detection of CFRD. Paediatr *Pulmonol.* 2014. 1 (49):S38-574.

[54] Clarke S F, Foster JR. A history of blood glucose meters and their role in self-monitoring of diabetes mellitus. *Br J Biomed Sci.* 2012;69 (2): 83-93.

[55] O'Riordan SMP, Hindmarsh P, Hill NR, et al. Validation of continuous glucose monitoring in children and adolescents with cystic fibrosis: a prospective cohort study. *Diabetes Care.* 2009;32(6):1020-22. doi:10.2337/dc08-1925.

[56] Khammar A, Stremler N, Dubus JC, Gross G, Sarles J, Reynaud R. Value of continuous glucose monitoring in screening for diabetes in cystic fibrosis. *Arch Pediatr.* 2009 December;16(12):1540-6. doi: 10.1016/j.arcped.2009.09.007. Epub 2009 Oct 24. French.

[57] Hameed S, Morton JR, Jaffé A, Field PI, Belessis Y, Yoong T, et al. Early glucose abnormalities in cystic fibrosis are preceded by poor weight gain. *Diabetes Care.* 2010;33(2):221-6.

[58] Sterescu AE, Rhodes B, Jackson R, Dupuis A, Hanna A, Wilson DC, et al. Natural history of glucose intolerance in patients with cystic fibrosis: ten-year prospective observation program. *J Pediatr.* 2010;156(4):613-7.

[59] Colomboa C, Ellemunter HB, Houwenc R, Munckd A, Taylor C, Wilschanski MF. Guidelines for the diagnosis and management of distal intestinal obstruction syndrome in cystic fibrosis patients. *J Cyst Fibro.* 2011; 10(Suppl 2):S24–S28.

[60] Leichsenring M, Rueckel B, Meissner P, Kratzer W. The variability of carbohydrate antigen 19-9 (CA 19-9) levels in cystic fibrosis patients. *J Cyst Fibro.* 2014; 13(Supplement 2):S95.

[61] Schwarzenberg SJ, Thomas W, Olsen TW, Grover T, Walk D, Milla C, Moran A. Microvascular complications in cystic fibrosis-related diabetes. *Diabetes Care.* 2007;30:1056–61.

[62] Perrin FMR, Serino W. Ischaemic heart disease – a new issue in cystic fibrosis? *J R Soc Med.* 2010;103:S44-S48.

[63] Simmonds NJ, Cullinan P, Hodson ME. Growing old with cystic fibrosis - the characteristics of long-term survivors of cystic fibrosis. *Respir Med.* 2009 April;103(4):629-35. doi: 10.1016/j.rmed.2008.10.011. Epub 2008 Nov 20.

[64] Rolon MA, Benali K, Munck A, Navarro J, Clement A, Tubiana-Rufi N, Czernichow P, Polak M. Cystic fibrosis-related diabetes mellitus: clinical impact of prediabetes and effects of insulin therapy. *Acta Paediatr.* 2001;90:860-67.

[65] Minicucci L, Haupt M, Casciaro R, De Alessandri A, Bagnasco F, Lucidi V, et al. Slow-release insulin in cystic fibrosis patients with glucose intolerance: a randomized clinical trial. *Pediatr Diabetes.* 2012;13(2):197-202.

[66] Dobson L, Hattersley AT, Tiley S, Elworthy S, Oades PJ, Sheldon CD. Clinical improvement in cystic fibrosis with early insulin treatment. *Arch Dis Child*. 2002;87(5): 430-31.

[67] Bizzarri C, Lucidi V, Ciampalini P, Bella S, Russo B, Cappa M. Clinical effects of early treatment with insulin glargine in patients with cystic fibrosis and impaired glucose tolerance. *J Endocrinol Invest*. 2006;29(3):RC1-4.

[68] Onady GM, Langdon LJ. Insulin versus oral agents in the management of Cystic Fibrosis Related Diabetes: a case based study. *BMC Endocr Disord*. 2006;6:4.

[69] Kongsuphol P, Cassidy D, Romeiras F, Schreiber R, Mehta A, Kunzelmann K. Metformin treatment of diabetes mellitus increases the risk for pancreatitis in patients bearing the CFTR-mutation S573C. *Cell Physiol Biochem*. 2010;25(4-5):389-96.

[70] Kentrup H, Bongers H, Spengler M, Kusenbach G, Skopnik H. Efficacy and safety of acarbose in patients with cystic fibrosis and impaired glucose tolerance. *Eur J Pediatr*. 1999;158(6):455-59.

[71] [Cochrane] Onady GM, Stolfi A. Insulin and oral agents for managing cystic fibrosis-related diabetes. *Cochrane Database Syst Rev*. 2013;7:CD004730.

[72] Balzer BW, Graham CL, Craig ME, Selvadurai H, Donaghue KC, Brand-Miller JC, et al. Low glycaemic index dietary interventions in youth with cystic fibrosis: a systematic review and discussion of the clinical implications. *Nutrients*. 2012;4(4):286-96.

[73] Hellman, J. Fischier, A. Hollsing. Incretin-based treatment of diabetes related to cystic fibrosis: a case study. *J Cyst Fibro*. 2014;13 (2):S126.

[74] Kelly A, Moran, A. Update on cystic fibrosis related diabetes. *J Cyst Fibro*. 2013;(12) 318-31.

[75] Ashworth, F., et al. The management of cystic fibrosis related diabetes. *Brit J Homecare* 1. 1999;136-140.

[76] Radike K, Molz K, Holl RW, Poeter B, Hebestreit H, Ballmann M. *Diabetes Care*. 2011 April;34(4):e43. doi: 10.2337/dc10-2286. No abstract available.

[77] Dwyer TJ, Elkins MR, Bye PTP. The role of exercise in maintaining health in cystic fibrosis. *Curr Opin Pulm Med*. 2011;17 (6): 455-60.

[78] [ClinicalTrials.gov [Internet]. Bethesda (MD): National Library of Medicine (US).2000 Feb 29 -. Identifier NCT02127957, Effects of an Exercise Program Among CF Patients With Dysglycemia (FKEX); 2014 Apr 18 [cited 2015 Feb 13]; [about 4 screens]. Available from: https://clinicaltrials.gov/ct2/show/NCT02127957.]

[79] Holstein, A, et al. Clinical implications of hepatogenous diabetes in liver cirrhosis. *J Gastroenterology Hepatol*. 2002;17(6): 677-81.

[80] Sc NN, Shoseyov D, Kerem E, Zangen DH. Patients with cystic fibrosis and normoglycemia exhibit glucose tolerance during pulmonary exacerbation. *J Cyst Fibro*. 2010; 9:199-204.

[81] Zeller, M., et al. Glycemia in acute coronary syndromes. *Diabetes Metabol* 2006;32: 2S42-2S47.

[82] ClinicalTrials.gov [Internet]. Bethesda (MD): National Library of Medicine (US). 2000 Feb 29 -. Identifier NCT00967798. Prevention of Cystic Fibrosis Diabetes. August 27, 2009 [cited February 13 2015] Available from: https://clinicaltrials.gov/ct2/show/NCT00967798

[83] ClinicalTrials.gov [Internet]. Bethesda (MD): National Library of Medicine (US). 2000 Feb 29 -. Identifier NCT01879228. Effect of Chronic Incretin-based Therapy in Cystic Fibrosis. June 12, 2013 [cited February 13 2015] Available from https://clinicaltrials.gov/ct2/show/NCT01879228

[84] [Pancreatic Safety of Incretin-Based Drugs — FDA and EMA Assessment. Amy G. Egan, M.D., M.P.H., Eberhard Blind, M.D., Ph.D., Kristina Dunder, M.D., Pieter A. de Graeff, M.D., B. Timothy Hummer, Ph.D., Todd Bourcier, Ph.D., and Curtis Rosebraugh, M.D., M.P.H. N Engl J Med 2014; 370:794-797].

Permissions

All chapters in this book were first published in CFLNR, by InTech Open; hereby published with permission under the Creative Commons Attribution License or equivalent. Every chapter published in this book has been scrutinized by our experts. Their significance has been extensively debated. The topics covered herein carry significant findings which will fuel the growth of the discipline. They may even be implemented as practical applications or may be referred to as a beginning point for another development.

The contributors of this book come from diverse backgrounds, making this book a truly international effort. This book will bring forth new frontiers with its revolutionizing research information and detailed analysis of the nascent developments around the world.

We would like to thank all the contributing authors for lending their expertise to make the book truly unique. They have played a crucial role in the development of this book. Without their invaluable contributions this book wouldn't have been possible. They have made vital efforts to compile up to date information on the varied aspects of this subject to make this book a valuable addition to the collection of many professionals and students.

This book was conceptualized with the vision of imparting up-to-date information and advanced data in this field. To ensure the same, a matchless editorial board was set up. Every individual on the board went through rigorous rounds of assessment to prove their worth. After which they invested a large part of their time researching and compiling the most relevant data for our readers.

The editorial board has been involved in producing this book since its inception. They have spent rigorous hours researching and exploring the diverse topics which have resulted in the successful publishing of this book. They have passed on their knowledge of decades through this book. To expedite this challenging task, the publisher supported the team at every step. A small team of assistant editors was also appointed to further simplify the editing procedure and attain best results for the readers.

Apart from the editorial board, the designing team has also invested a significant amount of their time in understanding the subject and creating the most relevant covers. They scrutinized every image to scout for the most suitable representation of the subject and create an appropriate cover for the book.

The publishing team has been an ardent support to the editorial, designing and production team. Their endless efforts to recruit the best for this project, has resulted in the accomplishment of this book. They are a veteran in the field of academics and their pool of knowledge is as vast as their experience in printing. Their expertise and guidance has proved useful at every step. Their uncompromising quality standards have made this book an exceptional effort. Their encouragement from time to time has been an inspiration for everyone.

The publisher and the editorial board hope that this book will prove to be a valuable piece of knowledge for researchers, students, practitioners and scholars across the globe.

List of Contributors

Dennis Wat
Liverpool Heart and Chest Hospital, Liverpool, United Kingdom

Michelle M. White, Fatma Gargoum, Niall Browne, Killian Hurley, Noel G. McElvaney and Emer P. Reeves
Respiratory Research Division, Department of Medicine, Royal College of Surgeons in Ireland, Education and Research Centre, Beaumont Hospital, Dublin, Ireland

Anne Bergougnoux and Caroline Raynal
Laboratory of Molecular Genetics, Montpellier Hospital, France

Magali Taulan-Cadars and Mireille Claustres
Montpellier University, France

Rosaria Casciaro, Federico Cresta, Federica Favilli and Laura Minicucci
Pneumology Unit - Cystic Fibrosis Center, IRCCS Giannina Gaslini, Genova, Italy

Terry W. Chin
Miller Children's Hospital, Long Beach, University of California, Irvine, USA

Alda Marques, Joana Cruz, Cristina Jácome and Ana Oliveira
Lab 3R - Respiratory Rehabilitation Research Laboratory, School of Health Sciences, University of Aveiro (ESSUA), Aveiro, Portugal
Center for Health Technology and Services Research (CINTESIS), School of Health Sciences, University of Aveiro, Aveiro, Portugal

Cormac McCarthy, Orla O'Carroll, Alessandro N. Franciosi and Noel G. McElvaney
Respiratory Research Division, Department of Medicine, Royal College of Surgeons in Ireland, Education and Research Centre, Beaumont Hospital, Dublin, Ireland

Michael Sebastian Daniel Kormann
University Children's Clinic Department of Pediatrics I, Pediatric Infectiology & Immunology, Translational Genomics and Gene Therapy in Pediatrics, University of Tübingen, Tübingen, Germany

Roberto Gambari, Giulia Breveglieri and Francesca Salvatori
Department of Life Sciences and Biotechnology, Biochemistry and Molecular Biology Section, University of Ferrara, Ferrara, Italy
Biotechnology Center, University of Ferrara, Ferrara, Italy

Alessia Finotti and Monica Borgatti
Department of Life Sciences and Biotechnology, Biochemistry and Molecular Biology Section, University of Ferrara, Ferrara, Italy

Paula Dyce, Gareth Huw Jones and Martin J Walshaw
Adult CF Centre, Liverpool Heart & Chest Hospital, United Kingdom

Index

www.ingramcontent.com/pod-product-compliance
Lightning Source LLC
LaVergne TN
LVHW080639210926
848485LV00003B/294
* 9 7 8 1 6 3 9 8 7 1 4 9 0 *